VOLUME EIGHTY SEVEN

ADVANCES IN PHARMACOLOGY

VOLUME EIGHTY SEVEN

ADVANCES IN PHARMACOLOGY

Pharmacological Advances in Natural Product Drug Discovery

Edited by

GUANHUA DU

Institute of Materia Medica, Chinese Academy of Medical Science and Peking Union Medical College, Beijing, China

Serial Editor

S.J. ENNA

University of Kansas Medical Center, Kansas City, KS, United States

Managing Editor

LYNN LeCOUNT

University of Kansas Medical Center, School of Medicine, Kansas City, KS, United States

ELSEVIER

ACADEMIC PRESS

An imprint of Elsevier

Academic Press is an imprint of Elsevier
50 Hampshire Street, 5th Floor, Cambridge, MA 02139, United States
525 B Street, Suite 1650, San Diego, CA 92101, United States
The Boulevard, Langford Lane, Kidlington, Oxford OX5 1GB, United Kingdom
125 London Wall, London, EC2Y 5AS, United Kingdom

First edition 2020

ISBN: 978-0-12-820185-5
ISSN: 1054-3589

For information on all Academic Press publications
visit our website at https://www.elsevier.com/books-and-journals

Publisher: Zoe Kruze
Editorial Project Manager: Shellie Bryant
Production Project Manager: Denny Mansingh
Cover Designer: Matthew Limbert

Typeset by SPi Global, India

Contents

Contributors

Giovanna Bermano
Centre for Natural Products in Health, School of Pharmacy & Life Sciences, Robert Gordon University, Aberdeen, United Kingdom

Xiaorui Cheng
Beijing Institute of Pharmacology and Toxicology; State Key Laboratory of Toxicology and Medical Countermeasures, Beijing, China

Guanhua Du
Institute of Materia Medica, Chinese Academy of Medical Science and Peking Union Medical College, Beijing, China

Lida Du
Department of Surgery, University of Toronto, Toronto, ON, Canada

Mengyue Fan
Tianjin University of Traditional Chinese Medicine, Tianjin, China

Lianhua Fang
Institute of Materia Medica, Chinese Academy of Medical Science and Peking Union Medical College, Beijing, China

Li Gao
Modern Research Center for Traditional Chinese Medicine, Shanxi University, Taiyuan, China

Xiumei Gao
Tianjin University of Traditional Chinese Medicine, Tianjin, China

Xiaoqiang Geng
State Key Laboratory of Natural and Biomimetic Drugs, Department of Pharmacology, School of Basic Medical Sciences, Peking University; Key Laboratory of Molecular Cardiovascular Sciences, Ministry of Education, Beijing, China

Chunyang He
Key Laboratory of Basic Pharmacology of Ministry of Education and Joint International Research Laboratory of Ethnomedicine of Ministry of Education; Generic Drug Research Center of Guizhou Province, School of Pharmacy, Zunyi Medical University, Zunyi, Guizhou, P.R. China

Franck Hennequart
R&D Department, Algaia, Saint-Lô, France

Nana Huang
The Second Hospital of Shandong University, Shandong University, Jinan, China

Yan Huang
Beijing Institute of Pharmacology and Toxicology; State Key Laboratory of Toxicology and Medical Countermeasures, Beijing, China

Xiaojiaoyang Li
Beijing University of Chinese Medicine, Beijing, China

Zhibin Lin
State Key Laboratory of Natural and Biomimetic Drugs, Department of Pharmacology, School of Basic Medical Sciences, Peking University; Key Laboratory of Molecular Cardiovascular Sciences, Ministry of Education, Beijing, China

Runping Liu
Beijing University of Chinese Medicine, Beijing, China

Xiao Liu
Tianjin University of Traditional Chinese Medicine, Tianjin, China

Mingsan Miao
Department of Medicine, Henan University of Chinese Medicine, Zhengzhou, China

David J. Newman
Newman Consulting LLC, Wayne, PA, United States

Guifen Qiang
Institute of Materia Medica, Chinese Academy of Medical Science and Peking Union Medical College, Beijing, China

Xuemei Qin
Modern Research Center for Traditional Chinese Medicine, Shanxi University, Taiyuan, China

Jingshan Shi
Key Laboratory of Basic Pharmacology of Ministry of Education and Joint International Research Laboratory of Ethnomedicine of Ministry of Education; Generic Drug Research Center of Guizhou Province, School of Pharmacy, Zunyi Medical University, Zunyi, Guizhou, P.R. China

Junke Song
Institute of Materia Medica, Chinese Academy of Medical Science and Peking Union Medical College, Beijing, China

Teodora Stoyanova
Centre for Natural Products in Health, School of Pharmacy & Life Sciences, Robert Gordon University, Aberdeen, United Kingdom

Limin Su
State Key Laboratory of Natural and Biomimetic Drugs, Department of Pharmacology, School of Basic Medical Sciences, Peking University; Key Laboratory of Molecular Cardiovascular Sciences, Ministry of Education, Beijing, China

Rong Sun
The Second Hospital of Shandong University; Advanced Medical Research Institute, Shandong University, Jinan; Tianjin University of Traditional Chinese Medicine, Tianjin, China

Cherry L. Wainwright
Centre for Natural Products in Health, School of Pharmacy & Life Sciences, Robert Gordon University, Aberdeen, United Kingdom

Shoubao Wang
Institute of Materia Medica, Chinese Academy of Medical Science and Peking Union Medical College, Beijing, China

Xiaoying Wang
Tianjin University of Traditional Chinese Medicine, Tianjin, China

Ze Wang
Generic Drug Research Center of Guizhou Province, School of Pharmacy, Zunyi Medical University, Zunyi, Guizhou, P.R. China

Chuxuan Wu
Modern Research Center for Traditional Chinese Medicine, Shanxi University, Taiyuan, China

Liling Xiang
Department of Medicine, Henan University of Chinese Medicine, Zhengzhou, China

Zhiyong Xiao
Beijing Institute of Pharmacology and Toxicology; State Key Laboratory of Toxicology and Medical Countermeasures, Beijing, China

Baoxue Yang
State Key Laboratory of Natural and Biomimetic Drugs, Department of Pharmacology, School of Basic Medical Sciences, Peking University; Key Laboratory of Molecular Cardiovascular Sciences, Ministry of Education, Beijing, China

Xiuying Yang
Institute of Materia Medica, Chinese Academy of Medical Science and Peking Union Medical College, Beijing, China

Yang Yang
Tianjin University of Traditional Chinese Medicine, Tianjin, China

Jianqin Zhang
Modern Research Center for Traditional Chinese Medicine, Shanxi University, Taiyuan, China

Li Zhang
Institute of Materia Medica, Chinese Academy of Medical Science and Peking Union Medical College, Beijing, China

Yongxiang Zhang
Beijing Institute of Pharmacology and Toxicology; State Key Laboratory of Toxicology and Medical Countermeasures, Beijing, China

Dandan Zhong
State Key Laboratory of Natural and Biomimetic Drugs, Department of Pharmacology, School of Basic Medical Sciences, Peking University; Key Laboratory of Molecular Cardiovascular Sciences, Ministry of Education, Beijing, China

Wenxia Zhou
Beijing Institute of Pharmacology and Toxicology; State Key Laboratory of Toxicology and Medical Countermeasures, Beijing, China

Preface

Historically, natural products, which are obtained primarily from animals and plants, were the only substances available for the treatment of disease. For millennia, empirical studies with such agents yielded useful therapeutics, many of which, or chemical derivatives thereof, are still in use today. Currently, there are thousands of compounds that were isolated from plant and animal materials that are reported to display therapeutic potential in the laboratory setting. With the advent of the de novo synthesis of drug candidates, high-throughput screening, and techniques for identifying drug targets, there is a growing demand for more fundamental pharmacological research on the biologically active constituents of traditional medicines. Work on the chemical, pharmacokinetic, and pharmacodynamic properties of purified natural products is now yielding critical information about their pharmacophores, sites of action, and clinical efficacy. Such data are stimulating interest in the role of natural products as a source for new medications. This volume of *Advances in Pharmacology* was assembled to highlight the value of natural products in drug discovery and to provide critical reviews of recent findings in this field.

I would like to give my warmest thanks to all the authors and reviewers for their contributions on the scientific aspects. My special thanks go to Dr. S.J. Enna, the Series Editor of *Advances in Pharmacology*, for his valuable guidance and comments. I also wish to thank Ms. Lynn LeCount in the *Advances in Pharmacology* Editorial Office for her great patience and improvements, and Dr. Ying Zhao in the Chinese Pharmacological Society Administrative Office for her assistance with the authors. Together with them, I hope this work serves as a source of inspiration, instruction, and ideas for pharmacologists, chemists, graduate students, and others involved in drug discovery.

Guanhua Du
December 11, 2019

CHAPTER ONE

Chemical and pharmacological research on the polyphenol acids isolated from Danshen: A review of salvianolic acids

Guanhua Du[a,*], Junke Song[a], Lida Du[b], Li Zhang[a], Guifen Qiang[a], Shoubao Wang[a], Xiuying Yang[a], Lianhua Fang[a]

[a]Institute of Materia Medica, Chinese Academy of Medical Science and Peking Union Medical College, Beijing, China

[b]Department of Surgery, University of Toronto, Toronto, ON, Canada

[*]Corresponding author: e-mail address: dugh@imm.ac.cn

Contents

Advances in Pharmacology, Volume 87
ISSN 1054-3589
https://doi.org/10.1016/bs.apha.2019.12.004

Abstract

Danshen, the dried root of *Salvia miltiorrhiza* Bge, is a common medicinal herb in Traditional Chinese Medicine, which has been used for the treatment of a number of diseases for thousands of years. More than 2000 years ago, the Chinese early pharmacy monograph "Shennong Materia Medica" recorded that Danshen could be used for the treatment of gastrointestinal diseases, cardiovascular diseases, certain gynecological diseases, etc. Since then, Danshen has been widely used clinically in many different prescriptions for many different diseases, especially for the treatment of cardiovascular diseases. Nowadays, many pharmacological studies about the water-soluble components from Danshen have been reported, especially salvianolic acids. It turned out that salvianolic acids showed strong anti-lipid peroxidation and anti-thrombic activities, and among them, SalAA and SalAB were the most potent. This review focused on the achievements in research of salvianolic acids regarding their bioactivities and pharmacological effects. These studies not only shed light on the water-soluble active components of Danshen and their mechanisms at the molecular level, but also provided theoretical information for the development of new medicines from Danshen for the treatment of cardiovascular and cerebrovascular diseases, inflammatory diseases, metabolic diseases, etc.

Abbreviations

14,15-EEZE	14,15-epoxyeicosa-5(*Z*)-enoic acid
AGEs	advanced glycation end products
AMPK	adenosine monophosphate activated protein kinase
Ang II	angiotensin II
BMPRII	bone morphogenetic protein receptor II
CaMKKβ	Ca^{2+}/calmodulin-dependent protein kinase kinase-β
CCL5	chemokine (C-C motif) ligand 5
Cdk5	cyclin-dependent kinase 5
ChREBP	carbohydrate response element-binding protein
DDAH	dimethylarginine dimethylaminohydrolase
EBI	early brain injury
EETs	epoxyeicosatrienoic acids
eNOS	endothelial nitric oxide synthase
ERK	extracellular signal regulated kinase
Gsk-3β	glycogen synthase kinase-3β
HFD	high fat diet
HPLC-MS	high-performance liquid chromatography mass spectrometry
HSC	hepatic stellate cell
I/R	ischemia-reperfusion
LDL	low-density lipoprotein
LOX-1	lectin-like oxidized low-density lipoprotein receptor-1
MAPK	mitogen-activated protein kinase
MCAO	middle cerebral artery occlusion
MDA	malondialdehyde

mPTP	mitochondrial permeability transition pore
MMP-9	matrix metalloproteinase-9
mTOR	mammalian target of rapamycin
NAD+	nicotinamide adenine dinucleotide
NADPH	reduced nicotinamide adenine dinucleotide phosphate
NLRP3	nod-like receptor family, pyrin domain containing 3
nNOS	neuronal nitric oxide synthase
Nox4	NADPH oxidase 4
Nrf2	NF-E2-related factor 2
OSCC	oral squamous cell carcinoma
PAH	pulmonary arterial hypertension
PGC-1α	peroxisome proliferator-activated receptor γ coactivator
PI3K	phosphoinositide 3-kinase
RAGEs	receptor for advanced glycation end products
ROS	reactive oxygen species
SalAA	salvianolic acid A
SalAB	salvianolic acid B
SalAC	salvianolic acid C
SERCA	sarco/endoplasmic reticulum Ca^{2+}-ATPase
SMDS	salvia miltiorrhiza depside salt
STAT	signal transducer and activator of transcription
TGFβ	transforming growth factor β
TRPM	transient receptor potential melastatin
TXNIP	thioredoxin-interacting protein
UUO	Unilateral ureteral obstruction
VEGF	vascular endothelial growth factor
VEGFR	vascular endothelial growth factor receptor

1. Introduction

Danshen, the dried root of *Salvia miltiorrhiza* Bge, is a common medicinal herb in Traditional Chinese Medicine, which has been used for the treatment of a number of diseases for thousands of years. More than 2000 years ago, the Chinese early pharmacy monograph "Shennong Materia Medica" recorded that Danshen could be used for the treatment of gastrointestinal diseases, cardiovascular diseases, certain gynecological diseases, etc. Since then, Danshen has been widely used clinically in many different prescriptions for many different diseases, especially for the treatment of cardiovascular diseases.

Since the 1930s, scientists have researched the ingredients of Danshen using modern chemical techniques and investigated bioactivities using modern pharmacological methods. Lipid-soluble ingredients have been isolated, such as Tanshinone I, Tanshinone II, cryptotanshinone, etc. At the same time, the pharmacological effects of lipid-soluble components were investigated. A number of new drugs based on Tanshinone have been developed.

Until the 1980s, Chinese scientists have researched the water-soluble components of Danshen, based on the traditional clinical application of Danshen preparation, which was used as a decoction. Since then, Chinese scientists have paid great attention to the chemical, pharmacological, and clinical research and uses of the water-soluble components of Danshen. Currently, at least 15 water-soluble chemical components have been isolated. These compounds have been named in sequence as salvianolic acids A, B, C, D, etc., by Professor L.N. Li.

All these salvianolic acids have the basic chemical structures of danshensu and caffeic acid and belong to polyphenol acid. The pharmacological study of these compounds demonstrated that most of the salvianolic acids have multiple biological activities, such as improving regional cerebral blood flow in the ischemic hemisphere without stale blood hypotension, and inhibiting platelet aggregation and thrombosis without hemorrhagic risk. So, salvianolic acids have been developed as an injection for the treatment of cerebral ischemic diseases.

In recent decades, research efforts have been focused on the discovery and development of new therapeutic agents from salvianolic acids because of their different molecules with special actions on diverse targets.

All the research results suggest that salvianolic acids are the main active components in Danshen, which has been used as medicine for the treatment of different diseases. The different salvianolic acids have special bioactivities and pharmacological effects on different animal disease models. For example, SalAA can inhibit aldose reductase activity and reduce in vivo and in vitro superoxidant stress- and hyperglycemia stress-induced injuries. And, SalAA has been developed as a drug for the treatment of diabetic peripheral neuropathy in clinical trials. Also, the different salvianolic acids have similar bioactivities such as antioxidation effects, anti-inflammation effects, etc. Therefore, salvianolic acids have been used clinically for the treatment of cerebral ischemia. This review focused on the achievements in research of salvianolic acids regarding their bioactivities and pharmacological effects. These studies not only shed light on the water-soluble active components of Danshen and their mechanisms at the molecular level, but also provided theoretical information for the development of new medicines from Danshen for the treatment of cardiovascular and cerebrovascular diseases, inflammatory diseases, metabolic diseases, etc.

2. Chemical properties of salvianolic acids

In the early 1980s, chemists and pharmacologists at the Institute of Materia Medica, Chinese Academy of Medical Sciences, began systematic studies of the water-soluble components of Danshen. Thirteen phenolic acids were isolated, among which salvianolic acids A, B, C, D, E, F, and G were new compounds (Li, 1997). During this period the Shanghai First Medical College and Shanghai Institute of Materia Medica successfully isolated protocatechuic aldehyde, danshensu, and danshen acid B and C from injections of Danshen. The Tanaka et al. isolated magnesium lithospermate B and ammonium-potassium lithospermate B from Danshen (Tanaka et al., 1989). At present, further phenolic acids have been isolated and identified (Gong et al., 2015; Lu & Foo, 2001, 2002; Tang et al., 2014; Zhang, Chen, Peng, Li, & Jiang, 2008), including nearly 20 kinds of compounds called salvianolic acids (Figs. 1 and 2).

The chemical structures of the water-soluble phenolic acids of Danshen are composed of C6C3 units. Danshensu, R-(+)-β-(3,4-dihydroxyphenyl)-lactic acid, is a simple monomeric compound, while most of the phenolic acids are depsides of danshensu and a caffeic acid derivative or caffeic acid dimer forming several kinds of skeletons. Similar to the free danshensu, the danshensu portion of these depsides also possesses an R configuration, while the carbon skeleton of the caffeic acid dimer might be recognized as neolignans. It is noteworthy that most of the lignans obtained naturally are liposoluble constituents. The water-soluble salvianolic acids possess a unique structure of a depside with free hydroxyls in the neolignan skeleton.

Salvianolic acid A and F are stilbene derivatives, and might be considered to be formed by decarboxylation of a caffeic acid dimer. In its acidic condition, it can be converted to a 2-arylbenzofurane, which is the skeleton of salvianolic acid C (SalAC). Salvianolic acid B (SalAB), lithospermic acid, and przewalskinic acid possess a 2-aryldihydrobenzofuranoid skeleton with

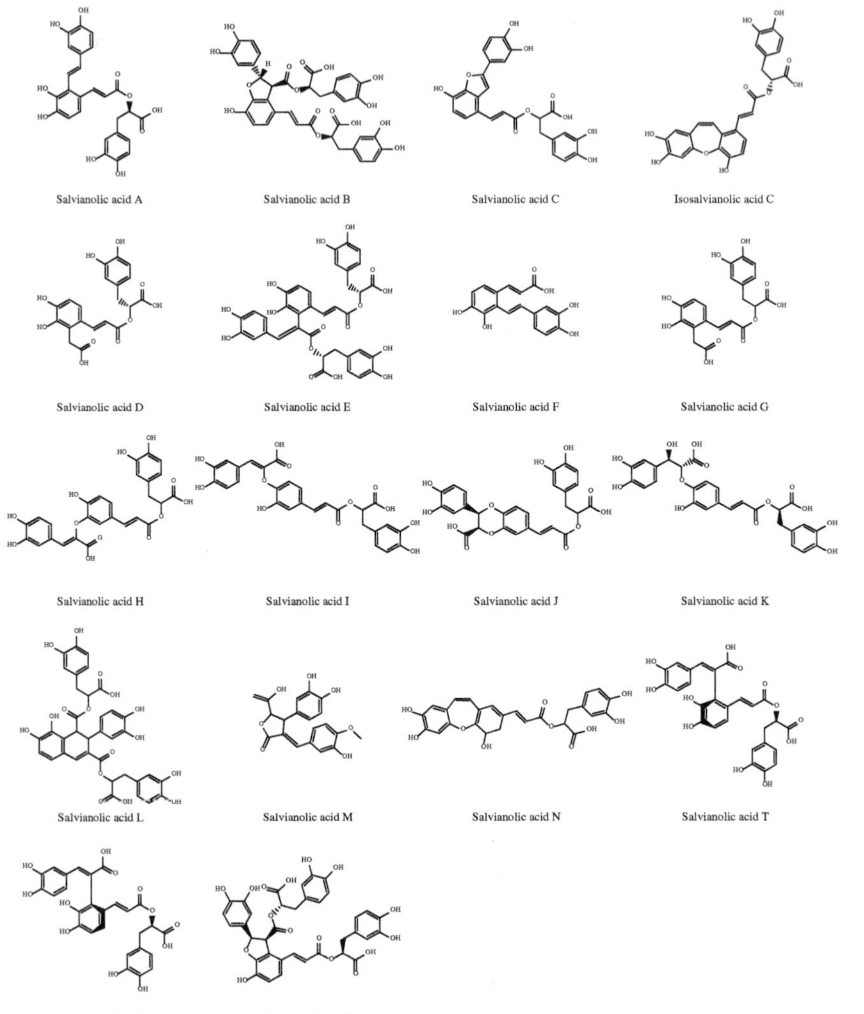

Fig. 1 Chemical structures of salvianolic acids.

2R,3R configuration and 2β-pseudoequatorial, 3β-pseudoaxial conformation. Salvianolic acid J has a 2-arylbenzodioxane skeleton, while salvianolic acid G and isosalvianolic acid C possess an unusual dibenzooxepin skeleton. Rosmarinic acid is a simple depside constructed of danshensu and caffeic acid, while salvianolic acid E is a dimer of rosmarinic acid cyclized to a 2-aryldihydrobenzofurane. Salvianolic acid H and I are regioisomeric compounds, which might be considered as polymerization products of rosmarinic acid and caffeic acid.

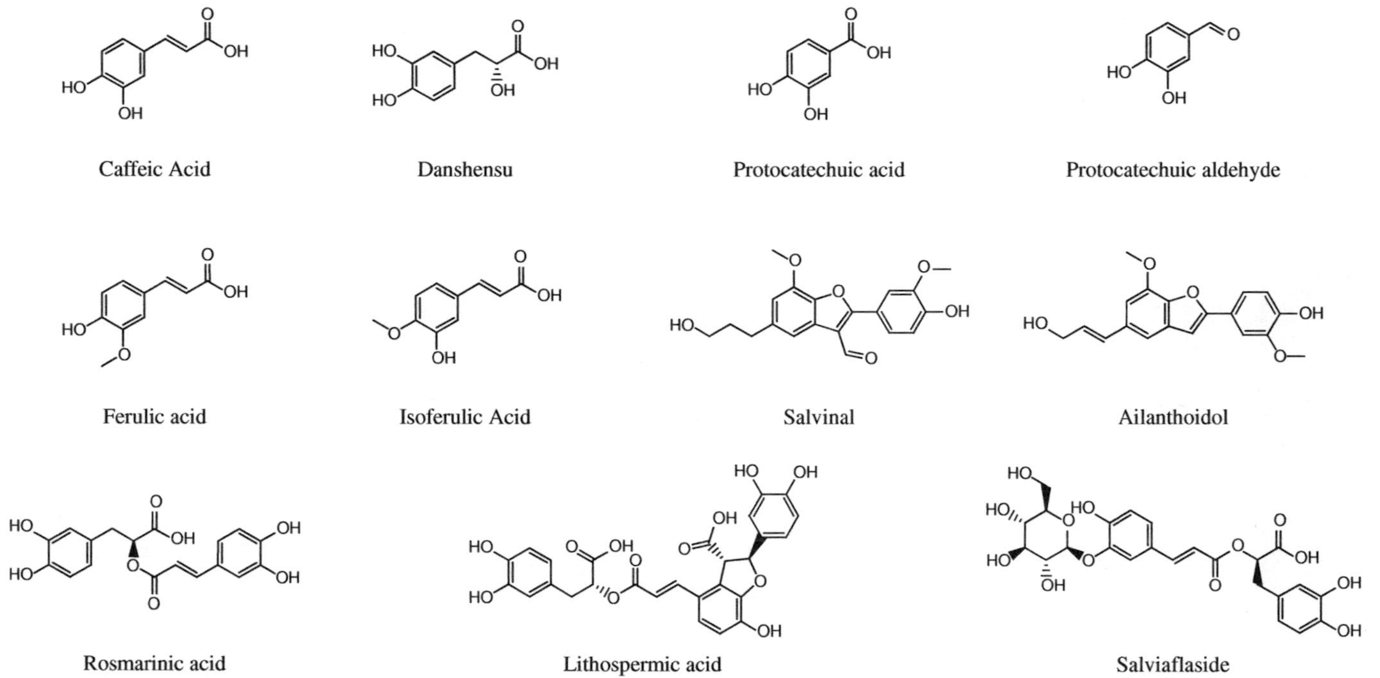

Fig. 2 Chemical structures of other phenolic acids in Danshen.

3. Pharmacological research on SalAA

SalAA, (2*R*)-3-(3,4-dihydroxyphenyl)-2-[(E)-3-[2-[(E)-2-(3,4-dihydroxyphenyl)ethenyl]-3,4-dihydroxyphenyl]prop-2-enoyl]oxypropanoic acid, a caffeic acid derivative, is one of the major water-soluble components in Danshen. SalAA has been reported to possess a wide range of pharmacological effects, including anti-inflammatory, antioxidative, antiplatelet, estrogenic, anticarcinogenic, and antifibrotic properties. In some respects, SalAA exerts more and special potent effects than other salvianolic acids in Danshen. It has been studied in clinical trials for the treatment of diabetic neuropathy.

3.1 Therapeutic effects of SalAA on diabetes and diabetic complications

The World Health Organization (WHO) predicts that by 2025 there will be 300 million people with diabetes. Diabetes is a metabolic disorder characterized by hyperglycemia followed by micro- and macrovascular complications. The therapeutic effect of SalAA on diabetes was investigated. Peripheral nerve dysfunction, pathological progression of hepatic fibrosis, vascular endothelial dysfunction, intestinal motility of diabetic rats and the potential protective mechanisms of SalAA against diabetes were studied (Hou et al., 2017; Qiang et al., 2015; Yu et al., 2012; Yu, Zhang, Yang, Li, & Du, 2016). Results showed that in both type 1 and type 2 diabetic animals, SalAA lowered fasting blood glucose and fed blood glucose in a dose-dependent manner, as well as reduced 24-h food and water intake. SalAA exhibited the antidiabetic effects in diabetic animal models through improving mitochondrial function, increasing ATP production, and decreasing MMP via the CaMKKβ/AMPK signaling pathway.

The pathophysiology of diabetic foot is complicated, involving neurological and blood flow abnormalities in the foot. In SalAA-treated rats, plantar pain withdrawal latency fell, limb grip strength increased, and motor nerve conduction velocity accelerated, suggesting that overall peripheral nerve function had improved (Yu et al., 2012). Treatment with SalAA increased the areas of medullary sheath and axis cylinder compared with the diabetic model group. SalAA treatment showed a trend toward upregulation of the density of myelinated fiber, although without significant difference compared with the model group.

The influence of SalAA on peripheral microcirculation and post-occlusive reactive hyperemia in diabetic rats improved the treatment of peripheral perfusion in diabetic rats. With regard to postocclusive reactive hyperemia, peak values and velocities decreased in diabetic rats, indicating the possible impairments in vascular endothelial structure or function. SalAA mitigated these effects in this study, suggesting that SalAA protects vascular endothelial cell function (Yang, Sun, et al., 2011).

Under many scenarios, the net effect of AMPK activation is to inhibit lipid and glycogen synthesis concomitant with the activation of fatty acid oxidation and glycolysis. Thus, AMPK switches the cell from energy storing to energy releasing under conditions when ATP is limited (Emerling et al., 2009). AMPK is also a stress-sensitive kinase that can be activated by a number of pathological stresses, including hypoxia, oxidative stress, glucose deprivation, exercise, and dietary hormones (Fogarty & Hardie, 2010). Activated AMPK stimulates glycolysis by coordinately promoting glucose uptake and glycolysis flux for stress adaptation. Upon binding to AMP, AMPK undergoes conformational change that facilitates the phosphorylation of the α-subunit. The β-subunit contains a glycogen-binding site that can regulate protein activation via intracellular glycogen levels (Polekhina et al., 2005). SalAA increases the phosphorylation level of AMPK, suggesting a positive activator of AMPK (Yu et al., 2012).

It has been demonstrated that SalAA inhibits binding between the SH_2 domains of Lck and Src and their phosphotyrosine-containing binding motif, which may be the molecular basis for the activation of AMPK by SalAA. AMPK activation increases PGC-1α expression/phosphorylation and AMPK requires PGC-1α activity to modulate the expression of several key players in mitochondrial and glucose metabolism (Jager, Handschin, St-Pierre, & Spiegelman, 2007). Through varied interactions, PGC-1α coordinately regulates gluconeogenesis, glycolysis, lipogenesis, peroxisomal and mitochondrial fatty acid oxidation, and mitochondrial respiration effectiveness (Chowdhury, Dobrowsky, & Fernyhough, 2011). It has been demonstrated that in human peripheral blood neutrophil and lymphocyte, the expression of PGC-1α correlated positively with that of Sirt3 to induce antioxidant defenses (Ferrer, Tauler, Sureda, Tur, & Pons, 2009). Sirt3, as a mitochondrial enzyme, mediates NAD^+-dependent deacetylation of target substrates, senses NAD^+ levels, and thus directly connects metabolic perturbations with transcriptional outputs (Kim et al., 2007). By increasing the expression of PGC-1α and Sirt3, SalAA could increase the mitochondrial function and improve insulin resistance in L6 myoblasts (Yu et al., 2012). Thus, the upregulation of PGC-1α and Sirt3 further suggests that SalAA exerts its protective effects through activation of the AMPK signaling pathway. It has been revealed that AMPK phosphorylates muscle neuronal NOS (nNOS) on Ser (Chen, McConell, et al., 2000). nNOS is an important nitric oxide (NO)-producing enzyme, which serves as a neuromodulator in a second messenger system for neuron-to-neuron communications. nNOS is also required for maintaining the normal peripheral nerve function and small sensory nerve fiber innervations. Therefore, the upregulated expression of nNOS may contribute to the protective effects of SalAA.

The administration of SalAA could significantly alleviate the lesions of hepatic steatosis and fibrosis by HE staining and reduced the content of collagen types I and III by Picro acid-Sirius red staining (Qiang et al., 2014), a method of estimating the degree of fibrosis (Nair, Diehl, Wiseman, Farr, & Perrillo, 2004). This is the first report in which SalAA could inhibit the formation of hepatic steatosis and fibrosis in type 2 diabetic rats and is different from the previous studies in CCl_4- or thioacetamide-induced hepatic fibrosis.

Endothelial dysfunction, elevated level of AGEs, and oxidative stress were present in diabetic rats. SalAA treatment attenuated this endothelial dysfunction concomitantly with markedly decreased oxidative stress and AGEs in aortas. This is the first in vivo study to assess the endothelial protective effect of SalAA in a type 2 diabetes model related to oxidative stress and AGEs. A couple of pathways, whose mechanisms are multifactorial, have been shown to augment oxidative stress during long-standing diabetes (Farhangkhoee et al., 2006; Khan, Farhangkhoee, & Chakrabarti, 2006). One mechanism increases flux through the mitochondrial electron transport chain leading to the production of superoxide anions. Other pathways include the generation of AGEs and autooxidation of glucose (Khan et al., 2006).

NO plays a key role in endothelial dysfunction. A high-fat diet leads to increased NOS expression to produce more NO to resist injury. Impaired antioxidative function by hypercholesterolemia leads to the production of more reactive oxygen species (ROS) and scavenging dysfunction, which secondarily induces the degradation of NO. Both NO and superoxide anions are the main mediators of oxidative damage. Diabetes led to decreased vasorelaxation and vasoconstrictor response in association with oxidative stress and increased MDA and total NOS, including endothelial nitric oxide synthase (eNOS) and iNOS activity. Treatment of diabetic animals with SalAA prevents diabetes-induced MDA and NOS upregulation and oxidative stress (Yang, Qiang, et al., 2011). AGE formation is enhanced by hyperglycemia and oxidative stress. Moreover, AGE produces ROS and increases oxidative stress by activation of nicotinamide adenine dinucleotide phosphate (NADPH) oxidase through AGE receptors (RAGEs). It was also shown that antioxidants not only reduce the formation of AGEs (Coughlan, Cooper, & Thomas, 2007), but also suppress AGE-mediated intracellular effects (Yamaji et al., 2005). Therefore, AGEs and oxidative stress are not independent but correlative. In conclusion, SalAA could protect against early vascular endothelial dysfunction induced by type 2 diabetes and this endothelial protective effect might be correlated with the downregulation of AGEs and NOS activity in aortas via its antioxidative property.

In addition, SalAA could accelerate the GI transit and increase the enteric neuronal population in diabetic rats by upregulating the expression of PGP9.5, a cytosolic ubiquitin carboxylterminal hydroxylase present in all neurons and nerve fibers (Beiswenger, Calcutt, & Mizisin, 2008). These results suggest that SalAA is a potential neuroprotective agent with the capacity to improve GI dysmotility caused by diabetic neuropathy.

In summary, SalAA protects diabetic rats against neuropathy and peripheral vascular circulation dysfunction, suggesting that SalAA is a potential agent capable of improving various deficits associated with this condition.

3.2 Cardiovascular activities of SalAA

It has been reported that in recent years, SalAA exerts therapeutic potential on hepatic protection, neural protection, cancer treatment, and other diseases, and the greatest clinical impact of SalAA is cardiovascular protection. Excessive accumulation of ROS leads to oxidative stress, which can cause ischemic cardiomyopathy in a direct or indirect way. Therefore, antioxidative stress is an important part of protecting against myocardial ischemic injury. SalAA represents a new class of natural antioxidants, with strong antioxidant activity due to a plurality of the phenolic hydroxyl group. There are many studies demonstrating the antioxidant role of SalAA. By using the patch clamp technique, SalAA reversed the inhibition of oxygen free radicals generated by xanthane/xanthane oxidase on the unitary currents of single potassium channel activity (Bao, 1993). SalAA could exert a protective effect against ischemia/reperfusion-induced cell damage in Langendorff-perfused rat hearts (Du, Qiu, & Zhang, 1995). The pharmacological and biological mechanisms underlying potential cardiovascular protection of SalAA were discussed and elucidated.

3.2.1 Protecting myocardial cells from apoptosis

Apoptosis is an important mechanism of myocardial cell death in the setting of acute myocardial ischemia and reperfusion. The results suggested that SalAA exerted an anti-apoptotic effect and improved cardiac function following I/R injury through the JNK/PI3K/Akt signaling pathway in this model (Chen, Xu, et al., 2016). SalAA could upregulate Bcl-2 expression and increase the phosphorylation of Akt, p42/p44 extracellular signal-related kinases (Erk1/2), and their related effectors to exert a marked protective effect on myocardial ischemia-reperfusion injury (Fan et al., 2012; Li et al., 2016). Recent studies demonstrated that SalAA inhibited cardiomyocyte apoptosis in response to I/R by the PI3K/Akt, GSK-3β, JNK, and ERK1/2 pathways, and by JNK-ERK1/2 crosstalk. The mechanisms for SalAA attenuating cardiomyocyte apoptosis during I/R injury through the p38MAPK, caspase, JAK/STAT, NF-κB, and LOX-1 signaling pathways need further illustration. There may be potential crosstalk between PI3K/Akt and JNK, and Akt/GSK-3beta and ERK1/2 in the process of SalAA against I/R-induced cardiomyocyte apoptosis (Qian, Wang, Xu, & Li, 2019).

3.2.2 Antiplatelet and antithrombotic effects

The antithrombotic effect might be related to its antiplatelet action and ability to modulate hemorheology without affecting the coagulation system. Pretreatment with SalAA on washed rat and human platelets significantly inhibited various agonists-stimulated platelet aggregation and caused an increase in cyclic adenosine monophosphate level in platelets activated by ADP (Fan et al., 2010). SalAA inhibited platelet activation via the inhibition of PI3K and attenuated arterial thrombus formation in vivo. These data suggested that SalAA may be developed as a novel therapeutic agent for the prevention of thrombotic disorders (Huang et al., 2010). A study showed that SalAA was protective against myocardial ischemia/reperfusion injury in rats by serving antiplatelet and anti-inflammation roles (Yuan, Xiang, et al., 2017).

3.2.3 Improvement of mitochondrial dysfunction

Mitochondrial respiratory dysfunction characterized by decreased respiratory control ratio and ADP/O was observed in isoproterenol-treated rats. Administration of SalAA for a period of 8 days significantly attenuated isoproterenol-induced cardiac dysfunction and myocardial injury and improved mitochondrial respiratory function. The results suggested that SalAA possessing antioxidant activity had a significant protective effect against isoproterenol-induced myocardial infarction (MI) (Wang et al., 2009). A study investigated the effects of SalAA on cardiomyocyte apoptosis and mitochondrial dysfunction in response to hypoxia/reoxygenation injury by determining the mitochondrial membrane potential ($\triangle\Psi m$) and mitochondrial permeability transition pore (mPTP). The results showed that SalAA prevented the loss of $\triangle\Psi m$ and inhibited the activation of mPTP, indicating the preservation of mitochondrial function (Li, Fan, Liu, & Liang, 2019). SalAA protected against adriamycin-induced heart mitochondrial toxicity of rats, while SalAA had no antagonizing effect on the antitumor activity of adriamycin (Lin, Liu, Liu, & Xu, 1992).

3.2.4 Endothelial cell protection

SalAA potentiated ischemia-induced neovascularization after 1-week post-operation compared to a vehicle-treated group. This effect could be attributed to an increased formation of VEGF, VEGFR-2, and MMP-9 as well as the promotion of numbers and functions of EPCs. These findings showed that SalAA has potent proangiogenic properties by promoting the expression of proangiogenic factors and the functions of EPCs, indicating that SalAA might contribute to protecting against coronary disease (Li, Duan, & Liu, 2014).

3.2.5 Acting on ion flux

The results showed that SalAA pretreatment alleviated cardiac dysfunction and Ca^{2+} overload induced by ATO in vivo and vitro. Moreover, SalAA increased sarco/endoplasmic reticulum Ca^{2+}-ATPase (SERCA) activity and expression, alleviated $[Ca^{2+}]$ ER depletion, and decreased ER stress-related protein expression. SalAA protects the heart from ATO-induced injury and its administration correlates with the modulation of SERCA, the recovery of Ca^{2+} homeostasis, and the downregulation of ER stress-mediated apoptosis (Wang, Zhang, et al., 2019).

3.2.6 Preventing cell migration, proliferation, and intimal hyperplasia

SalAA inhibited angiotensin II (Ang II)-induced proliferation of human umbilical vein endothelial cells via reducing the expression levels of phospho-Src and phospho-Akt (473), thereby attenuating the production of ROS (Yang et al., 2012). SalAA ameliorated pulmonary arterial remodeling in MCT-induced pulmonary arterial hypertension (PAH) rats most likely via activating the BMPRII-Smad pathway and inhibiting apoptosis. Thus, SalAA may have therapeutic potential for patients at high risk of PAH (Chen, Yuan et al., 2016). A study indicated that SalAA treatment can protect human pulmonary arterial endothelial cells from endoMT induced by hypoxia, which may be performed via the inhibition on

ROS production and further through the downstream effectors of BMPRs or TGFβR, including Smads, ERK, and ROCK/cofilin pathways (Yuan, Chen, Zhang, Fang, & Du, 2017).

3.2.7 Inhibiting left ventricular remodeling

Cardiac fibrosis is a deleterious consequence of hypertension that may further advance to heart failure, and increased matrix metalloproteinase-9 (MMP-9) contributes to the underlying mechanism. The results indicated that SalAA is a novel inhibitor of MMP-9, thus playing an inhibitory role in hypertensive fibrosis (Jiang et al., 2013).

3.2.8 Other mechanisms

Intensified research has demonstrated that inflammation was involved in the process of MI, endothelium injury, atherosclerosis, and cardiovascular hypertrophy. In lipopolysaccharide (LPS)-stimulated RAW264.7 cells, SalAA exhibited its anti-inflammatory effect via the p38-HO-1 pathway, reduced transfer of NF-κB to the nuclei, and thus reduced production of inflammatory mediators (Huang et al., 2013). The variations of dimethylarginines in plasma and tissues were induced by the inhibition of DDAH activity and their leakage in the infarct zone after MI. SalAA exerted beneficial effects in MI by decreasing plasma and tissue dimethylarginine levels via restoring DDAH activity (He et al., 2013). In WT mice, SalAA targeted transgelin and had a protective effect on myocardium but did not have the same protective effect on transgelin$^{-/-}$ mice. SalAA stabilized the transgelin-actin complex, modulated the reorganization of the actin cytoskeleton, facilitated F-actin bundling, further enhanced the contractility and blood flows of coronary arteries, and improves outcomes of myocardial ischemia (Zhong et al., 2018).

3.3 Cerebrovascular activities of SalAA

3.3.1 Preserving the integrity of the blood-brain barrier

SalAA blocked inflammatory responses by impairing NF-κB signaling, thereby limiting inflammation/nitrosative stress and preserving the integrity of the blood-brain barrier (Chien et al., 2016). Granulocyte adherence has been proven to be a principal cause of ischemia-reperfusion injury. A study demonstrated that the inhibition of granulocyte adherence was one of the targets of SalAA in the treatment of ischemic stroke. Meanwhile, SalAA inhibited granulocyte adherence by decreasing the expression of ICAM-1 in BMEC (Jiang et al., 2011).

3.3.2 Promoting neurogenesis

SalAA also concomitantly promoted neurogenesis-related protein expression by compromising GSK3beta/Cdk5 activity to enhance the expression levels of β-catenin/DCX and Bcl-2 for neuroprotection (Chien et al., 2016).

3.3.3 Neuroprotective effects

Studies indicated that the ameliorating effect of SalAA on learning and memory impairment caused by cerebral ischemia-reperfusion may be related to its antioxidant activity (Du & Zhang, 1997; Feng et al., 2017). In a study, an experimental stroke model induced by photothrombosis in the unilateral frontal cortex of rats was used to investigate whether SalAA has long-term protective effects on ischemia-induced sensorimotor and memory deficits in behavioral tests. The results indicated that a single SalAA treatment improved the cortical ischemia-induced sensorimotor deficits during a 15-day cylinder test period, and alleviated ischemia-induced sustained spatial memory impairments during the 2-month dependent Morris Water Maze tests. Overall, SalAA might have therapeutic potential for the treatment of memory deficits associated with ischemic stroke (Jiao et al., 2017). Oxidative stress and inflammation play an important role in the pathogenesis of early brain injury (EBI) following subarachnoid hemorrhage (SAH). A study indicated that SalAA ameliorated EBI and provides neuroprotection after SAH in rat models via its antioxidative, anti-inflammatory, and anti-apoptotic effects (Gu et al., 2017).

3.3.4 Soluble epoxide hydrolase inhibition

Epoxyeicosatrienoic acids (EETs) and their regulating enzyme-soluble epoxide hydrolase (sEH) have been associated with ischemic stroke. The results showed that SalAA treatment ameliorated neurological deficits and reduced infarct volume. Notably, the beneficial effects of SalAA were attenuated by coadministration of (14,15-epoxyeicosa-5(*Z*)-enoic acid (14,15-EEZE)), a putative selective EETs antagonist. Furthermore, SalAA increased the 14,15-EET levels in the blood and brain of sham and middle cerebral artery occlusion (MCAO) rats. Assay for hydrolase activity showed that 1 and 3 mg/kg of SalAA significantly diminished brain sEH activity of MCAO rats. A fluorescent assay in vitro indicated that SalAA could inhibit recombinant human sEH activity in a concentration-dependent manner ($IC_{50} = 1.62\,\mu mol/L$). Immunohistochemical analysis showed that SalAA at the doses of 1 and 3 mg/kg significantly decreased sEH protein expression in the hippocampus CA1 region of MCAO rats. In conclusion, cerebral protection of SalAA was mediated, at least in part, via inhibiting sEH to increase EETs levels (Wang et al., 2012).

3.4 Other activities of SalAA

3.4.1 Antitumor

Numerous data indicate that SalAA treatment has a potent antitumor effect. SalAA treatment significantly decreased A549 cell growth by upregulating the phosphatase and tensin homolog protein level, while consistently downregulating Akt phosphorylation (Bi, Chen, Yuan, Jiang, & Chen, 2013). SalAA could reverse paclitaxel resistance through suppressing transgelin 2 expression by mechanisms involving attenuation of PI3K/Akt pathway activation and ABC transporter upregulation. These results not only provided insight into the potential application of SalAA in reversing paclitaxel resistance, thus facilitating the sensitivity of breast cancer chemotherapy, but also highlighted a potential role of transgelin 2 in the development of paclitaxel resistance in breast cancer (Cai et al., 2014). A study found that SalAA-downregulated lung cancer multidrug resistance gene *MDR1* was likely to be affected by the miRNA expression and regulation of target genes (Chen, Bi, et al., 2016). The metastasis of oral squamous cell carcinoma (OSCC) is one of the most important causes of cancer-related deaths. Some findings suggested that SalAA inhibited the invasion and migration of OSCC by inhibiting the c-Raf/MEK/ERK pathways that control MMP-2 expression (Fang et al., 2018).

3.4.2 Effects on Alzheimer's disease

The effects of SalAA on the treatment of Alzheimer's disease (AD) were investigated. SalAA significantly inhibited $A\beta_{42}$ self-aggregation and disaggregates preformed $A\beta_{42}$ fibrils, reduced metal-induced $A\beta_{42}$ aggregation through chelating metal ions, and blocked the formation of ROS in SH-SY5Y cells. SalAA protected cells against $A\beta_{42}$-induced toxicity. Furthermore, SalAA, possibly because of the effects of decreasing toxicity effects of Aβ species, alleviated Aβ-induced paralysis in transgenic *Caenorhabditis elegans*. Circular dichroism experiments and molecular dynamic simulations demonstrated that SalAA inhibited $A\beta_{42}$ self-aggregation through binding to the C-terminus of $A\beta_{42}$, and therefore stabilizing the $A\beta_{42}$-helical conformations. Altogether, the data showed that SalAA, as the multifunctional agent, was likely to be a promising therapeutic for AD (Cao et al., 2013).

3.4.3 *Effects against liver injury and fibrosis*

SalAA protected against HFD-induced NAFLD by ameliorating hepatic lipid accumulation and inflammation, and these protective effects might be partially due to regulation of the TXNIP/NLRP3 and TXNIP/ChREBP pathways (Ding et al., 2016). Secretion from the peroxidative-injured hepatocyte could stimulate HSC activation, and SalAA could decrease activation by alleviation of hepatocyte peroxidation (Hu, Liu, et al., 2000; Hu, Wang, et al., 2000). SalAA showed marked effects against liver injury and fibrosis, associated with its anti-lipid peroxidation actions (Hu et al., 1997). SalAA inhibited PDGF-BB-activated HSC proliferation, partially through apoptosis induction (Lin, Lee, Huang, & Huang, 2006; Liu et al., 2000). SalAA could prevent the pathological progression of hepatic fibrosis in HFD-fed and STZ-induced diabetic rats involving the reduction of oxidative stress, the suppression of α-SMA and TGF-β1 expression, as well as the exertion of anti-apoptotic and mitochondria-protective effects (Qiang et al., 2014). SalAA could reduce liver fibrosis through the regulation of PI3K/AKT/mTOR, Bcl-2/Bax, and caspase-3/cleaved caspase-3 signaling pathways (Wang, Song, et al., 2019).

3.4.4 *Preventing galactose-induced cataract*

SalAA has been demonstrated to have efficient antioxidative and free radical scavenging effects. In a study, the preventive effects of SalAA on galactose-induced cataract in rats were investigated. These results indicated that SalAA could prevent galactose-induced cataract by antioxidation and inhibition of aldose reductase (Du, Qiu, Tian, & Zhang, 1995).

3.4.5 *Protection against nephropathy*

As a multifunctional agent, SalAA had favorable renoprotection in doxorubicin-induced nephropathy. The anti-inflammation, antioxidation, amelioration of podocyte injury, improvement of hemorheology, and hypolipidemic properties may constituent an important part of its therapeutic effects. All these indicated that SalAA was likely to be a promising agent for NS (Fan et al., 2015; Hou et al., 2017).

3.4.6 *Antiallergic effect*

The effects of SalAA on allergic asthma were investigated using rat RBL-2H3 mast cells and female BALB/c mice. SalAA did not inhibit antigen-induced degranulation of mast cells. Administration of SalAA decreased the number of immune cells, particularly eosinophils in allergic asthma-induced mice. Histological studies showed that SalAA reduced mucin production and inflammation in the lungs. Administration of SalAA reduced the expression and secretion of Th2 cytokines (IL-4 and IL-13) in the bronchoalveolar lavage fluid and lung tissues of mice with ovalbumin-induced allergic asthma. These findings provided evidence that SalAA might be a potential antiallergic therapeutic (Heo & Im, 2019).

3.4.7 Effects on systemic lupus erythematosus

The effects of SalAA on systemic lupus erythematosus (SLE) were investigated in BALB/c mice subjected to pristane. SalAA treatment caused a significant reduction in the levels of anti-Sm autoantibodies and reduced renal histopathological changes and pathological effects. SalAA treatment also significantly inhibited the phosphorylation of IKK, IκB, and NF-κB in renal tissues of lupus mice. The results suggested that SalAA alleviates renal injury in pristane-induced SLE in BALB/c mice through inhibition of phosphorylation of IKK, IκB, and NF-κB (Lin et al., 2017).

4. Pharmacological research on SalAB

SalAB is one of the water-soluble components isolated from Danshen. It has been demonstrated that SalAB possessed extensive pharmacological activities, including antioxidative stress, antiplatelet aggregation, and anti-ischemia (Du, Qiu, & Zhang, 2000; Huang & Zhang, 1992). Furthermore, SalAB exerts protective effects on cardiovascular diseases, metabolic diseases, ischemic cerebrovascular diseases, neurodegenerative disorders, and lung injury as well.

4.1 The protective effects of SalAB on cardiovascular diseases

It has been suggested that oral administration of SalAB (25 mg/kg/day) for 11 days lowered systolic blood pressure by 30% and improved impaired endothelium-dependent relaxation and contraction in Ang II (1.2 mg/kg/day)-infused hypertensive C57BL/6J mice. They further demonstrated that SalAB downregulated the expression of AT1 receptors, NADPH oxidase subunits (Nox-2 and Nox-4), and nitrotyrosine in arteries of Ang II-infused mice or in Ang II-treated HUVECs. Hence, vasoprotective and antioxidative effects might be involved in the antihypertensive action of SalAB (Ling et al., 2017). Pan et al. observed that 4-week intraperitoneal injection of SalAB at 40 mg/kg/day exhibited cardioprotective effects by inhibiting postinfarction cardiac hypertrophy and infarction size, and improving cardiac function in MI C57 mice through the eNOS/NO pathway (Pan et al., 2011). Also, oral administration of SalAB (10, 20, 30 mg/kg) significantly improved heart function and decreased infarct size in acute myocardial ischemia-reperfusion injury rats through antioxidation, anti-inflammation, and anti-apoptosis (Qiao & Xu, 2016). Moreover, 2-week oral administration of SalAB (240 mg/kg/day) alleviated transverse aortic constriction surgery-induced heart failure by increasing cardiac systolic function via inactivating the ERK1/2/GATA4 signaling pathway after pressure overload in mice (Yu, Chen, et al., 2016). Taken together, SalAB protected against cardiovascular diseases.

4.2 The neuroprotective effects of SalAB

Our previous studies have demonstrated that SalAB protected against the cerebral transient ischemia-induced learning and memory dysfunctions and cerebral ischemia-reperfusion-induced brain injury by reducing lipid peroxides, scavenging free radicals, and improving energy metabolism (Chen, Du, & Zhang, 2000; Du et al., 2000). More recently, Jiang et al. found that SalAB exerted a neuroprotective effect in a mouse model of cerebral ischemia and reperfusion injury established by bilateral carotid artery occlusion for 30 min followed by 24-h reperfusion. A 22.5 mg/kg injection of SalAB rescued neuronal loss in the hippocampal CA1 region through a mitochondria-dependent antioxidative effect and anti-apoptosis activity (Jiang et al., 2015). In addition, the neuroprotective effects of SalAB on neurodegenerative disorders were observed in AD and Parkinson's disease (PD) animal models. Subchronic administration of SalAB at 10 mg/kg for 7 days significantly ameliorated the $A\beta_{25-35}$ peptide-induced memory impairment in the passive avoidance task, and also reduced the number of activated microglia and astrocytes via anti-inflammation and antioxidation in $A\beta_{25-35}$ peptide-induced AD mice (Lee et al., 2013). SalAB attenuated toxin-induced neuronal injury via Nrf2-dependent glial cell-mediated protective activity in MPTP-induced PD mice after intraperitoneal administration of SalAB at 50 mg/kg twice a day for 6 days (Zhou et al., 2014). Additionally, Chen et al. reported that 15-day injection of SalAB (25 mg/kg) attenuated brain damage and inflammation after traumatic brain injury in mice by suppressing inflammatory reaction (Chen et al., 2011). In summary, SalAB represents a promising candidate for the prevention and treatment of ischemic cerebrovascular disease and neurodegenerative disorders.

4.3 SalAB is beneficial to metabolic diseases

Oral administration of SalAB (20, 40 mg/kg) for 3 weeks exhibited antidiabetic effects with decreased blood glucose and improved glucose tolerance in multiple low-dose streptozotocin-induced diabetic rats through stimulating insulin secretion. However, only 40 mg/kg of SalAB increased the number and area of pancreatic islets by anti-apoptosis and antioxidation (Raoufi et al., 2015). Huang et al. also observed antidiabetic effects of SalAB in type 2 diabetic rats induced by a high-fat diet and streptozotocin; however, the dose of SalAB they used was 100 and 200 mg/kg with a reduction of blood glucose by 23.8% and 21.7%, respectively (Huang et al., 2015). Apart from antidiabetic effects, SalAB possessed hypolipidemic activity, and attenuated insulin resistance and oxidative stress as well (Huang et al., 2015). Further mechanism study suggested that AMPK pathway regulation was involved in the antidiabetic and hypolipidemic effects of SalAB in db/db mice (Huang et al., 2016). Furthermore, the anti-obesity property of SalAB was demonstrated by reduction of body weight gain and fat mass, as well as prevention of dyslipidemia in high-fat diet-induced obesity mice (An et al., 2019; Wang et al., 2014). Collectively, SalAB may serve as a potential therapeutic approach for metabolic diseases.

4.4 SalAB protects against lung injury

The novel protective effects of SalAB on lung injury have been reported. Yang et al. demonstrated that SalAB protected against acute lung injury by downregulating the expression of channel kinase TRPM6 and TRPM7 in an LPS-induced sepsis rat model (Yang, Liu, Li, Sui, & Liu, 2018). Other research also suggested that intragastrical treatment of SalAB (200, 400 mg/kg) protected against paraquat-induced pulmonary injury and pulmonary fibrosis through mediating Nrf2/Nox4 redox balance and TGF-β1/Smad3 signaling (Liu et al., 2016). Interestingly, Zhang et al. reported that intraperitoneal injection of SalAB exhibited a protective effect on cigarette smoke-induced lung injury by attenuating lung inflammation in mice. Its possible mechanism was associated with activating Nrf-2 and inhibiting NF-κB activation (Zhang, Zhang, & Li, 2015).

4.5 Other pharmacological effects of SalAB

SalAB exerted antifibrotic effects in CCL_4-induced liver fibrosis mice and unilateral ureteral obstruction (UUO)-induced renal fibrosis mice (Li, Zhang, He, et al., 2017; Yu et al., 2015). In addition, it is interesting that SalAB was demonstrated to successfully reverse multidrug resistance in nude mice bearing colon cancer cells (Guo et al., 2018). Further investigation is needed to evaluate the pharmacological effects and assess the underlying mechanisms of SalAB.

5. Other salvianolic acids and total salvianolic acids

5.1 Salvianolic acid C

In recent years, the pharmacological effects of SalAC have been reported. In UUO rats, SalAC (12.5 mg/kg/day) improved renal and tubular function by inhibiting kidney secretion of inflammatory cytokines CCL5 and CXCL10 (Li, Gu, Fu, & Zhao, 2015). Results showed that SalAC inhibited the activities of MMP-2 and MMP-9 significantly, and 20 mg/kg/day SalAC (i.p., a week) ameliorated the progression of aortic aneurysm in $ApoE^{-/-}$ mice (Wu et al., 2016). SalAC also inhibited LPS-mediated inflammatory response and NF-κB nuclear translocation via the activation of AMPK/Nrf2 signaling both in vivo (5, 10, and 20 mg/kg/day doses in rats) and in vitro (0.1, 1, and 5 μM in BV2 microglia cells) (Song et al., 2018). Xanthine oxidase serves as an important drug target for gout, a common form of inflammatory arthritis. SalAC showed a potent xanthine oxidase inhibitory effect with an IC_{50} of 5.84 ± 0.18 μM (Tang & Zhao, 2019). Acetaminophen overdose is one of the reasons for acute liver damage. SalAC (5, 10, and 20 mg/kg/day, i.p.) for 6 days in mice protected against APAP-induced liver injury by inhibiting mitochondrial oxidative stress, inflammation, and apoptosis via the Keap 1/Nrf2/HO-1 signaling pathway (Wu et al., 2019).

5.2 Pharmacology, toxicity and therapeutic effect of total salvianolic acids

Salvianolic acids are important components of the water-soluble components of Danshen. There are a great variety of salvianolic acids, which have similar basic organic acid structure with phenolic hydroxyls and similar pharmacological actions. Salvianolic acids have many activities such as antioxidation, improving microcirculation, and antiplatelet aggregation, and promoting tissue repair.

5.2.1 Protection against ischemic stroke

Substantial studies have reported that salvianolic acids protect against cerebral ischemia injury (Hou et al., 2016; Tang et al., 2014). Total salvianolic acid 12.5–25 mg/kg had the effect of anticerebral ischemia in MCAO in rats, including decreasing the infarction area and cerebral edema. Mechanism study also demonstrated that total salvianolic acids (10 and 30 mg/kg, i.p.) enhance cerebral angiogenesis and promote neurological recovery after ischemic stroke (Li, Zhang, Cui, et al., 2017; Zhang et al., 2017), which may be related with attenuated inflammation in microglia (23 and 46 mg/kg, i.p.) (Zhuang et al., 2017) and inactivation of NADPH oxidase through a signaling pathway implicating AMPK/Akt/PKC (1.67 mg/kg, i.v.) (Tang et al., 2014), etc.

5.2.2 Actions on cardiovascular diseases

Salvianolic acids have protective actions on the in vitro perfused rat heart against injury caused by ischemia-reperfusion, and can decrease the incidence rate of ventricular fibrillation, alleviate the level of destruction to the ultrastructure of myocardium, and reduce the content of MDA in tissues. Total salvianolic acid injection (8 mg/kg/h, i.v.) attenuated I/R-induced myocardial injury (Huang et al., 2019).

5.2.3 Protective actions on learning and memory

Studies using cerebral ischemia experimental animal models (mice and rats) have shown that salvianolic acids (3–10 mg/kg, i.v.) have protective actions on the brain, and against injury caused by cerebral ischemia and ischemia-reperfusion, manifested by reducing the area of ischemic brain, decreasing the content of MDA, alleviating the ethological disorders caused by cerebral ischemia, and significantly improving the disorders in memory functions (Chen, Du, et al., 2000; Du et al., 2000; Du & Zhang, 1997). Total salvianolic acids (30 and 60 mg/kg/day, i.p.) induced a remarkable amelioration of learning and memory impairments in APPswe/PS1dE9 mice through the regulation of $A\beta_{42}$, $A\beta_{40}$, carbohydrate, and vitamin metabolites in the hippocampus and LDL-C and CHOL in the plasma (Shen et al., 2017). Study also showed that total salvianolic acids (20 mg/kg, i.v.) balance brain functional network topology in rat hippocampi overexpressing miR-30e (Li et al., 2018). Combination therapy of salvianolic acid (40 mg/kg) and fluoxetine (20 mg/kg) can alleviate depression-like symptoms and cognitive deficit induced by chronic stress (Yu, An, et al., 2016).

5.2.4 Other effects

Salvianolic acids have strong antioxidation actions. It has been shown by in vivo and in vitro experiments that salvianolic acids can scavenge oxygen free radicals and inhibit the peroxide reactions of lipids. These actions have been proved by different researchers under different experimental conditions (Petersen & Simmonds, 2003). Research proved that 5–50 mg/kg total acid could inhibit lipid peroxidation of microsomes from liver induced by the Fe^{2+}-cys system; scavenge superoxide anion produced by the xanthine/xanthine oxidase system; and scavenge free hydroxyl radicals produced by the Fe^{2+}-H_2O_2 system; the inhibition was 98.7%, 75.2%, and 98.99%, respectively. Total salvianolic acids were more effective than vitamin E at the same dose. It has been shown by experimental results that salvianolic acids can protect blood vessel endothelial cells against injury caused by oxidative stress (Ren, Du, & Zhang, 2003) and high glucose-induced endothelial injury (Zhai et al., 2019). Studies showed that salvianolic acids (<1 μmol/L) can increase the activity of Na^+-K^+ ATPase. Salvianolic acids have significant influence on the aggregation of platelets (Tang, Ren, Zhang, & Du, 2002; Yu & Xu, 1994). A study found that salvianolic acids (50 mg/kg, i.g.) improve liver lipid metabolism in ovariectomized rats via blocking STAT-3/SREBP1 signaling (Chen et al., 2018). Salvianolic acids (20 mg/kg, i.g.) have an inhibitory effect on the rheumatoid arthritis of collagen-induced arthritis model rats (Sun, Zhao, Liu, Sun, & Li, 2018).

5.3 Clinical studies of salvianolic acids

Clinical indications of salvianolic acids include the treatment of stroke, nephropathy, etc. (Yan et al., 2017). There are two types of salvianolic acid drugs approved for clinical use: Salvia miltiorrhiza depside salt (SMDS) for infusion and salvianolic acids for injection, which is made by separating the effective components of water-soluble phenolic acids. The effect of salvianolic acids on acute cerebral infarction was investigated in several clinical studies. The studies indicated that salvianolic acids may improve the neurological dysfunction of patients with acute stroke, which may be explained by the increased perfusion of hypoperfused brain tissues (Peng, Liu, Meng, Zhang, & Yu, 2018; Yang, Ju, Li, & Yun, 2018). The effects of salvianolic acids on cardiovascular disease were also investigated. A system review showed that the combined use of salvianolate injection and western medicine in the treatment of unstable angina pectoris can achieve a better effect (Zhang, Wu, Liu, Zhang, & Zhang, 2016).

5.4 Safety studies of salvianolic acids

The safety of salvianolic acids has been reported recently, which provides toxicological data as well as references for the research and development of salvianolic acid-related drugs. Adverse reactions of salvianolic acid injections mainly include allergic reactions, bleeding, etc. In the toxicological study of SMDS, the median lethal dose (LD_{50}) was 1.49 g/kg. Long-term tests on beagle dogs indicated that doses of <80 mg/kg were safe, and doses of 320 mg/kg were toxic (Chang et al., 2014). A system review of the safety of salvianolate injection showed that many rare, serious adverse events were not seen in the clinical application of salvianolate injection (Chen, Xie, Liao, & Wang, 2016). A prospective, multicenter, cohort study showed that SMDS was well tolerated in the general population. The incidences of adverse events, adverse drug events, and adverse drug reactions were 6.40%, 1.57%, and 0.79%, respectively. Adverse drug events included rash, pruritus, erythemas, headache, dizziness, palpitations, increased transaminases, positive fecal occult blood, increased international normalized ratio, increased blood bilirubin, increased blood creatinine, and abnormal platelet count (Yan et al., 2017).

6. Pharmacokinetic research on salvianolic acids

Salvianolic acids are the main active components in Danshen. To study the pharmacokinetics of these compounds is important for understanding their pharmacodynamics and developing new drugs. There have been many studies on the pharmacokinetics of salvianolic acids that have reported the results of their absorption, distribution, metabolism, and excretion in different animals.

6.1 The pharmacokinetics of SalAA

SalAA has been reported for its pharmacokinetic properties in rats, dogs, and monkeys. At present, the detection of SalAA in plasma samples is mainly by high-performance liquid chromatography (HPLC) or high-performance liquid chromatography tandem mass spectrometry (HPLC-MS).

The pharmacokinetic parameters of SalAA after intravenous injection have been studied in rats by HPLC. Male Sprague–Dawley (SD) rats (220–250 g, $n=5$) were injected intravenously with 5 mL/kg of Danshen (4 mg/kg of SalAA). The results showed that the $t_{1/2\alpha}$ of SalAA was 0.139 ± 0.035 h, $t_{1/2\beta}$ was 1.346 ± 0.307 h, $AUC_{0-4\ h}$ was 25.142 ± 6.858 mg h L^{-1}, $AUC_{0-\infty}$ was 38.014 ± 8.219 mg h L^{-1}, CL was 0.105 ± 0.022 L kg h^{-1}, MRT was 1.145 ± 0.391 h. Further analysis showed that SalAA was rapidly eliminated and distributed to tissues

(Hou, Peng, & Chao, 2007). Other experiments were carried out in SD rats after oral doses of 5, 10, and 20 mg/kg, and an intravenous dose of 50 μg/kg. The absolute bioavailability of SalAA after oral administration in SD rats was calculated to be 0.39–0.52% (Sun, Song, et al., 2018).

The pharmacokinetic parameters of SalAA in rats were determined after oral administration of 100 mg/kg of SalAA by HPLC-MS. The pharmacokinetic parameters were analyzed by a noncompartmental model. Results showed that the AUC of SalAA was 698 ± 129 ngh/mL, the $t_{1/2}$ was 3.29 h, and 9 h after administration, the plasma concentration was below 30 ng/mL (Pei et al., 2008).

Sun et al. studied the bioavailability and dose proportionality of SalAA after oral administration in beagle dogs using HPLC-MS. After oral administration of 5, 10, and 20 mg/kg and intravenous administration of 50 μg/kg of SalAA, the C_{max} was calculated to be 14.38, 28.95, and 38.18 mg/L for 5, 10, and 20 mg/kg doses, respectively. The AUC for three doses was 38.77, 81.47, and 130.33 mg/L h, respectively. The bioavailability of SalAA in beagle dogs was 1.42%, and the pharmacokinetic parameters appeared to be approximately dose proportional, but did not meet the statistical criteria (Sun et al., 2013). Song et al. developed a rapid, simple, sensitive, and accurate HPLC-MS method for the determination of SalAA in monkey plasma and studied the pharmacokinetics after intravenous injection. Results showed that the AUC values were 3.316 ± 0.871, 5.754 ± 2.150, and 13.761 ± 2.825 mg/L h for 2.5, 5.0, and 10.0 mg/kg doses in rhesus monkeys. Furthermore, this study showed that SalAA revealed linear pharmacokinetics at 2.5, 5, and 10 mg/kg doses administered by intravenous injection (Song, Zhang, Zhang, et al., 2015). Table 1 summarizes the pharmacokinetic parameters of SalAA.

The metabolites of SalAA in rat plasma after i.v. administration of 20 mg/kg of SalAA, including SalAA-monoglucuronide, monomethyl-SalAA-monoglucuronide, monomethyl-SalAA, dimethyl-SalAA, and dimethyl-SalAA-monoglucuronide, were studied. The results suggested that SalA was mainly metabolized through methylation and glucuronidation pathways (Shen, Wang, Xu, Liu, & Chao, 2009). In another experiment, the metabolites of SalAA were studied both in vivo and in vitro. The results showed that SalAA was rapidly metabolized into 3-*O*-methyl-SalAA, 3′-*O*-methyl-SalAA, 3,3″-*O*-dimethyl-SalAA, and 3′,3″-*O*-dimethyl-SalAA through methylation catalyzed by catechol-*O*-methyltransferase. These methylation products all showed high antioxidant potency (Xu et al., 2014).

Table 1 Pharmacokinetics (PK) of salvianolic acid A in reported studies.

Species	Route	Dose SalAA	PK parameters	Important information and references
SD rat	i.v.	4 mg/kg (Danshen injection)	$t_{1/2\alpha}$: 0.139 ± 0.035 h $t_{1/2\beta}$: 1.346 ± 0.307 h AUC_{0-4h}: 25.142 ± 6.858 mg h L^{-1} $AUC_{0-\infty}$: 38.014 ± 8.219 mg h L^{-1} CL: 0.105 ± 0.022 L kg h^{-1} MRT: 1.145 ± 0.391 h	Rapidly eliminated and distributed to tissues (Hou et al., 2007). The absolute bioavailability in SD rats is 0.39–0.52% (Sun, Song, et al., 2018)
	p.o.	5 mg/kg	$t_{1/2}$: 1.96 h C_{max}: 31.53 μg/L AUC_{0-t}: 105.93 μg/L h	
	p.o.	10 mg/kg	$t_{1/2}$: 1.72 h C_{max}: 57.39 μg/L AUC_{0-t}: 167.18 μg/L h	
	p.o.	20 mg/kg	$t_{1/2}$: 1.79 h C_{max}: 111.91 μg/L AUC_{0-t}: 317.11 μg/L h	
	i.v.	50 μg/kg	$t_{1/2}$: 6.16 h C_{max}: 578.89 μg/L AUC_{0-t}: 204.57 μg/L h	
Wistar rat	p.o.	100 mg/kg	$t_{1/2}$: 3.29 h C_{max}: 318 ± 189 ng/mL AUC: 698 ± 129 ng h/mL	After administration for 9 h, the plasma concentration of SalAA was below 30 ng/mL (Pei et al., 2008)
Dog	p.o.	5 mg/kg	$t_{1/2}$: 3.25 ± 3.13 h C_{max}:14.38 ± 9.12 μg/L AUC_{0-t}: 38.77 ± 40.04 μg/L h	Bioavailability in beagle dogs: 1.42% The PK parameters are approximately dose proportional, but do not meet the statistical criteria (Sun et al., 2013)
	p.o.	10 mg/kg	$t_{1/2}$: 1.20 ± 0.44 h C_{max}: 28.95 ± 12.25 μg/L AUC_{0-t}: 81.47 ± 32.95 μg/L h	
	p.o.	20 mg/kg	$t_{1/2}$: 3.00 ± 0.79 h C_{max}: 38.18 ± 19.08 μg/L AUC_{0-t}: 130.33 ± 95.53 μg/L h	
	i.v.	50 μg/kg	$t_{1/2}$: 0.05 ± 0.00 h C_{max}: 186.94 ± 51.45 μg/L AUC_{0-t}: 22.17 ± 6.59 μg/L h	

Table 1 Pharmacokinetics (PK) of salvianolic acid A in reported studies.—Cont'd

Species	Route	Dose SalAA	PK parameters	Important information and references
Monkey	i.v.	2.5 mg/kg	$t_{1/2}$: 0.474 ± 0.110 h C_{max}: 28.343 ± 6.426 mg/L AUC: 3.316 ± 0.871 mg/L h	SalAA revealed linear pharmacokinetics at 2.5, 5, and 10 mg/kg doses in monkeys (Song et al., 2018)
	i.v.	5 mg/kg	$t_{1/2}$: 0.540 ± 0.331 h C_{max}: 45.679 ± 12.301 mg/L AUC: 5.754 ± 2.150 mg/L h	
	i.v.	10 mg/kg	$t_{1/2}$: 0.421 ± 0.236 h C_{max}: 113.293 ± 24.360 mg/L h AUC: 13.761 ± 2.825 mg/L h	

AUC, area under concentration-time curve; *CL*, total body clearance; C_{max}, maximum concentration; *MRT*, mean residence time; $t_{1/2}$, half-life; t_{max}, time for maximum concentration.

6.2 The pharmacokinetics of SalAB

The pharmacokinetics of SalAB has been studied in rats and the results showed that the absolute bioavailability of SalAB is 0.022%. The reason for the poor bioavailability of SalAB has been researched and it was found that there was still 60% of given SalAB remaining in the gut after 4 h administration orally (Zhang, Akao, Nakamura, Duan, et al., 2004). The pharmacokinetics of magnesium SalAB in beagle dogs was also studied after intravenously injected with 3, 6, and 12 mg/kg. The plasma concentration of SalAB was measured by triple quadrupole mass spectrometry, and the pharmacokinetic parameters were calculated and analyzed by DAS software. The dynamic process of SalAB after intravenous injection in beagle dogs was estimated to be a two-compartment model. Results showed that the distribution and elimination of SalAB were fast. The $t_{1/2\alpha}$ values were 2.2, 2.7, and 2.9 min and $t_{1/2\beta}$ values were 43, 42, and 42 min, respectively (Li et al., 2004). After intravenous injection of 100 mg/kg SalAB, the concentration of SalAB in bile increased rapidly and steadily, and the SalAB in the bile reached the highest value at 30 min. The concentration of SalAB in bile is higher than that in plasma at many time points. This suggested that the hepatobiliary elimination of SalAB may involve active transport

(Chen, Jaw, Shiao, & Tsai, 2005). Studies have shown that the urinary excretion rate of SalAB is <0.16%. At the same time, 24 h after oral administration of 10 and 50 mg/kg SalAB, the recovery of SalAB from the gastrointestinal tract was 41.2% and 23.3%, respectively.

In addition, Caco-2 cell studies have shown that SalAB has lower cell membrane permeability. The bioavailability of SalAB after oral administration is about 5%. The poor bioavailability of SalAB may be related to its poor absorption or fast metabolic clearance (Kim et al., 2005). Rats were given 100 mg/kg of SalAB intravenously and 500 mg/kg of SalAB orally. The AUC values were 5030 ± 565 and 582 ± 222 min μg/mL, respectively. The oral bioavailability of SalAB was calculated to be 2.3% (Wu et al., 2006). Three groups of rabbits were treated with SalAB. Intravenous doses were 2.62 and 5.25 mg/kg, respectively. Oral dose was 105 mg/kg. The pharmacokinetic parameters of intravenous injection were fitted by a two-compartment model, and the pharmacokinetic parameters of oral administration were fitted with a one-compartment model. The bioavailability of SalAB was calculated to be 5.6% (Ma & Wang, 2007). The pharmacokinetic parameters showed a rapid elimination of SalAB after intravenous injection of 10, 20, and 40 mg/kg doses. The concentrations of SalAB in three doses were about 100 times lower at 4 h than that at 3 min (Han et al., 2009). Zhao et al. reported that the total bile elimination of SalAB was reduced significantly by pre-administration with rifampicin 15 min prior due to the inhibition of organic anion transporting polypeptide-mediated influx (Zhao et al., 2012). Table 2 summarizes the reported pharmacokinetics of SalAB.

A number of strategies have been adopted to improve the bioavailability of SalAB. The SalAB in phospholipid complex-loaded nanoparticles was increased compared with free SalAB. The relative bioavailability was increased to 286% (Peng et al., 2008). Zhou et al. used sodium caprate to increase the intestinal absorption and bioavailability of SalAB (Zhou, Chow, & Zuo, 2009). The $t_{1/2}$ values of SalAB in beagle dogs were increased by 5.8- and 17.5-fold when encapsulated into conventional and PEGylated liposomes, respectively. The AUC_{0-t} values were increased by 6.7- and 13.3-fold (Zhang et al., 2012). Chitosan nanoparticles can enhance the absorption of SalAB. The $AUC_{0-\infty}$ of the SalAB-3 kDa chitosan nanoparticles was 16.03-fold higher than that of free SalAB (Jin, Zhang, Li, Liang, & Jia, 2016).

There are three *O*-methylated metabolites in rat serum that have been found by LC/MS/MS method. The bile excretion rates of SalAB and its

Table 2 Pharmacokinetics (PK) of salvianolic acid B in reported studies.

Species	Route	Dose SalAB	PK parameters	Key information and references
Wistar rat	i.v.	4 mg/kg Mg-SalAB	$t_{1/2\alpha}$: 12.3 ± 2.14 min $t_{1/2\beta}$: 128 ± 4.68 min AUC: 87.8 ± 10.9 μg/mL min V_{ss}: 7.60 ± 1.03 L/kg MRT: 137 ± 3.71 min CL_t: 55.52 ± 7.1 mL/min/kg	The oral bioavailability of Mg-SalAB is 0.022%
		20 mg/kg Mg-SalAB	$t_{1/2\alpha}$: 22.7 ± 4.29 min $t_{1/2\beta}$: 176 ± 30.4 min AUC: 1130 ± 329 μg/mL min V_{ss}: 3.61 ± 1.16 L/kg MRT: 141 ± 23.4 min CL_t: 23.5 ± 6.0 mL/min/kg	About 65% was left in the gastrointestinal tract 4 h after oral administration (Zhang, Akao, Nakamura, Duan, et al., 2004)
	p.o.	100 mg/kg Mg-SalAB	AUC: 1.26 ± 0.36 μg/mL min C_{max}: 0.041 ± 0.007 μg/mL t_{max}: 20 ± 5.47 min	
Dog	i.v.	3 mg/kg Mg-SalAB	$t_{1/2\alpha}$: 2.2 ± 0.2 min $t_{1/2\beta}$: 43 ± 9 min AUC: 109 ± 24 μg/mL min MRT: 16.3 ± 3.8 min CL_t: 28 ± 5 mL/min/kg	Linear pharmacokinetics of C_0 and AUC after i.v. administration
		6 mg/kg Mg-SalAB	$t_{1/2\alpha}$: 2.7 ± 0.5 min $t_{1/2\beta}$: 42 ± 7 min AUC: 248 ± 55 μg/mL min CL_t: 26 ± 7 mL/min/kg	Distributed and eliminated quickly in beagle dogs (Li et al., 2004)
		12 mg/kg Mg-SalAB	$t_{1/2\alpha}$: 2.9 ± 0.3 min $t_{1/2\beta}$: 42 ± 10 min AUC: 582 ± 84 μg/mL min CL_t: 21 ± 3 mL/min/kg	
SD rat	i.v.	100 mg/kg	Blood: $t_{1/2\beta}$: 53 ± 15 min AUC: 1340 ± 167 μg/mL min CL_t: 79 ± 9 mL/min/kg	The concentration of SalAB in bile increased rapidly and reached the highest value at 30 min
			Bile: C_{max}: 85.2 ± 12.7 μg/mL T_{max}: 30 ± 0 μg/mL $t_{1/2\beta}$: 9 ± 1 min AUC: 2080 ± 278 μg/mL min	The concentration of SalAB in bile is higher than that in blood plasma (Chen et al., 2005)

Continued

Table 2 Pharmacokinetics (PK) of salvianolic acid B in reported studies.—Cont'd

Species	Route	Dose SalAB	PK parameters	Key information and references
SD rat	i.v.	10 mg/kg	$t_{1/2}$: 136 ± 63.3 min AUC: 702 ± 84.4 μg/mL min V_{ss}: 343 ± 224 mL/kg MRT: 30.9 ± 15.3 min CL: 15.4 ± 4.8 mL/min/kg	The oral bioavailability of SalAB is about 5% in SD rats
	i.v.	50 mg/kg	$t_{1/2}$: 103 ± 33.1 min AUC: 4963 ± 1088 μg/mL min V_{ss}: 298 ± 111 mL/kg MRT: 31.8 ± 9.3 min CL: 10.5 ± 2.3 mL/min/kg	SalAB in the gastrointestinal tract was 23.3% after oral administration of 50 mg/kg for 24 h Lower permeability of SalAB in Caco-2 cells (Kim et al., 2005)
	p.o.	50 mg/kg	$t_{1/2}$: 128 ± 55.2 min AUC: 247 ± 488 μg/mL min T_{max}: 45.0 ± 46.2 min C_{max}: 8.93 ± 19.6 μg/mL CL: 0.38 ± 0.47 mL/min/kg	
SD rat	i.v.	100 mg/kg	$t_{1/2}$: 105 ± 19 min AUC: 5030 ± 565 μg/mL min C_{max}: 910 ± 380 μg/mL	The oral bioavailability of SalAB is 2.3% in SD rats (Wu et al., 2006)
	p.o.	500 mg/kg	$t_{1/2}$: 248 ± 11 min AUC: 582 ± 222 μg/mL min C_{max}: 1.5 ± 0.5 μg/mL	
Rabbit	i.v.	2.62 mg/kg	$t_{1/2}$: 2.57 ± 1.38 h AUC: 2658 ± 837 μg/L h CL: 1.05 ± 0.33 L/h/kg	The oral bioavailability of SalAB is 5.6% in rabbits (Ma & Wang, 2007)
	i.v.	5.25 mg/kg	$t_{1/2}$: 3.07 ± 1.86 h AUC: 5478 ± 1670 μg/L h CL: 0.94 ± 0.27 L/h/kg	
	p.o.	105 mg/kg	$t_{1/2}$: 7.08 ± 2.47 h AUC: 5135 ± 788 μg/L h T_{max}: 2.50 ± 1.73 h C_{max}: 645 ± 450 μg/L CL: 0.98 ± 0.28 L/h/kg	

AUC, area under concentration-time curve; *CL*, total body clearance; C_{max}, maximum concentration; *Mg-SalAB*, magnesium SalAB; *MRT*, mean residence time; $t_{1/2}$, half-life; t_{max}, time for maximum concentration; V_{ss}, apparent volume of distribution at steady state.

three metabolites were 0.36%, 1.91%, 2.07%, and 0.91%, respectively, and the total recovery was calculated to be 5.24% (Li et al., 2007).

Another two metabolites of SalAB were found in rat urine: 3-(3-hydroxyphenyl)-propionic acid and *trans*-cinnamoylglycine. Four metabolites were found in bile, including 3,3″,3‴-*O*-tri-methyl-SalAB, 3-*O*-monomethyl-SalAB, 3,3″-*O*-dimethyl-SalAB, and 3,3‴-*O*-dimethyl-SalAB. In feces, five metabolites were found, including (*s*)-3-(3,4-dihydroxyphenyl) lactic acid, danshensu, salvianolic acid R, salvianolic acid S, and salvianolic acid T (Xu et al., 2007). There was no metabolite found in antibiotic-treated rats, indicating an important role of intestinal bacteria in the metabolism of SalAB. Zhang et al. also identified four metabolites in bile after intravenous injection of SalAB in rats. These four metabolites included 3-*O*-monomethyl-SalAB, 3,3‴-*O*-dimethyl-SalAB, 3,3″-*O*-dimethyl-SalAB, and 3,3″,3‴-*O*-trimethyl-SalAB, which are all potent antioxidants. The enzyme responsible for the biotransformation is catechol *o*-methyltransferase. It was also found that over 90% of the dose was excreted into bile and not into urine within 2 h after administration (Zhang, Akao, Nakamura, Hattori, et al., 2004).

6.3 The pharmacokinetics of other salvianolic acids

6.3.1 Salvianolic acid C

Song et al. developed and validated a sensitive and reliable LC-ESI-MS method for the determination of SalAC in rat plasma. This validated method was successfully applied to pharmacokinetic study after oral and intravenous administration of SalAC to rats. The absolute oral bioavailability of SalAC was 0.29% ± 0.05% (Song et al., 2016).

6.3.2 Salvianolic acid D

A two-compartmental model was employed to study the pharmacokinetics of salvianolic acid D (SalAD) in rats by Song et al. The plasma concentrations of SalAD at 2 min ($C_{2\ min}$) were 5756.06 ± 719.61, 11,073.01 ± 1783.46, and 21,077.58 ± 5581.97 μg/L for 0.25, 0.5, and 1 mg/kg intravenous injection, respectively. The C_{max} was 333.08 ± 61.21 μg/L for 4 mg/kg oral administration of SalAD. The AUC was 14,384.379 ± 8443.184, 22,813.369 ± 11,860.823, 46,406.122 ± 27,592.645, and 8201.740 ± 4711.961 μg/L h for intravenous injection (0.25, 0.5, 1 mg/kg) and oral administration (4 mg/kg), respectively. The bioavailability of SalAD was calculated to be 4.159% ± 0.517% (Song, Zhang, Sun, et al., 2015).

Salvianolic acids usually have both good water and lipid solubility. They are mainly metabolized through methylation and glucuronidation in vivo and in vitro. Due to the large number of phenolic hydroxyl groups in these compounds, phase II reactions are more likely to occur, and a large number of metabolites will be produced by the arrangement and combination of metabolic reactions at different phenolic hydroxyl group positions. A thorough understand of their metabolism and the activities of their metabolites contributes to the drug development of these compounds. Interestingly, the methylated metabolites of SalAA also showed high antioxidant potency. Although the oral bioavailability of these parent drugs was relatively low, they and their metabolites play pharmacological roles together.

7. Conclusion

The salvianolic acids isolated from Danshen have been researched and developed as drugs for a long time. Total salvianolic acids have been used as an injection for the treatment of cerebral ischemia and stroke and have achieved significant therapeutic effects in clinical practice in China. Some of the compounds, such as SalAA, have also been developed as drugs based on their special pharmacological actions. All the results show that the salvianolic acids are the effective components in Danshen. The different salvianolic acids, even though they have similar phenol acid structures, could exert respective pharmacological actions.

There is much research information on salvianolic acids regarding their bioactivities and pharmacological effects. The information includes basic research for mechanisms and molecular targets and pharmacological research to investigate the effects for the treatment of different diseases such as cardiovascular and cerebral vascular diseases, inflammatory diseases, metabolic diseases, etc. Salvianolic acids might be developed as drugs for the treatment of a number of diseases. The key scientific point for drug development from salvianolic acids is the therapeutic effects evaluation for the ideal indication.

Conflict of interest statement

The authors have no conflicts of interest to declare.

References

An, T., Zhang, J., Lv, B., Liu, Y., Huang, J., Lian, J., et al. (2019). Salvianolic acid B plays an anti-obesity role in high fat diet-induced obese mice by regulating the expression of mRNA, circRNA, and lncRNA. *PeerJ*, 7, e6506.

Bao, G. (1993). Inhibition of oxygen free radicals in potassium channels of cardiac myocytes and the action of salvianolic acid A. *Zhongguo Yi Xue Ke Xue Yuan Xue Bao*, *15*(5), 320–324.

Beiswenger, K. K., Calcutt, N. A., & Mizisin, A. P. (2008). Epidermal nerve fiber quantification in the assessment of diabetic neuropathy. *Acta Histochemica*, *110*(5), 351–362.

Bi, L., Chen, J., Yuan, X., Jiang, Z., & Chen, W. (2013). Salvianolic acid A positively regulates PTEN protein level and inhibits growth of A549 lung cancer cells. *Biomedical Reports*, *1*(2), 213–217.

Cai, J., Chen, S., Zhang, W., Zheng, X., Hu, S., Pang, C., et al. (2014). Salvianolic acid A reverses paclitaxel resistance in human breast cancer MCF-7 cells via targeting the expression of transgelin 2 and attenuating PI3 K/Akt pathway. *Phytomedicine*, *21*(12), 1725–1732.

Cao, Y. Y., Wang, L., Ge, H., Lu, X. L., Pei, Z., Gu, Q., et al. (2013). Salvianolic acid A, a polyphenolic derivative from Salvia miltiorrhiza bunge, as a multifunctional agent for the treatment of Alzheimer's disease. *Molecular Diversity*, *17*(3), 515–524.

Chang, Y., Zhang, W., Xie, Y., Xu, X., Sun, R., Wang, Z., et al. (2014). Postmarketing safety evaluation: Depside salt injection made from Danshen (Radix Salviae Miltiorrhizae). *Journal of Traditional Chinese Medicine*, *34*(6), 749–753.

Chen, F. Y., Bi, L., Qian, L., Gao, J., Jiang, Y. C., & Chen, W. P. (2016). Identification of multidrug resistance gene MDR1 associated microRNA of salvianolic acid A reversal in lung cancer. *Zhongguo Zhong Yao Za Zhi*, *41*(17), 3279–3284.

Chen, Y. H., Du, G. H., & Zhang, J. T. (2000). Salvianolic acid B protects brain against injuries caused by ischemia-reperfusion in rats. *Acta Pharmacologica Sinica*, *21*(5), 463–466.

Chen, Y. F., Jaw, I., Shiao, M. S., & Tsai, T. H. (2005). Determination and pharmacokinetic analysis of salvianolic acid B in rat blood and bile by microdialysis and liquid chromatography. *Journal of Chromatography A*, *1088*(1–2), 140–145.

Chen, T., Liu, W., Chao, X., Zhang, L., Qu, Y., Huo, J., et al. (2011). Salvianolic acid B attenuates brain damage and inflammation after traumatic brain injury in mice. *Brain Research Bulletin*, *84*(2), 163–168.

Chen, Z. P., McConell, G. K., Michell, B. J., Snow, R. J., Canny, B. J., & Kemp, B. E. (2000). AMPK signaling in contracting human skeletal muscle: Acetyl-CoA carboxylase and NO synthase phosphorylation. *American Journal of Physiology-Endocrinology and Metabolism*, *279*(5), E1202–E1206.

Chen, Z. W., Xie, Y. M., Liao, X., & Wang, G. Q. (2016). Systematic review on safety of Salvianolate injection. *Zhongguo Zhong Yao Za Zhi*, *41*(19), 3686–3695.

Chen, Q., Xu, T., Li, D., Pan, D., Wu, P., Luo, Y., et al. (2016). JNK/PI3K/Akt signaling pathway is involved in myocardial ischemia/reperfusion injury in diabetic rats: Effects of salvianolic acid A intervention. *American Journal of Translational Research*, *8*(6), 2534–2548.

Chen, Y. C., Yuan, T. Y., Zhang, H. F., Wang, D. S., Yan, Y., Niu, Z. R., et al. (2016). Salvianolic acid A attenuates vascular remodeling in a pulmonary arterial hypertension rat model. *Acta Pharmacologica Sinica*, *37*(6), 772–782.

Chen, J., Yue, J., Liu, J., Liu, Y., Jiao, K. L., Teng, M. Y., et al. (2018). Salvianolic acids improve liver lipid metabolism in ovariectomized rats via blocking STAT-3/SREBP1 signaling. *Chinese Journal of Natural Medicines*, *16*(11), 838–845.

Chien, M. Y., Chuang, C. H., Chern, C. M., Liou, K. T., Liu, D. Z., Hou, Y. C., et al. (2016). Salvianolic acid A alleviates ischemic brain injury through the inhibition of inflammation and apoptosis and the promotion of neurogenesis in mice. *Free Radical Biology & Medicine*, *99*, 508–519.

Chowdhury, S. K., Dobrowsky, R. T., & Fernyhough, P. (2011). Nutrient excess and altered mitochondrial proteome and function contribute to neurodegeneration in diabetes. *Mitochondrion*, *11*(6), 845–854.

Coughlan, M. T., Cooper, M. E., & Thomas, M. C. (2007). Can you reduce your AGE? Strategies to prevent AGE accumulation in diabetes. *Drug Discovery Today: Therapeutic Strategies*, *4*(1), 85–92.

Ding, C., Zhao, Y., Shi, X., Zhang, N., Zu, G., Li, Z., et al. (2016). New insights into salvianolic acid A action: Regulation of the TXNIP/NLRP3 and TXNIP/ChREBP pathways ameliorates HFD-induced NAFLD in rats. *Scientific Reports*, *6*, 28734.

Du, G. H., Qiu, Y., Tian, Y. E., & Zhang, J. T. (1995). Prevention of galactose-induced cataractogenesis in rats by salvianolic acid A. *Yao Xue Xue Bao*, *30*(8), 561–566.

Du, G. H., Qiu, Y., & Zhang, J. T. (1995). Protective effect of salvianolic acid A on ischemia-reperfusion induced injury in isolated rat heart. *Yao Xue Xue Bao*, *30*(10), 731–735.

Du, G. H., Qiu, Y., & Zhang, J. T. (2000). Salvianolic acid B protects the memory functions against transient cerebral ischemia in mice. *Journal of Asian Natural Products Research*, *2*(2), 145–152.

Du, G. H., & Zhang, J. T. (1997). Protective effects of salvianolic acid A against impairment of memory induced by cerebral ischemia-reperfusion in mice. *Chinese Medical Journal*, *110*(1), 65–68.

Emerling, B. M., Weinberg, F., Snyder, C., Burgess, Z., Mutlu, G. M., Viollet, B., et al. (2009). Hypoxic activation of AMPK is dependent on mitochondrial ROS but independent of an increase in AMP/ATP ratio. *Free Radical Biology & Medicine*, *46*(10), 1386–1391.

Fan, H. Y., Fu, F. H., Yang, M. Y., Xu, H., Zhang, A. H., & Liu, K. (2010). Antiplatelet and antithrombotic activities of salvianolic acid A. *Thrombosis Research*, *126*(1), e17–e22.

Fan, H., Yang, L., Fu, F., Xu, H., Meng, Q., Zhu, H., et al. (2012). Cardioprotective effects of salvianolic acid a on myocardial ischemia-reperfusion injury in vivo and in vitro. *Evidence-based Complementary and Alternative Medicine*, *2012*, 508938.

Fan, H. Y., Yang, M. Y., Qi, D., Zhang, Z. K., Zhu, L., Shang-Guan, X. X., et al. (2015). Salvianolic acid A as a multifunctional agent ameliorates doxorubicin-induced nephropathy in rats. *Scientific Reports*, *5*, 12273.

Fang, C. Y., Wu, C. Z., Chen, P. N., Chang, Y. C., Chuang, C. Y., Lai, C. T., et al. (2018). Antimetastatic potentials of salvianolic acid A on oral squamous cell carcinoma by targeting MMP-2 and the c-Raf/MEK/ERK pathway. *Environmental Toxicology*, *33*(5), 545–554.

Farhangkhoee, H., Khan, Z. A., Kaur, H., Xin, X., Chen, S., & Chakrabarti, S. (2006). Vascular endothelial dysfunction in diabetic cardiomyopathy: Pathogenesis and potential treatment targets. *Pharmacology & Therapeutics*, *111*(2), 384–399.

Feng, S. Q., Aa, N., Geng, J. L., Huang, J. Q., Sun, R. B., Ge, C., et al. (2017). Pharmacokinetic and metabolomic analyses of the neuroprotective effects of salvianolic acid A in a rat ischemic stroke model. *Acta Pharmacologica Sinica*, *38*(11), 1435–1444.

Ferrer, M. D., Tauler, P., Sureda, A., Tur, J. A., & Pons, A. (2009). Antioxidant regulatory mechanisms in neutrophils and lymphocytes after intense exercise. *Journal of Sports Sciences*, *27*(1), 49–58.

Fogarty, S., & Hardie, D. G. (2010). Development of protein kinase activators: AMPK as a target in metabolic disorders and cancer. *Biochimica et Biophysica Acta*, *1804*(3), 581–591.

Gong, J., Ju, A., Zhou, D., Li, D., Zhou, W., Geng, W., et al. (2015). Salvianolic acid Y: A new protector of PC12 cells against hydrogen peroxide-induced injury from Salvia officinalis. *Molecules*, *20*(1), 683–692.

Gu, X., Zheng, C., Zheng, Q., Chen, S., Li, W., Shang, Z., et al. (2017). Salvianolic acid A attenuates early brain injury after subarachnoid hemorrhage in rats by regulating ERK/P38/Nrf2 signaling. *American Journal of Translational Research*, *9*(12), 5643–5652.

Guo, P., Wang, J., Gao, W., Liu, X., Wu, S., Wan, B., et al. (2018). Salvianolic acid B reverses multidrug resistance in nude mice bearing human colon cancer stem cells. *Molecular Medicine Reports*, *18*(2), 1323–1334.

Han, D. E., Gao, Z. D., Zhao, D., Wang, L., Li, N., Li, T. T., et al. (2009). Liquid chromatography mass spectrometry for the determination of salvianolic acid B, a natural compound from the herb Danshen in rat plasma and application to pharmacokinetic study. *Biomedical Chromatography*, *23*(10), 1073–1078.

He, H., Li, X., Wang, H., Zhang, W., Jiang, H., Wang, S., et al. (2013). Effects of salvianolic acid A on plasma and tissue dimethylarginine levels in a rat model of myocardial infarction. *Journal of Cardiovascular Pharmacology*, *61*(6), 482–488.

Heo, J. Y., & Im, D. S. (2019). Anti-allergic effects of salvianolic acid A and tanshinone IIA from Salvia miltiorrhiza determined using in vivo and in vitro experiments. *International Immunopharmacology*, *67*, 69–77.

Hou, Y. Y., Peng, J. M., & Chao, R. B. (2007). Pharmacokinetic study of salvianolic acid A in rat after intravenous administration of Danshen injection. *Biomedical Chromatography*, *21*(6), 598–601.

Hou, B., Qiang, G., Zhao, Y., Yang, X., Chen, X., Yan, Y., et al. (2017). Salvianolic acid A protects against diabetic nephropathy through ameliorating glomerular endothelial dysfunction via inhibiting AGE-RAGE signaling. *Cellular Physiology and Biochemistry*, *44*(6), 2378–2394.

Hou, S., Zhao, M. M., Shen, P. P., Liu, X. P., Sun, Y., & Feng, J. C. (2016). Neuroprotective effect of salvianolic acids against cerebral ischemia/reperfusion injury. *International Journal of Molecular Sciences*, *17*(7), 1190.

Hu, Y. Y., Liu, P., Liu, C., Xu, L. M., Liu, C. H., Zhu, D. Y., et al. (1997). Actions of salvianolic acid A on CCl4-poisoned liver injury and fibrosis in rats. *Zhongguo Yao Li Xue Bao*, *18*(5), 478–480.

Hu, Y. Y., Liu, C. H., Wang, R. P., Liu, C., Liu, P., & Zhu, D. Y. (2000). Protective actions of salvianolic acid A on hepatocyte injured by peroxidation in vitro. *World Journal of Gastroenterology*, *6*(3), 402–404.

Hu, Y., Wang, R., Zhang, X., Liu, C., Liu, C., Liu, P., et al. (2000). Effects of carbon tetrachloride-injured hepatocytes on hepatic stellate cell activation and salvianolic acid A preventive action in vitro. *Zhonghua Gan Zang Bing Za Zhi*, *8*(5), 299–301.

Huang, J., Qin, Y., Liu, B., Li, G. Y., Ouyang, L., & Wang, J. H. (2013). In silico analysis and experimental validation of molecular mechanisms of salvianolic acid A-inhibited LPS-stimulated inflammation, in RAW264.7 macrophages. *Cell Proliferation*, *46*(5), 595–605.

Huang, M., Wang, P., Xu, S., Xu, W., Xu, W., Chu, K., et al. (2015). Biological activities of salvianolic acid B from Salvia miltiorrhiza on type 2 diabetes induced by high-fat diet and streptozotocin. *Pharmaceutical Biology*, *53*(7), 1058–1065.

Huang, D. D., Wei, X. H., Mu, H. N., Pan, C. S., Li, Q., Hu, B. H., et al. (2019). Total Salvianolic acid injection prevents ischemia/reperfusion-induced myocardial injury via antioxidant mechanism involving mitochondrial respiratory chain through the upregulation of Sirtuin1 and Sirtuin3. *Shock*, *51*(6), 745–756.

Huang, Z. S., Zeng, C. L., Zhu, L. J., Jiang, L., Li, N., & Hu, H. (2010). Salvianolic acid A inhibits platelet activation and arterial thrombosis via inhibition of phosphoinositide 3-kinase. *Journal of Thrombosis and Haemostasis*, *8*(6), 1383–1393.

Huang, Y. S., & Zhang, J. T. (1992). Antioxidative effect of three water-soluble components isolated from Salvia miltiorrhiza in vitro. *Yao Xue Xue Bao*, *27*(2), 96–100.

Huang, M. Q., Zhou, C. J., Zhang, Y. P., Zhang, X. Q., Xu, W., Lin, J., et al. (2016). Salvianolic acid B ameliorates hyperglycemia and dyslipidemia in db/db mice through the AMPK pathway. *Cellular Physiology and Biochemistry*, *40*(5), 933–943.

Jager, S., Handschin, C., St-Pierre, J., & Spiegelman, B. M. (2007). AMP-activated protein kinase (AMPK) action in skeletal muscle via direct phosphorylation of PGC-1alpha. *Proceedings of the National Academy of Sciences of the United States of America*, *104*(29), 12017–12022.

Jiang, B., Li, D., Deng, Y., Teng, F., Chen, J., Xue, S., et al. (2013). Salvianolic acid A, a novel matrix metalloproteinase-9 inhibitor, prevents cardiac remodeling in spontaneously hypertensive rats. *PLoS One*, *8*(3), e59621.

Jiang, Y. F., Liu, Z. Q., Cui, W., Zhang, W. T., Gong, J. P., Wang, X. M., et al. (2015). Antioxidant effect of salvianolic acid B on hippocampal CA1 neurons in mice with cerebral ischemia and reperfusion injury. *Chinese Journal of Integrative Medicine*, *21*(7), 516–522.

Jiang, M., Wang, X. Y., Zhou, W. Y., Li, J., Wang, J., & Guo, L. P. (2011). Cerebral protection of salvianolic acid A by the inhibition of granulocyte adherence. *The American Journal of Chinese Medicine*, *39*(1), 111–120.

Jiao, C. X., Zhou, H., Yang, C. X., Ma, C., Yang, Y. X., Mao, R. R., et al. (2017). Protective efficacy of a single salvianolic acid A treatment on photothrombosis-induced sustained spatial memory impairments. *Neuropsychiatric Disease and Treatment*, *13*, 1181–1192.

Jin, X., Zhang, S. B., Li, S. M., Liang, K., & Jia, Z. Y. (2016). Influence of chitosan nanoparticles as the absorption enhancers on salvianolic acid B in vitro and in vivo evaluation. *Pharmacognosy Magazine*, *12*(45), 57–63.

Khan, Z. A., Farhangkhoee, H., & Chakrabarti, S. (2006). Towards newer molecular targets for chronic diabetic complications. *Current Vascular Pharmacology*, *4*(1), 45–57.

Kim, H. H., Kim, J., Ji, H. Y., Kim, Y. C., Sohn, D. H., Lee, B. M., et al. (2005). Pharmacokinetics of lithospermic acid B isolated from Salvia miltiorrhiza in rats. *Journal of Toxicology and Environmental Health, Part A*, *68*(23–24), 2239–2247.

Kim, D., Nguyen, M. D., Dobbin, M. M., Fischer, A., Sananbenesi, F., Rodgers, J. T., et al. (2007). SIRT1 deacetylase protects against neurodegeneration in models for Alzheimer's disease and amyotrophic lateral sclerosis. *The EMBO Journal*, *26*(13), 3169–3179.

Lee, Y. W., Kim, D. H., Jeon, S. J., Park, S. J., Kim, J. M., Jung, J. M., et al. (2013). Neuroprotective effects of salvianolic acid B on an Aβ25–35 peptide-induced mouse model of Alzheimer's disease. *European Journal of Pharmacology*, *704*(1), 70–77.

Li, L. N. (1997). Water soluble active components of Salvia miltiorrhiza and related plants. *Journal of Chinese Pharmaceutical Sciences*, *6*(2), 57–64.

Li, Y. J., Duan, C. L., & Liu, J. X. (2014). Salvianolic acid A promotes the acceleration of neovascularization in the ischemic rat myocardium and the functions of endothelial progenitor cells. *Journal of Ethnopharmacology*, *151*(1), 218–227.

Li, X. L., Fan, J. P., Liu, J. X., & Liang, L. N. (2019). Salvianolic acid a protects neonatal cardiomyocytes against hypoxia/reoxygenation-induced injury by preserving mitochondrial function and activating Akt/GSK-3beta signals. *Chinese Journal of Integrative Medicine*, *25*(1), 23–30.

Li, J., Gu, T., Fu, X., & Zhao, R. (2015). Effect of salvianolic acid A and C compatibility on inflammatory cytokines in rats with unilateral ureteral obstruction. *Journal of Traditional Chinese Medicine*, *35*(5), 564–570.

Li, Q., Wang, L., Li, X. Y., Chen, X., Lu, B., Cheng, L., et al. (2018). Total salvianolic acid balances brain functional network topology in rat hippocampi overexpressing miR-30e. *Frontiers in Neuroscience*, *12*, 448.

Li, L., Xu, T., Du, Y., Pan, D., Wu, W., Zhu, H., et al. (2016). Salvianolic acid A attenuates cell apoptosis, oxidative stress, Akt and NF-kappaB activation in angiotensin-II induced murine peritoneal macrophages. *Current Pharmaceutical Biotechnology*, *17*(3), 283–290.

Li, X. C., Yu, C., Sun, W. K., Liu, G. Y., Jia, J. Y., & Wang, Y. P. (2004). Pharmacokinetics of magnesium lithospermate B after intravenous administration in beagle dogs. *Acta Pharmacologica Sinica*, *25*(11), 1402–1407.

Li, X., Yu, C., Wang, L., Lu, Y., Wang, W., Xuan, L., et al. (2007). Simultaneous determination of lithospermic acid B and its three metabolites by liquid chromatography/tandem mass spectrometry. *Journal of Pharmaceutical and Biomedical Analysis*, *43*(5), 1864–1868.

Li, Y., Zhang, X., Cui, L., Chen, R., Zhang, Y., Zhang, C., et al. (2017). Salvianolic acids enhance cerebral angiogenesis and neurological recovery by activating JAK2/STAT3 signaling pathway after ischemic stroke in mice. *Journal of Neurochemistry*, *143*(1), 87–99.

Li, J., Zhang, C., He, W., Qiao, H., Chen, J., Wang, K., et al. (2017). Coordination-driven assembly of catechol-modified chitosan for the kidney-specific delivery of salvianolic acid B to treat renal fibrosis. *Biomaterials Science*, *6*(1), 179–188.

Lin, Y. L., Lee, T. F., Huang, Y. J., & Huang, Y. T. (2006). Antiproliferative effect of salvianolic acid A on rat hepatic stellate cells. *The Journal of Pharmacy and Pharmacology*, *58*(7), 933–939.

Lin, T. J., Liu, G. T., Liu, Y., & Xu, G. Z. (1992). Protection by salvianolic acid A against adriamycin toxicity on rat heart mitochondria. *Free Radical Biology & Medicine*, *12*(5), 347–351.

Lin, Y., Yan, Y., Zhang, H., Chen, Y., He, Y., Wang, S., et al. (2017). Salvianolic acid A alleviates renal injury in systemic lupus erythematosus induced by pristane in BALB/c mice. *Acta Pharmaceutica Sinica B*, 7(2), 159–166.

Ling, W. C., Liu, J., Lau, C. W., Murugan, D. D., Mustafa, M. R., & Huang, Y. (2017). Treatment with salvianolic acid B restores endothelial function in angiotensin II-induced hypertensive mice. *Biochemical Pharmacology*, *136*, 76–85.

Liu, B., Cao, B., Zhang, D., Xiao, N., Chen, H., & Li, G.-q., Wei, L.Q. (2016). Salvianolic acid B protects against paraquat-induced pulmonary injury by mediating Nrf2/Nox4 redox balance and TGF-β1/Smad3 signaling. *Toxicology and Applied Pharmacology*, *309*, 111–120.

Liu, C. H., Liu, P., Hu, Y. Y., Xu, L. M., Tan, Y. Z., Wang, Z. N., et al. (2000). Effects of salvianolic acid-A on rat hepatic stellate cell proliferation and collagen production in culture. *Acta Pharmacologica Sinica*, *21*(8), 721–726.

Lu, Y., & Foo, L. Y. (2001). Salvianolic acid L, a potent phenolic antioxidant from Salvia officinalis. *Tetrahedron Letters*, *42*(46), 8223–8225.

Lu, Y., & Foo, L. Y. (2002). Polyphenolics of salvia—A review. *Phytochemistry*, *59*(2), 117–140.

Ma, Y., & Wang, T. (2007). A solid-phase extraction method for high-performance liquid chromatographic determination of salvianolic acid B in rabbit plasma: Application to pharmacokinetic study. *Biomedical Chromatography*, *21*(2), 217–220.

Nair, S., Diehl, A. M., Wiseman, M., Farr, G. H., Jr., & Perrillo, R. P. (2004). Metformin in the treatment of non-alcoholic steatohepatitis: A pilot open label trial. *Alimentary Pharmacology & Therapeutics*, *20*(1), 23–28.

Pan, C., Lou, L., Huo, Y., Singh, G., Chen, M., Zhang, D., et al. (2011). Salvianolic acid B and tanshinone IIA attenuate myocardial ischemia injury in mice by NO production through multiple pathways. *Therapeutic Advances in Cardiovascular Disease*, *5*(2), 99–111.

Pei, L., Bao, Y., Wang, H., Yang, F., Xu, B., Wang, S., et al. (2008). A sensitive method for determination of salvianolic acid A in rat plasma using liquid chromatography/tandem mass spectrometry. *Biomedical Chromatography*, *22*(7), 786–794.

Peng, Q., Gong, T., Zuo, J., Liu, J., Zhao, D., & Zhang, Z. (2008). Enhanced oral bioavailability of salvianolic acid B by phospholipid complex loaded nanoparticles. *Pharmazie, 63*(9), 661–666.

Peng, J. W., Liu, Y., Meng, G., Zhang, J. Y., & Yu, L. F. (2018). Effects of salvianolic acid on cerebral perfusion in patients after acute stroke: A single-center randomized controlled trial. *Experimental and Therapeutic Medicine, 16*(3), 2600–2614.

Petersen, M., & Simmonds, M. S. (2003). Rosmarinic acid. *Phytochemistry, 62*(2), 121–125.

Polekhina, G., Gupta, A., van Denderen, B. J., Feil, S. C., Kemp, B. E., Stapleton, D., et al. (2005). Structural basis for glycogen recognition by AMP-activated protein kinase. *Structure, 13*(10), 1453–1462.

Qian, W., Wang, Z., Xu, T., & Li, D. (2019). Anti-apoptotic effects and mechanisms of salvianolic acid A on cardiomyocytes in ischemia-reperfusion injury. *Histology and Histopathology, 34*(3), 223–231.

Qiang, G., Yang, X., Shi, L., Zhang, H., Chen, B., Zhao, Y., et al. (2015). Antidiabetic effect of Salvianolic acid A on diabetic animal models via AMPK activation and mitochondrial regulation. *Cellular Physiology and Biochemistry, 36*(1), 395–408.

Qiang, G., Yang, X., Xuan, Q., Shi, L., Zhang, H., Chen, B., et al. (2014). Salvianolic acid a prevents the pathological progression of hepatic fibrosis in high-fat diet-fed and streptozotocin-induced diabetic rats. *The American Journal of Chinese Medicine, 42*(5), 1183–1198.

Qiao, Z., & Xu, Y. (2016). Salvianolic acid B alleviating myocardium injury in ischemia reperfusion rats. *African Journal of Traditional, Complementary, and Alternative Medicines, 13*(4), 157–161.

Raoufi, S., Baluchnejadmojarad, T., Roghani, M., Ghazanfari, T., Khojasteh, F., & Mansouri, M. (2015). Antidiabetic potential of salvianolic acid B in multiple low-dose streptozotocin-induced diabetes. *Pharmaceutical Biology, 53*(12), 1803–1809.

Ren, D. C., Du, G. H., & Zhang, J. T. (2003). Inhibitory effect of salvianolic acids on endothelial cells damage induced by hydrogen peroxide. *Chinese Journal of Pharmacology and Toxicology, 17*(5), 333–337.

Shen, L., Han, B., Geng, Y., Wang, J., Wang, Z., & Wang, M. (2017). Amelioration of cognitive impairments in APPswe/PS1dE9 mice is associated with metabolites alteration induced by total salvianolic acid. *PLoS One, 12*(3), e0174763.

Shen, Y., Wang, X., Xu, L., Liu, X., & Chao, R. (2009). Characterization of metabolites in rat plasma after intravenous administration of salvianolic acid A by liquid chromatography/time-of-flight mass spectrometry and liquid chromatography/ion trap mass spectrometry. *Rapid Communications in Mass Spectrometry, 23*(12), 1810–1816.

Song, J., Zhang, W., Sun, J., Xu, X., Zhang, X., Zhang, L., et al. (2015). Pharmacokinetic study of salvianolic acid D after oral and intravenous administration in rats. *Acta Pharmaceutica Sinica B, 5*(3), 246–253.

Song, J., Zhang, W., Sun, J., Zhang, X., Xu, X., Zhang, L., et al. (2016). Determination of salvianolic acid C in rat plasma using liquid chromatography-mass spectrometry and its application to pharmacokinetic study. *Biomedical Chromatography, 30*(3), 376–383.

Song, J., Zhang, W., Wang, J., Yang, H., Zhao, X., Zhou, Q., et al. (2018). Activation of Nrf2 signaling by salvianolic acid C attenuates NFkappaB mediated inflammatory response both in vivo and in vitro. *International Immunopharmacology, 63*, 299–310.

Song, J. K., Zhang, W., Zhang, W. K., Feng, Z. Y., Xie, T., & Du, G. H. (2015). Pharmacokinetics of salvianolic acid A after single intravenous administration in rhesus monkey. *Yao Xue Xue Bao, 50*(9), 1142–1147.

Sun, J., Song, J., Zhang, W., Jing, F., Xu, W., Leng, P., et al. (2018). Some pharmacokinetic parameters of salvianolic acid A following single-dose oral administration to rats. *Pharmaceutical Biology, 56*(1), 399–406.

Sun, J., Zhang, L., Song, J., Tian, S., Huang, C., Feng, Z., et al. (2013). Pharmacokinetic study of salvianolic acid A in beagle dog after oral administration by a liquid chromatography-mass spectrometry method: A study on bioavailability and dose proportionality. *Journal of Ethnopharmacology, 148*(2), 617–623.

Sun, Y., Zhao, D., Liu, Z., Sun, X., & Li, Y. (2018). Inhibitory effect of salvianolic acid on inflammatory mediators of rats with collagen-induced rheumatoid arthritis. *Experimental and Therapeutic Medicine, 16*(5), 4037–4041.

Tanaka, T., Morimoto, S., Nonaka, G. I., Nishioka, I., Yokozawa, T., Chung, H. Y., et al. (1989). Magnesium and ammonium-potassium lithospermates B, the active principles having a uremia-preventive effect from Salvia miltiorrhiza. *Chemical & Pharmaceutical Bulletin, 37*(2), 340–344.

Tang, H., Pan, C. S., Mao, X. W., Liu, Y. Y., Yan, L., Zhou, C. M., et al. (2014). Role of NADPH oxidase in total salvianolic acid injection attenuating ischemia-reperfusion impaired cerebral microcirculation and neurons: Implication of AMPK/Akt/PKC. *Microcirculation: The Official Journal of the Microcirculatory Society, Inc, 21*(7), 615–627.

Tang, M. K., Ren, D. C., Zhang, J. T., & Du, G. H. (2002). Effect of salvianolic acids from Radix Salviae miltiorrhizae on regional cerebral blood flow and platelet aggregation in rats. *Phytomedicine, 9*(5), 405–409.

Tang, H., & Zhao, D. (2019). Investigation of the interaction between salvianolic acid C and xanthine oxidase: Insights from experimental studies merging with molecular docking methods. *Bioorganic Chemistry, 88*, 102981.

Wang, S. B., Pang, X. B., Zhao, Y., Wang, Y. H., Zhang, L., Yang, X. Y., et al. (2012). Protection of salvianolic acid A on rat brain from ischemic damage via soluble epoxide hydrolase inhibition. *Journal of Asian Natural Products Research, 14*(11), 1084–1092.

Wang, R., Song, F., Li, S., Wu, B., Gu, Y., & Yuan, Y. (2019). Salvianolic acid A attenuates CCl4-induced liver fibrosis by regulating the PI3K/AKT/mTOR, Bcl-2/Bax and caspase-3/cleaved caspase-3 signaling pathways. *Drug Design, Development and Therapy, 13*, 1889–1900.

Wang, S. B., Tian, S., Yang, F., Yang, H. G., Yang, X. Y., & Du, G. H. (2009). Cardioprotective effect of salvianolic acid A on isoproterenol-induced myocardial infarction in rats. *European Journal of Pharmacology, 615*(1–3), 125–132.

Wang, P., Xu, S., Li, W., Wang, F., Yang, Z., Jiang, L., et al. (2014). Salvianolic acid B inhibited PPARγ expression and attenuated weight gain in mice with high-fat diet-induced obesity. *Cellular Physiology and Biochemistry, 34*(2), 288–298.

Wang, R., Zhang, J., Wang, S., Wang, M., Ye, T., Du, Y., et al. (2019). The cardiotoxicity induced by arsenic trioxide is alleviated by salvianolic acid a via maintaining calcium homeostasis and inhibiting endoplasmic reticulum stress. *Molecules, 24*(3), 543.

Wu, Y. T., Chen, Y. F., Hsieh, Y. J., Jaw, I., Shiao, M. S., & Tsai, T. H. (2006). Bioavailability of salvianolic acid B in conscious and freely moving rats. *International Journal of Pharmaceutics, 326*(1–2), 25–31.

Wu, C. T., Deng, J. S., Huang, W. C., Shieh, P. C., Chung, M. I., & Huang, G. J. (2019). Salvianolic acid C against acetaminophen-induced acute liver injury by attenuating inflammation, oxidative stress, and apoptosis through inhibition of the Keap1/Nrf2/HO-1 signaling. *Oxidative Medicine and Cellular Longevity, 2019*, 9056845.

Wu, P., Han, N., Yu, H., Wang, L., Li, X., Dong, Z., et al. (2016). Amelioration of salvianolic acid C on aortic structure in apolipoprotein E-deficient mice treated with angiotension II. *Life Sciences, 166*, 75–81.

Xu, M., Guo, H., Han, J., Sun, S. F., Liu, A. H., Wang, B. R., et al. (2007). Structural characterization of metabolites of salvianolic acid B from Salvia miltiorrhiza in normal and antibiotic-treated rats by liquid chromatography-mass spectrometry. *Journal of Chromatography. B, Analytical Technologies in the Biomedical and Life Sciences, 858*(1–2), 184–198.

Xu, H., Li, Y., Che, X., Tian, H., Fan, H., & Liu, K. (2014). Metabolism of salvianolic acid A and antioxidant activities of its methylated metabolites. *Drug Metabolism and Disposition*, *42*(2), 274–281.

Yamaji, K., Wang, Y., Liu, Y., Abeyama, K., Hashiguchi, T., Uchimura, T., et al. (2005). Activated protein C, a natural anticoagulant protein, has antioxidant properties and inhibits lipid peroxidation and advanced glycation end products formation. *Thrombosis Research*, *115*(4), 319–325.

Yan, Y. Y., Yang, Y. H., Wang, W. W., Pan, Y. T., Zhan, S. Y., Sun, M. Y., et al. (2017). Post-marketing safety surveillance of the Salvia Miltiorrhiza depside salt for infusion: A real world study. *PLoS One*, *12*(1), e0170182.

Yang, N. Z., Ju, A. C., Li, X., & Yun, X. H. (2018). Salvianolate injection in the treatment of acute cerebral infarction: A systematic review and a meta-analysis. *Medicine*, *97*(47), e12374.

Yang, L. L., Li, D. Y., Zhang, Y. B., Zhu, M. Y., Chen, D., & Xu, T. D. (2012). Salvianolic acid A inhibits angiotensin II-induced proliferation of human umbilical vein endothelial cells by attenuating the production of ROS. *Acta Pharmacologica Sinica*, *33*(1), 41–48.

Yang, C. W., Liu, H., Li, X. D., Sui, S. G., & Liu, Y. F. (2018). Salvianolic acid B protects against acute lung injury by decreasing TRPM6 and TRPM7 expressions in a rat model of sepsis. *Journal of Cellular Biochemistry*, *119*(1), 701–711.

Yang, X. Y., Qiang, G. F., Zhang, L., Zhu, X. M., Wang, S. B., Sun, L., et al. (2011). Salvianolic acid A protects against vascular endothelial dysfunction in high-fat diet fed and streptozotocin-induced diabetic rats. *J Asian Nat Prod Res*, *13*(10), 884–894.

Yang, X. Y., Sun, L., Xu, P., Gong, L. L., Qiang, G. F., Zhang, L., et al. (2011). Effects of salvianolic scid A on plantar microcirculation and peripheral nerve function in diabetic rats. *Eur J Pharmacol*, *665*(1-3), 40–46.

Yu, L., An, C., Jia, L., Li, Y., Chen, Q., Zhen, F., et al. (2016). Combination therapy of salvianolic acid and fluoxetine improves the cognitive function of rats with chronic stress-induced depression. *World Neurosurgery*, *86*, 173–180.

Yu, J., Chen, R., Tan, Y., Wu, J., Qi, J., Zhang, M., et al. (2016). Salvianolic acid B alleviates heart failure by inactivating ERK1/2/GATA4 signaling pathway after pressure overload in mice. *PLoS One*, *11*(11), e0166560.

Yu, F., Lu, Z., Chen, B., Wu, X., Dong, P., & Zheng, J. (2015). Salvianolic acid B-induced microRNA-152 inhibits liver fibrosis by attenuating DNMT1-mediated Patched1 methylation. *Journal of Cellular and Molecular Medicine*, *19*(11), 2617–2632.

Yu, W. G., & Xu, L. N. (1994). Effect of acetylsalvianolic acid A on platelet function. *Yao xue xue bao = Acta pharmaceutica Sinica*, *29*(6), 412–416.

Yu, X., Zhang, L., Yang, X., Huang, H., Huang, Z., Shi, L., et al. (2012). Salvianolic acid a protects the peripheral nerve function in diabetic rats through regulation of the AMPK-PGC1α-Sirt3 axis. *Molecules*, *17*(9), 11216–11228.

Yu, X. Y., Zhang, L., Yang, X. Y., Li, X. T., & Du, G. H. (2016). Salvianolic acid A improves intestinal motility in diabetic rats through antioxidant capacity and upregulation of nNOS. *Journal of Digestive Diseases*, *17*(7), 441–447.

Yuan, T., Chen, Y., Zhang, H., Fang, L., & Du, G. (2017). Salvianolic acid A, a component of Salvia miltiorrhiza, attenuates endothelial-mesenchymal transition of HPAECs induced by hypoxia. *The American Journal of Chinese Medicine*, *45*(6), 1185–1200.

Yuan, X., Xiang, Y., Zhu, N., Zhao, X., Ye, S., Zhong, P., et al. (2017). Salvianolic acid A protects against myocardial ischemia/reperfusion injury by reducing platelet activation and inflammation. *Experimental and Therapeutic Medicine*, *14*(2), 961–966.

Zhai, J., Qu, X., Zhang, Y., Gao, H., Tao, L., Song, Y., et al. (2019). Salvianolic acid inhibits the effects of high glucose on vascular endothelial dysfunction by modulating the Sirt1-eNOS pathway. *Journal of Biochemical and Molecular Toxicology*, *33*(2), e22245.

Zhang, Y., Akao, T., Nakamura, N., Duan, C. L., Hattori, M., Yang, X. W., et al. (2004). Extremely low bioavailability of magnesium lithospermate B, an active component from Salvia miltiorrhiza, in rat. *Planta Medica*, *70*(2), 138–142.

Zhang, Y., Akao, T., Nakamura, N., Hattori, M., Yang, X. W., Duan, C. L., et al. (2004). Magnesium lithospermate B is excreted rapidly into rat bile mostly as methylated metabolites, which are potent antioxidants. *Drug Metabolism and Disposition*, *32*(7), 752–757.

Zhang, Z. F., Chen, H. S., Peng, Z. G., Li, Z. R., & Jiang, J. D. (2008). A potent anti-HIV polyphenol from Salvia yunnanensis. *Journal of Asian Natural Products Research*, *10*(3–4), 273–277.

Zhang, L., Han, L., Sun, X., Gao, D., Qin, J., & Wang, J. (2012). The use of PEGylated liposomes to prolong the circulation lifetime of salvianolic acid B. *Fitoterapia*, *83*(4), 678–689.

Zhang, D., Wu, J., Liu, S., Zhang, X., & Zhang, B. (2016). Salvianolate injection in the treatment of unstable angina pectoris: A systematic review and meta-analysis. *Medicine*, *95*(51), e5692.

Zhang, Y., Zhang, X., Cui, L., Chen, R., Zhang, C., Li, Y., et al. (2017). Salvianolic acids for injection (SAFI) promotes functional recovery and neurogenesis via sonic hedgehog pathway after stroke in mice. *Neurochemistry International*, *110*, 38–48.

Zhang, D. F., Zhang, J., & Li, R. (2015). Salvianolic acid B attenuates lung inflammation induced by cigarette smoke in mice. *European Journal of Pharmacology*, *761*, 174–179.

Zhao, D., Gao, Z. D., Han, D. E., Li, N., Zhang, Y. J., Lu, Y., et al. (2012). Influence of rifampicin on the pharmacokinetics of salvianolic acid B may involve inhibition of organic anion transporting polypeptide (Oatp) mediated influx. *Phytotherapy Research*, *26*(1), 118–121.

Zhong, W., Sun, B., Gao, W., Qin, Y., Zhang, H., Huai, L., et al. (2018). Salvianolic acid A targeting the transgelin-actin complex to enhance vasoconstriction. *eBioMedicine*, *37*, 246–258.

Zhou, L., Chow, M. S., & Zuo, Z. (2009). Effect of sodium caprate on the oral absorptions of danshensu and salvianolic acid B. *International Journal of Pharmaceutics*, *379*(1), 109–118.

Zhou, J., Qu, X. D., Li, Z. Y., Wei, J., Liu, Q., Ma, Y. H., et al. (2014). Salvianolic acid B attenuates toxin-induced neuronal damage via Nrf2-dependent glial cells-mediated protective activity in Parkinson's disease models. *PLoS One*, *9*(7), e101668.

Zhuang, P., Wan, Y., Geng, S., He, Y., Feng, B., Ye, Z., et al. (2017). Salvianolic acids for injection (SAFI) suppresses inflammatory responses in activated microglia to attenuate brain damage in focal cerebral ischemia. *Journal of Ethnopharmacology*, *198*, 194–204.

CHAPTER TWO

Pharmacological properties of tanshinones, the natural products from *Salvia miltiorrhiza*

Xiaoying Wang, Yang Yang, Xiao Liu, Xiumei Gao*
Tianjin University of Traditional Chinese Medicine, Tianjin, China
*Corresponding author: e-mail address: gaoxiumei@tjutcm.edu.cn

Contents

Abstract

Danshen (Cai, et al. 2016) is the dry root and rhizome of the herbaceous plant *Salvia miltiorrhiza* Bge. of family labiatae, a perennial plant that is native to China and Japan. The primary modern clinical applications of Danshen are for heart disease, chronic hepatitis, early cirrhosis, cerebral ischemia and pulmonary heart disease. Emerging evidence from cellular, animal, and clinical studies has begun to illuminate the pharmacological attributes of the primary lipophilic tanshinones from Danshen, which include tanshinone I, tanshinone II, cryptotanshinone and dihydrotanshinone, etc. Tanshinones offer the properties of anti-oxidation, anti-inflammation, antitumor,

Advances in Pharmacology, Volume 87
ISSN 1054-3589
https://doi.org/10.1016/bs.apha.2019.10.001

phytoestrogenic activity, vasodilation, neuroprotection, regulate metabolic function and other pharmacological advances. This chapter will review the discovery of the pharmacodynamic mechanism and pharmacokinetic studies of tanshinones and Danshen for further clinical applications.

Abbbreviations

Akt	protein kinase B
AR	androgen receptor
AST	glutamic oxalate transaminase
ATP	adenosine triphosphate
Aβ	amyloid β-protein
Bad	Bcl2 associated agonist of cell death
Bax	B-cell lymphoma-2 associated x protein
Bcl-2	B-cell lymphoma-2
Caspase-3	cysteine aspartic protease-3
Caspase-9	cysteine aspartic protease-9
CAT	catalase
CCNB1	cyclin b1
CCND1	cyclin d1
CD40	Cd 40 molecule
CK	creatine kinase
CLIC1	intracellular chloride ion channel 1
COX-2	cyclooxygenase-2
DOX	doxorubicin
eNOS	endothelial nitric oxide synthase
EPCs	endothelial progenitor cells
ERK1/2	extracellular regulated protein kinase 1/2
ER-α	endoplasmic reticulum α
GPER	G protein-coupled estrogen receptor
GREB1	growth regulation by estrogen in breast cancer 1
GSH	glutathione
GSH-Px	glutathione peroxidase
HDL	high density lipoprotein
Hmgb1	high mobility group box-1 protein
HLMs	human liver microsomes
HO-1	heme oxygense 1
HPV	human papillomavirus
H2O2	hydrogen peroxide
ICAM-1	intercellular cell adhesion molecule-1
IL-6	interleukin-6
IL-1β	interleukin-1 beta
iNOS	inducible nitric oxide synthase
LDH	lactate dehydrogenase
LDL	low-density lipoprotein
MAPK	mitogen-activated protein kinase
MDA	malondialdehyde
MDM2	murine double minute 2

MI	myocardial infraction
MMP-2	matrix metalloproteinase 2
MMP-9	matrix metalloproteinase 9
MRP1	multidrug resistance-associated protein 1
MSC	mesenchymal stem cells
MT1A	metallothionein 1a
NAD(P)H	nicotinamide adenine dinucleotide phosphate
NF-κB	nuclear transcription factor-kb signaling pathway
NO	nitric oxide
NQO1	NAD(P)H: quinone oxidoreductase 1
Nrf-2	nuclear factor erythroid-2 related factor
NSCLC	non-small cell lung cancer
ox-LDL	oxidized low-density lipoprotein
PCNA	proliferating cell nuclear antigen
PHGDH	phosphoglycerate dehydrogenase
PGI2	prostacyclin
PPARγ	peroxisome proliferator activated receptor γ
PTEN	phosphatase and tensin homolog deleted on chromosome ten
PXR	pregnane x receptor
ROS	reactive oxygen species
SMCs	synovial mesenchymal cells
SOD	increase superoxide dismutase
STAT3	signal transducer and activator of transcription
T-AOC	total antioxidant capacity
TNF-α	tumor necrosis factor α
T-NOS	total nitric oxide synthase
TXA2	thromboxane A2
UGT1A9	UDP-glucuronosyltransferase 1A9
VCAM-1	vascular cell adhesion molecule 1
VSMCs	vascular smooth muscle cells

1. Introduction

Danshen (*Salvia miltiorrhiza* Bge.) originated from *Salvia miltiorrhiza*, a plant in the Labiatae family, and its medicinal parts include the dry roots and rhizomes of plants. It was published for the first time approximately 2000 years ago during the Eastern Han Dynasty in "The Herbal Classic of Sheng Nong." Danshen operates by increasing blood flow and dissipating stasis, inducing menstruation to relieve menalgia, improving heart and blood function (Commission, C. P, 2015), and it is mainly used to treat cardiovascular and cerebrovascular diseases, osteoporosis, hepatitis, cirrhosis, chronic renal failure, pain and insomnia due to neurasthenia.

The history of phytochemical research of *S. miltiorrhiza* could date back to the 1930s (Xu et al., 2009). More than 200 compounds from Danshen have been isolated and identified to date. The chemical compositions of this herb can be classified into two categories: hydrophilic phenolic compounds and lipid-soluble diterpenoid compounds, which are the main pharmacological activities for *S. miltiorrhiza* (Kakisawa, Hayashi, Okazaki, & Ohashi, 1968). The tanshinones in *Salvia miltiorrhiza* mainly are diterpenoid quinones, which could be classified into two series, one is the phenanthro [1,2-*b*] furan-10,11-diones, the other is the phenanthrol [3,2-*b*] furan-7, 11-diones. Tanshinone IIA from *S. miltiorrhiza* was first isolated and identified by the Japanese scholar Nakao in 1934. With the development of phytochemical separation technology, more than 40 tanshinones have been isolated from *S. miltiorrhiza* to date. Studies have found that these compounds mainly include tanshinone I, tanshinone IIA, tanshinone IIB, cryptotanshinone, hydroxytanshinone, dihydrotanshinone I, methyltanshinone, miltirone, tanshindiol, przewatanshinquinone, tanshinlactone, isotanshinone I, isotanshinone IIA and neotanshinone (Pang et al., 2016). Some tanshinones have widely pharmacological activities, such as anti-oxidation, anti-inflammatory, anti-myocardial ischemia, anti-atherosclerosis, scavenging free radical and decrease blood lipid (Cheng, 2006). Fig. 1 shows the top six tanshinones with significant pharmacological activities.

Among all bioactive constituents from Danshen, tanshinones have been intensively investigated world widely in the past decade (Du, 2018).

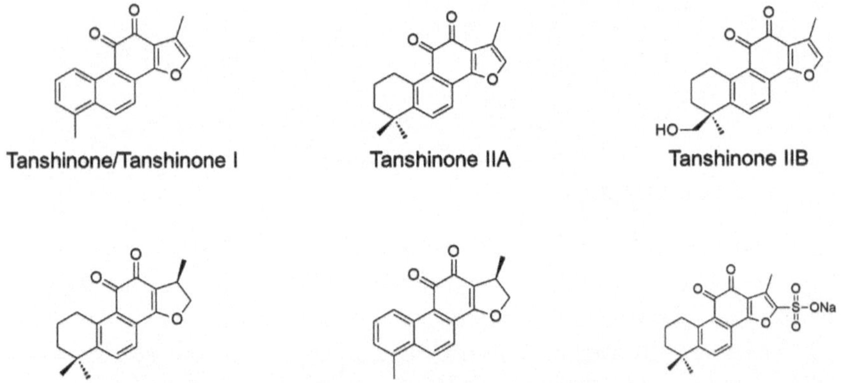

Fig. 1 Six tanshinones with significant pharmacological activities (Tanshinone I, Tanshinone IIA, Tanshinone IIB, Cryptotanshinone, Dihydrotanshinone I and tanshinlactone).

As increasingly more attention is directed toward the biological activities and therapeutic potential of tanshinones, it is necessary to review them to a further use in clinical application.

2. Pharmacodynamic mechanism of tanshinones

Tanshinones have been brought into focus due to their remarkable activities in the clinical use in cardiovascular diseases, cerebrovascular diseases, cancers and metabolic diseases treatment. Tanshinones have been found to possess extensive pharmacological activities, such as their antioxidation, anti-inflammation, antitumor, phytoestrogenic activity, vasodilation, neuroprotection, regulate metabolic function and other properties in the treatment with multi-diseases.

2.1 Antioxidation

Oxidative stress is a potential reason for multiple pathological disorders. Antioxidants could protect against the disorders by keeping reactive species in check (Shu, Hu, Huang, Huang, & Zhang, 2016). Tanshinones showed dramatical benefit on the treatment with cardiovascular and cerebrovascular diseases, espacilly in myocardial ischemia, atherosclerosis and cerebral ischemia. Tanshinone IA, tanshinone IIA, tanshinone IIB, cryptotanshinone and dihydrotanshinone I were found to act as antioxidants.

2.1.1 Antioxidant activity in myocardial ischemia

Myocardial ischemia is a cardiac dysfunction caused by a sharp decrease in blood flow to cardiac tissue, causes to a sudden decrease in oxygen supply to the heart (Liu, Liu, Wu, & Chai, 2007). Some studies have shown that tanshinones can improve the left ventricular function of myocardial infarction animals, reduce the size of myocardial infarction, and have significant anti-myocardial ischemia effects. Tanshinones can contributed prevention of cardiac injury development. It's benefit appeared relatively early post myocardial ischemia (Wang et al., 2011). Several tanshinones are a good scavenger of oxygen free radicals, which can inhibit lipid peroxidation in the myocardial cell membrane during myocardial ischemia and reperfusion, prevent calcium influx, and alleviate the damage to the myocardial cell membrane.

Tanshinone IA can reduce the myocardial infarction area in rats of myocardial ischemia-reperfusion injury; significantly decrease the serum levels of glutamic oxalate transaminase (AST), lactate dehydrogenase (LDH), malondialdehyde (Shu et al., 2016), increase superoxide dismutase (SOD) and glutathione peroxidase (GSH-Px), which can also pass through the blood, thereby inhibiting the lipid peroxidation process, alleviating the damage of free radicals to myocardial cells, and improving the antioxidant capacity of myocardium and thus exerting a protective effect against myocardial ischemia/reperfusion injury (Han, 2011). The oxidation metabolism of free radicals and anti-free radicals in the human body maintains a dynamic equilibrium under normal conditions. However, excessive production of free radicals or decreased antioxidant capacity can lead to imbalance. It has been reported that tanshinone can inhibit the activation of NADH/NADPH oxidase on cell membranes, increase SOD activity, scavenge oxygen free radicals and inhibit lipid peroxidation, thereby exerting a protective effect for vascular endothelial cells. In vitro experiments have shown that the SOD content of human umbilical vein endothelial cells damaged by oxidation increased significantly after treatment with tanshinone IA. Tanshinone IIA and tanshinone IIB were also reported to show antioxidant effect (Li, Wang, Li, Hao, & Zheng, 2006). Tanshinone IIA pretreatment significantly increased the viability and morphological changes of H9c2 cells damaged by doxorubicin (DOX), decreased the production of reactive oxygen species and increased the level of GSH in cells (Guo et al., 2018). Tanshinone IIA could increase SOD and GSH-Px activities and decrease MDA, and inducible nitric oxide synthase (iNOS) levels in a rat ischemia-reperfusion model (Li et al., 2015). Tanshinone IIA derivatives can be enriched in mitochondria and inhibit succinate dehydrogenase activity more effectively, while is closely related to ischemia/reperfusion leading oxidative damage (Zhao et al., 2019). Cryptotanshinone could enhance superoxide dismutase activity in a rat model of coronary artery ligation (Liu et al., 2017). Sodium tanshinone IIA sulfonate demonstrates a good protective effect during myocardial ischemia-reperfusion in rabbits. After administration, it can significantly reduce the production of MDA in the myocardium, as well as the release of myocardial creatine kinase (Kubli et al., 2013). Experiments have shown that sodium tanshinone IA sulfonate demonstrates an obvious scavenging effect on superoxide anion free radicals and hydrogen peroxide (Tao, Wang, Liu, & Fang, 1996).

Reactive oxygen species (Kubli et al., 2013) is also a key antioxidant target of tanshinones with a process of regulated pathways. Tanshinone IA can inhibit the increase in ROS content in human aortic vascular smooth muscle cells induced by hydrogen peroxide and angiotensin I by upregulating the activity of nuclear factor erythroid-2 related factor

(Nrf-2) (Lin, Wang, Liu, Yang, & Han, 2006; Zhang & Wang, 2007). Dihydrotanshinone I induces transient ROS production by reversibly inhibiting mitochondrial respiratory complex I, thereby stabilizing hypoxia induction factor -1 alpha (HIF-1α) (Jiang et al., 2019). Sodium tanshinone IIA sulfonic acid pretreatment on experimental myocardial ischemia/reperfusion and the protective effects of oxidative stress, and is associated with an increased activity of heme oxygense 1 (HO-1) (Wei, Li, Ji, Hu, & Ji, 2014).

In recent years, it has been reported that oxidative stress and accumulation of intracellular reactive oxygen species can induce autophagy of mitochondria and remove damaged mitochondria under stress conditions such as ischemia, hypoxia and nutrient deficiency (Lin & Kuang, 2014). Mitochondrial autophagy is closely related to myocardial injury after myocardial ischemia (Kubli et al., 2013). Ischemia and hypoxia can lead to the dysfunction of mitochondria, which leads to the expression of reactive oxygen species and apoptotic proteins, and further aggravate the damage. Therefore, early autophagy and timely removal of damaged mitochondria are beneficial to mitigate cell damage (Dianat, Sadeghi, Badavi, Panahi, & Taheri Moghadam, 2014). Studies have shown that tanshinone IIA can regulated autophagy to alleviate neuronal damage induced by ischemia, suggesting that tanshinone IIA has the activity of regulating autophagy after ischemia (Zhu, Tang, Wang, & Han, 2017). Tanshinone IIA can inhibit the occurrence of myocardial mitochondrial autophagy in myocardial infraction (MI) rats. Combined with the previous reports, it is suggested that the effect of tanshinone IIA on enhancing cardiac function and reducing myocardial injury may be related to the inhibition of mitochondrial autophagy (Wang, Liu, & Du, 2019).

2.1.2 Antioxidant activity in atherosclerosis

Atherosclerosis is an important pathological basis for cardiovascular diseases. The occurrence and development of atherosclerosis are caused by many factors, including local inflammation of arterial wall and abnormal lipid metabolism. During the early stage of atherosclerosis, the main pathological changes include low-density lipoprotein (LDL) oxidation, macrophage uptake of oxidized low-density lipoprotein (ox-LDL) and migration of macrophages to endothelial cells, resulting in foam cells and lipid streaks. Therefore, inhibiting the oxidation of LDL plays an important role in the prevention and early treatment of atherosclerosis (Lusis, 2000). Tanshinone can decrease the contents of ox-LDL, ROS and MDA in the serum of atherosclerotic model rats and increase the level of SOD. Tanshinone IA can reduce lipid oxidation in the early stage of atherosclerosis and prevent foam cells from occurring (Tang et al., 2007). In a New Zealand white rabbit atherosclerosis model, tanshinone IA can reduce the expression of CD 40 molecule (CD40), matrix metalloproteinase 2 (MMP-2), matrix metalloproteinase 9 (MMP-9), vascular cell adhesion molecule 1 (VCAM-1) and interleukin-1 beta (IL-1β) in plaque, thereby inhibiting plaque formation, increasing plaque stability and preventing plaque rupture (Fang et al., 2008). Tanshinone IIA could inhibit plaque calcification in atherosclerosis rats by inhibiting oxidative stress. Later studies have indicated that it could also decrease the activity and gene expression of NADPH oxidase, as well as the production of ROS. Tanshinone IIA promoted cholesterol efflux and improves lipid accumulation in macrophages by Omentin-1/ABCA1pathway to reduce the development ofatherosclerosis (Tan et al., 2019). Inhibitory effect of tanshinone IIA on atherosclerosis in apolipoprotein *E*-deficient (ApoE −/−) mice, reduce inflammatory factor levels, inhibit apoptosis of vascular smooth muscle cells (VSMCs), reduce MMP-2 and MMP-9, consistent with ox-LDL-induced macrophage proliferation and migration (Wang, Ge, Cheng, & Zhao, 2017). In vitro and in vivo research has confirmed that tanshinone IIA sodium sulfonate can reduce the expression of intracellular chloride ion channel 1 (CLIC1), promote antioxidant defense systems, and inhibit lipid peroxidation and inflammation levels, thereby playing a beneficial role in anti-atherosclerosis (Zhu et al., 2017).

2.1.3 Antioxidant activity in cerebral ischemia

Studies have shown that tanshinones can alleviate infarct size, reduce edema and improve neurological function of rats with cerebral ischemia. Oxidative stress plays a critical role in cerebral ischemia/reperfusion. The protective mechanism of to tanshinone on cerebral ischemia-reperfusion s is to up-regulate the expression of the anti-apoptotic gene, down-regulate the expression of the pro-apoptotic protein gene, and enhance ability of glutathione peroxidase to scavenge oxygen free radicals (Wang, Sun, et al., 2019).

Tanshinone I can significantly reduce the dysfunction of muscle movement, motor function and spatial learning and memory impairment in neonatal model of hypoxic-ischemic brain damage, which mechanism is related to increasing the yield of antioxidants, including total antioxidant capacity (T-AOC), glutathione (GSH), SOD and catalase (CAT), decrease prooxidant production which included hydrogen peroxide (H_2O_2), total nitric oxide synthase (T-NOS) and iNOS (Dai, Liu, & Dong, 2017).

Tanshinone IIA can significantly protect the neurological function in focal cerebral ischemia rats, reduce the water content of brain tissue, and reduce the content of cyclooxygenase-2 (COX-2) and its downstream products thromboxane B2 (TXA2) and prostacyclin (PGI2) in a dose-dependent manner (Dong et al., 2012). One report have shown that tanshinone IA can significantly improve brain edema after focal cerebral ischemia, increase SOD activity, reduce the MDA content, inhibit the expression of nitric oxide (NO) and inducible nitric oxide synthase, and exert brain protection by inhibiting oxidative stress, promoting oxygen free radical metabolism and reducing free radical levels (Ren & Du, 2018).

2.2 Anti-inflammation

Cytokines and chemokine-induced inflammatory responses can cause a variety of inflammatory diseases, and anti-inflammatory is a very important therapeutic strategy. Tanshinone IIA and cryptotanshinone reveal anti-inflammation activities (Chen et al., 2001), the related clinical usage including but not limited to the treatment of ischemia, cancer and atherosclerosis.

The result showed that tanshinone IIA could inhibit the expression of inflammatory cytokines and TLR2, NF-κB, ICAM-1 protein, suggesting that tanshinone IIA could inhibit inflammatory response by blocking TLR2/NF-kappa B signaling pathway (Li & Zhou, 2018). Tanshinone IIA could regulate a range of cytokine production and miRNAs by reducing the TLR4-NF-κB signaling pathway in LPS-induced RAW264.7 cells (Fan et al., 2016). Tanshinone IIA reduced the expression of VCAM-1 and intercellular cell adhesion molecule-1 (ICAM-1) in tumor necrosis factor α (TNF-α) induced endothelial progenitor cells (EPCs) by inhibit nuclear transcription factor-kappa B signaling pathway (NF-κB) (Yang et al., 2016). According to the changes of a series of atherosclerosis-associated inflammatory markers secreted by endothelial cells and synovial mesenchymal cells (SMCs), a co-culture cell model was used to prove that tanshinone IIA showed significant inhibition on atherosclerosis related inflammatory response (Li, Bonneton, Chen, & Laudet, 2015). In two types of persistent pain caused by cancer, tanshinone IIA inhibited the expression of inflammatory factors like IL-1β, TNF-α and interleukin-6 (IL-6), to relieve persistent pain and sudden pain caused by tumors (Hao et al., 2016). It has been reported that the protective effect of tanshinone IIA on myocardial ischemia-reperfusion injury may be through inhibiting the increase of ROS induced by reperfusion, thereby reducing the expression of High mobility group box-1 protein (Hmgb1) and inhibiting inflammatory reaction (Hu et al., 2015). Cryptotanshinone also has significant anti-myocardial ischemia effects by inhibit the release of pro-inflammatory cytokines, reduce the infiltration of neutrophils, and block the activation of NF-κB (Jin et al., 2009). In addition, cryptotanshinone also has anti-inflammatory properties through a variety of mechanisms including inhibit NF-κB and proliferation of mitogen-activated protein kinase (MAPK) signaling pathways. (Tang et al., 2011).

2.3 Mitochondrial apoptosis

Apoptosis occurs normally during development and aging which is a homeostasis mechanism to maintain the populations in tissues (Elmore, 2007). The machinery of apoptosis is complex and involves many signaling pathways. Caspase-3 is the ultimate executor of cell apoptosis, which activity is of great significance to cell apoptosis. (Huang et al., 2018). In the process of mitochondrial apoptosis, Caspase-9 is activated and cascade reactions including Caspase-3 are initiated to promote the transfer of Cytochrome C and Smac from mitochondrial inner membrane to cytoplasm (Fitzwalter & Thorburn, 2017; Kiraz, Adan, Yandim, & Baran, 2016). Mitochondrial damage, such as mitochondrial oxidative stress and mitochondrial calcium overload, triggers caspase-9-related mitochondrial apoptosis pathway (Zong, Rabinowitz, & White, 2016). It also controls other apoptotic events, such as endoplasmic reticulum stress, inflammatory response (Nambiar et al., 2019), metabolic reprogramming (Pan & Kupper, 2018) and autophagy (Lin et al., 2018).

Researchers detected that the levels of mitochondrial B-cell lymphoma-2 associated x protein (Bax) and Bak protein increased gradually after the administrat of breast cancer MCF-7 cells with different concentrations of total tanshinone, but the expression of total Bax and Bak protein did not change significantly. This further indicated that total tanshinone induced MCF-7 cell apoptosis through mitochondrial pathway (Li, Kong, Dou, & Zheng, 2019). Tanshinone inhibits the proliferation of non-small cell lung cancer (NSCLC) in a dose-dependent manner and induces apoptosis in early and late stages. In addition, tanshinone reduced the expression of B-cell lymphoma-2 (Bcl-2) and Bcl-xL and increased the Bax. The results also indicated that tanshinone IIA could increase the expression of PTEN and decrease the phosphorylation of Akt (protein kinase B) in THR 308 and SER 473 domains. More importantly, mitochondria are the potential target of tanshinone IIA (Jieensinue et al., 2018). Tanshinone IIA has potential beneficial effects on A/R injury. Zhang et al. demonstrated that the mechanism may be related to up-regulation of 14-3-3η and transfer of Bcl-2 to mitochondria, thereby preventing mPTP from opening, inhibiting ROS bursts, reducing cyt c release, avoiding the activation caspase-3 and preventing cell apoptosis (Zhang et al., 2018).

2.4 Antitumor

Tanshinone IIA, cryptotanshinone and tanshinone I are the main antitumor ingredients of *Salvia miltiorrhiza*. The antitumor mechanisms of tanshinone IIA are as follows: (1) inhibiting the growth and proliferation of cancer cells, (2) inducing apoptosis, (3) inducing cell cycle arrest, and (4) inhibiting the invasion, migration and metastasis of cancer cells. The report shown that tanshinone IIA alone is not cytotoxic to these gastric cells, and the enhanced antitumor effect of doxorubicin on drug-resistant gastric cancer cells is caused by tanshinone IIA. It possible mechanism is to inhibit multidrug resistance-associated protein 1 (MRP1) function, enhance cell cycle arrest, increase apoptosis, induce autophagic cell death, and enhance the antitumor effect of tanshinone IIA on drug-resistant gastric cancer cells (Di Cesare Mannelli et al., 2018). Studies demonstrated that Tanshinone IIA combined with Nutlin-3 showed a synergistic antileukemia effect by regulate p53 gene and AKT/mTOR pathways, thus the combination of tanshinone IIA and small molecule murine double minute 2 (MDM2) antagonists might be a hopeful approach for the handling of acute leukemia (Xu et al., 2018). The gastric cancer cells 7901 survival rate decreased and that the apoptotic rate increased by tanshinone IIA-P188; however, the cell death rate remained at a low level, indicating that tanshinone IIA-P188 could induce the apoptosis ability of gastric cancer cells (Wang, Sun, et al., 2019). Tanshinone IIA also promoted mitochondrial division by activating JNK-MFF signaling pathway, dose-dependent promotion of SW837 colorectal cancer cell death, damaged cell migration and inhibition of cancer cell proliferation (Jieensinue et al., 2018).

Cryptotanshinone can inhibit human papillomavirus (HPV) E6 protein in cervical cancer and also increase the expression of p53 and p21 protein (Ye, Xu, & Zhong, 2010). It can also inhibit the phosphorylation of tyrosine 705 residue of signal transduction and transcription activator (stat3), down-regulate the expression of cyclin D1 (CCND1) and survivin, and also inhibit the proliferation of cancer cells (Lu et al., 2013). In addition, cryptotanshinone inhibits the epithelial-mesenchymal transition of breast cancer cells by inhibiting the transcriptional activity of NF-κB (Zhu et al., 2014).

Tanshinone IA has demonstrated significant inhibitory effects on the human digestive system (e.g., liver cancer, gastric cancer, colon cancer), reproductive system (cervical cancer, ovarian cancer), and urinary system (such as prostate cancer) (Wang et al., 2015). For example, tanshinone IA can induce the expression of bcl2 associated agonist of cell death (Dianat et al., 2014) and metallothionein 1A (MT1A) mRNA by increasing the intracellular calcium level of hepatocellular carcinoma cells and then induce the apoptosis of hepatocellular carcinoma cells.

Neo-tanshinlactone has a significant inhibitory effect on two ER-positive human breast cancer cell lines, 10 times stronger than tamoxifen citrate and 20 times more selective (Wang et al., 2004). Tanshinlactones and some related structural modification chemicals have been reported to induce nuclear division, lead to cell cycle arrest and caspase-dependent apoptosis in MCF-7 cells (Sashidhara et al., 2010). For example, Neo-tanshinlactone analog 1J leaded to active Chk2 and p53, caused DNA lysis-mediated apoptosis in different breast cancer cells, which may be a potential clue to future breast cancer treatment (Banerji et al., 2017).

2.5 Phytoestrogenic activity

Plant-derived molecules with estrogen rings (phytoestrogens) have been a focus of research due to the discovery of their effectiveness in alleviating symptoms of endogenous hormonal disorder diseases and cardiovascular conditions. It was first reported in 2009 that tanshinone IIA could be used as a latent selective estrogen receptor modulator in the treatment of inflammation-related neurodegenerative diseases and cardiovascular diseases without increasing the hazard of breast cancer. (Fan et al., 2009). Because of the structural similarity between tanshinones and endogenous hormone substances, it was reasonably speculated that the biological activities of phytoestrogen tanshinones may be brought to bind the nuclear receptors (Li, Bonneton, et al., 2015). Tanshinone I, tanshinone IIA, cryptotanshinone and dihydrotanshinone could act as agonists of human estrogen receptor α by transactivation of estrogen response element in MCF-7 cells, which could intervene in the reproduction, development, homeostasis and metabolism of cancer cells (Zhang et al., 2019). In relation to myocardium, tanshinone IIA treatment of cardiac fibroblasts significantly inhibited collagen I deposition and increased the production of new elastic fibers. Furthermore, the anti-collagen and elastic effects of tanshinone II can only occur after selective activation of G protein-coupled estrogen receptor (GPER). This subsequently led to the activation of the pka/creb phosphorylation pathway, which reversely regulates the transcription of collagen I and elastin genes (Mao, Wang, Zhang, & Hinek, 2014).

It has been reported that tanshinones could activate pregnane X receptor (PXR) (Gao et al., 2012), peroxisome proliferator activated receptor γ (PPARγ) (Guasch et al., 2013), and androgen receptor (AR). Tanshinones have been revealed to possess the potential to cure benign prostatic hyperplasia, prostate cancer and breast cancer; these intractable diseases are induced and influenced by endogenous hormones (Wang et al., 2015; Yu, Zhou, Mu, de Lima Lopes, & Luo, 2014). As the main receptors of phytoestrogens, estrogen receptors have been studied for their ability by binding active components of *Salvia miltiorrhiza* (Dasgupta, Lonard, & O'Malley, 2014). In a rat model of estrogen/androgen -induced prostatic hyperplasia, tanshinone IIA could inhibit the increasing thickness of prostatic smooth muscle layer, the expression of proliferating cell nuclear antigen (PCNA) in prostatic epithelial cells, down-regulated expression of AR, cyclin B1 (CCNB1) and CCND1, which showed the outcome in preventing disease progression (Wang et al., 2015). Acetyltanshinone IIA could inhibit the cell growth of estrogen receptor-positive breast cancer cells and reduce the transcription of an ER-responsive gene, growth regulation by estrogen in breast cancer 1 (GREB1). Furthermore, its therapeutic efficacy is superior to tamoxifen, a frequently used anti-breast cancer drug (Yu et al., 2014). In vitro and in vitro studies have shown that the effect of tanshinone IIA could be inhibited by estrogen receptor antagonist, suggesting a clear contribution of ER. Meanwhile, tanshinone IIA it could enhanced endothelial nitric oxide synthase (eNOS) mRNA expression and NO production as estrogen (Fan et al., 2011). A clinical evidence has revealed that the incidence of cardiovascular disease morbidity dramatically increases in postmenopausal women and could be alleviated by *Salvia miltiorrhiza* (Weng et al., 2013).

2.6 Vasodilation

Improving vascular endothelial function has important clinical significance in the diagnosis, treatment and prevention of cardiovascular diseases. Some studies have shown that tanshinone components play a significant role in promoting vasodilation. The release of NO synthesized by vascular endothelial cells into smooth muscle cells can promote vasodilation. Fluorescence imaging technology has demonstrated that tanshinone IA can promote the release of NO from human vascular endothelial cells. Tanshinone IA can alleviate the inhibitory effect of angiotensin I on NO secretion in vascular endothelial cells (Li et al., 2007). In addition, dihydrotanshinone can affect the concentration of calcium ions in cells, thereby regulating the calcium channels in aortic vascular smooth muscle cells and playing a role in vasodilation (Lam, Yeung, Chan, & Or, 2008). Tanshinone IIA can promote vasodilation activity by activate estrogen receptor signaling pathway, increase the expression of eNOS, NO production, phosphorylation of extracellular regulated protein kinase 1/2 (ERK1/2) and Ca^{2+} mobilization (Fan et al., 2011).

2.7 Neuroprotection

Tanshinone IIA, Tanshinone I and cryptotanshinone showed neuroprotective activity. Tanshinone I and cryptotanshinone have significant inhibitory effects in five majors slipophilic diterpenes derived from Danshen with gliosis induced transient cerebral ischemia injury in gerbils (Park et al., 2012).

It has been shown that tanshinone IIA can significantly promote the progress of cognitive dysfunction in diabetic rats which can reduce the cognitive impairment and development induced by diabetes mellitus and improve learning and memory by inhibiting the apoptosis induced by ER stress activation (Chen, Bi, Chen, Zhang, & Xu, 2018). A meta-analysis showed tanshinone IIA had a weak effect on inflammation following spinal cord injury (Koushki, Latifi, Norouzi Javidan, & Matin, 2015). Some researchers have proved that tanshinone IIA-incubated mesenchymal stem cells (MSC) could treat amyloid β-protein (Aβ) caused neuroinflammation (Huang et al., 2019). It was found that Tanshinone IIA-MSCs could show a better neuroprotective effect and a lower toxic protein production than MSCs alone by regulated neuroinflammatory-associated cytokines and promoted the survival of hippocampal neurons. Tanshinone IIA can improve the ratio of Bcl-2 and Bax induced by oAβ1–42, which can prevent cytochrome C from translocating into cytoplasmic mitochondria, reducing oAβ1–42-induced cleavage cysteine aspartic protease-9 (caspase-9), inhibiting caspase-3/7 activity, meanwhile increasing mitochondrial membrane potential (MMP) and adenosine triphosphate (ATP) content (Yang et al., 2019). It has been reported that tanshinone IIA inhibits apoptosis of hippocampal neurons in diabetic rats by inhibiting endoplasmic reticulum stress activation. (Chen et al., 2018). Tanshinone IIA also can protected mitochondrial membrane potential from damage, reduced the transfer of cytochrome *c* from mitochondria to the cytoplasm and the activation of Caspase-9 and Caspase-3 (Zhang et al., 2015). Tanshinone IIA PEGylated nanoparticles were also investigated on neuroprotective effects by regulating the MAPK pathway involved in the neuroinflammatory cascade of stroke (Liu, Ye, An, Pan, & Ji, 2013).

Protective effect of tanshinone I on ischemic injury of CA1 pyramidal neurons induced by transient cerebral ischemia. The mechanism is based on anti-oxidation and increasing neurotrophic factors. Pretreatment with Tanshinone I could inhibit ischemia-induced neuronal death in CA1 by regulating endogenous inflammatory cytokines (Park et al., 2014).

2.8 Regulate metabolic function

The first report of tanshinone IIA could improve nerve functions in diabetic rats was published in 2009, which protect effect was better on the early stage of diabetic nephropathy (Kim, Jung, & Lee, 2009). Recent researches mainly focus on the complex diseases together with diabetes, for example, ischemia and renal injury. A study suggested that TSN preconditioning can reduce the infarct size after ischemia/reperfusion in diabetic rats, with the decrease of cardiac apoptosis and inflammation, regulate PI3K/AKT pathway to improve cardiac dysfunction (Zhang et al., 2010). Tanshinone IIA could inhibit high glucose induced renal proximal tubular fibrosis (Cao et al., 2017). Sodium tanshinone IIA sulfonate has shown obvious antioxidation effects on the kidneys of diabetic rats in a dose-dependent manner. Meanwhile, sodium tanshinone IIA sulfonate can regulate lipid metabolism disorder, reduce the urinary protein excretion rate and alleviate diabetic kidney damage in diabetic rats (Chen et al., 2017).

The antioxidant activity of tanshinone IIA was reported to contribute to reduce lipid peroxidation in liver cells (Cao, Liu, Wang, & Xu, 1996).

Combine with atorvastatin, tanshinone IIA showed a dramatically effect on atherosclerosis (Xu et al., 2014). With a rat model of hyperlipidemia, tanshinone IIA was proved to reduce liver lipid deposition. Although it does not affect blood lipid levels, but lowers the level of middle sub-components in high density lipoprotein (HDL) and increases the level of HDL large sub-components, accordingly regulating cholesterol intake and excretion (Jia et al., 2016).

2.9 Other pharmacological advances

Osteoporosis manifests as a reduction in bone mass. Tanshinone has been shown to affect osteoclast differentiation; however, the role of tanshinone in osteoporosis suggests that tanshinone effectively inhibits ovx-induced osteoporosis and bone marrow mesenchymal stem cell senescence by upregulating phosphoglycerate dehydrogenase (PHGDH). (Wang, Cheng, Zhang, Wang, & Wang, 2019).

Radiotherapy not only directly acts on cell DNA to cause cell damage but also causes small vessel occlusion, which leads to vascular remodeling within the scope of radiotherapy and the local hypoxic environment. It can not only change the radiosensitivity of tumor cells but also leads to necrosis of normal tissue cells due to hypoxia. In previous studies of ischemia-reperfusion injury, tanshinone IIA effectively improved the ischemia-hypoxia state of normal tissues and protected nerve function (Dong et al., 2012; Lin, Lu, Huang, & Wang, 2013). It has been found that the survival fraction of HT-22 cultured hippocampal neuron cells irradiated with sodium tanshinone IIA sulfonate combined with radiation in vitro was significantly higher than that in the simple irradiation group (Ren & Du, 2018).

3. Pharmacokinetics of tanshinones

After drug metabolism, many types of metabolites and toxic side effects can be produced. By studying the metabolic regularity of plasma, urine, bile and feces in animals, analyzing the metabolic pathways and products of active ingredients of drugs, and studying the pharmacodynamics and toxicology of maternal drugs and metabolites, we can clarify the biotransformation process of drugs in the body, find and discover new effective substances, and modify the structure of toxic and side-effect products.

This method can not only avoid the toxic side effects but also obtain good pharmacodynamics and provide an enough theoretical basis for rational clinical drug use.

3.1 Absorption and distribution

Cai et al.'s (2016) determined four kinds of tanshinones-tanshinone IIA, dihydrotanshinone I, tanshinone I, and cryptotanshinone by the method of UPLC-TQ/MS and applied them to evaluate the pharmacokinetics of plasma in normal and chronic renal failure (CRF) rat, they found that pharmacokinetic characteristics of four tanshinones in CRF rats were different. The results showed that extract of *Salvia miltiorrhiza* could decrease the Cmax and $AUC_{0\text{–}t}$ of tanshinone IIA, tanshinone I, cryptotanshinone, and CLz/F increased in model group. Nevertheless, after intragastric administration of a combination of ethanol extract and water extract, the Cmax and AUC0–t of the four tanshinones were up-regulated, while CLz/F was down-regulated. In the Zeng's et al. (2015) study of the pharmacokinetics of cryptotanshinone in rats at single and multiple doses, blood was taken from rats that had been fasted before intragastric administration. Blood was taken from the fundus venous sinus of the rats. The concentration of cryptotanshinone in plasma was determined by LC-MS/MS. The results showed that there was no significant difference between single and multiple doses of cryptotanshinone, indicating that there was no risk of cryptotanshinone accumulation in vivo.

Wang et al.'s was determined successfully in rats of plasma concentrations for tanshinone IIA, notably, the concentration-time curve of tanshinone IIA was multi-peak pattern (Wang et al., 2014). The HPLC-MS/MS method developed by Li et al. (2017) has been successfully used to determine the plasma concentrations of 11 components after oral administration of NXTC at doses of 0.5 and 1.5 gkg^{-1}, respectively. It was indicated that the T1/2 values of cryptotanshinone and tanshinone IIA shown that the action time of cryptotanshinone and tanshinone IIA in vivo was significantly longer than that of other components. The distribution of tanshinone IIA in the gastrointestinal tract of normal mice showed that the tanshinone IIA profiles in the GI including stomach, duodenum, jejunum and ileum and colon tissue homogenates at 0.25, 2 and 12 h after oral tanshinone IIA administration. It is noteworthy that the tanshinone IIA level in the gastrointestinal tract was relatively high (Wang et al., 2017).

3.2 Metabolism and excretion

The metabolites of tanshinone I, dihydrotanshinone I, tanshinone IIA and cryptotanshinone in rats were systematically identified by LC-DAD-SEI-MS^n (Dai et al., 2009), and the results showed that after the biotransformation of tanshinone I and dihydrotanshinone I in rats, 16 phase I metabolites and 4 phase II metabolites could be identified. Two main metabolic pathways of tanshinones were summarized: (1) dehydrogenation, hydroxylation, furan ring cleavage and oxidation reactions from tanshinone; and (2) tanshinone was first metabolized into dihydrotanshinone and then into its components (dehydrogenation, hydroxylation, pyrolysis and oxidation of furan rings on the substrates). Phase II metabolites mainly form glucuronic acid conjugates and sulfate esterification conjugates. The drug metabolism plays a great role in drug clearance and directly affects systemic drug exposure. Researchers studied the bile excretion and intrahepatic transformation of tanshinone. It was found that tanshinone IIA, tanshinone I and cryptotanshinone could be excreted through the liver through bile (Luo, Sheng, Zhang, Xu, & Wei, 1983). A LC-ESI-MS^n method has been established to identify metabolites in rat bile samples after intravenous injection of dihydrotanshinone I (Wang et al., 2010). The results showed that 15 phase I metabolites and 2 phase II metabolites were detected in rats bile. Determination of phase I metabolites in bile of rats after intravenous injection of seven tanshinones (tanshinone IIA, sodium tanshinone IIA sulfonate, cryptotanshinone I, 15, 16-dihydrotanshinone I, tanshinone IIB, shikonin and tanshinone I) by the use of HPLC/MS^n (Sun et al., 2007). A total of 33 metabolites were detected, suggesting that tanshinone IIA was primarily metabolized by hydroxylation and dehydrogenation and that tanshinone IIB was primarily hydroxylated.

Hydroxylated metabolite of tanshinone I were observed in rat liver microsomes, and O-glucuronidation tanshinone I was also found in rat urine (Liu, Wu, Wang, & Cai, 2007), and dehydrogenation, hydroxylation, furan ring cleavage, as well as oxidation were the main pathways of tanshinone I phase I biotransformation of tanshinone in rat bile (Wang et al., 2010). In Li et al.'s study (Li et al., 2019), they used human liver microsomes preparations to determine major metabolites of tanshinone I by HPLC-UV and Q-Trap mass spectrometer. Six metabolites were detected, which indicated that hydroxylation, reduction and glucuronidation were the main pathways for tanshinones I biotransformation.

In addition, a research used LC-MS^n technology to study the metabolites of tanshinone IIB in plasma after sublingual administration of Compound Danshen Dropping Pills (Cai et al., 2016; Zheng et al., 2007). The results showed that tanshinone IIB could easily lose hydroxymethyl in vivo. A study about the metabolites of cryptotanshinone in rats showed that the metabolites of cryptotanshinone in urine and bile were cryptotanshinone, tanshinone IIA, tanshinone IIA hydroxylation products and the combination of tanshinone IIA and glutamic acid (Xie & Shen, 1983). The excretion of cryptotanshinone in rat bile was higher than that in urine.

In vitro and in vivo studies indicated that the predominant metabolic pathway of tanshinone IIA was NAD(P)H: quinone oxidoreductase 1 (NQO1)-mediated quinone reduction and subsequent gelation, and UDP-glucuronosyltransferase 1A9 (UGT1A9) played an important role in this process (Zhang, Cao, Wang, Yuan, & Fang, 2017). When gave tanshinone to miniature pigs, the plasma results showed that cryptotanshinone was dehydrogenated after the actions of blood and liver enzymes, and the main metabolite was tanshinone IIA (Xue et al., 1999). The metabolites of tanshinone IIA in zebrafish were analyzed using high-performance liquid chromatography/IT-MS^n (Wei et al., 2012). It was showed that the main metabolites of tanshinone IIA in zebrafish were monohydroxylation, dihydroxylation and dehydrogenation products. Another study also found that the metabolite of cryptotanshinone in rat plasma was tanshinone IIA (Song, Hang, Zhang Zh, Du, & Chen, 2005). There is one research evaluated for the liver microsomes of rat on metabolic stability, indicating that tanshinone IIA may inhibit the activities of CYP450 (Wang, Zhang, Wang, Yu, & Yuan, 2016).

4. Conclusion

In conclusion, tanshinones, the liposolubility components of *Salvia miltiorrhiza* have important pharmacological activities in cardiovascular, cerebrovascular, cancer and other effects (Fig. 2). At present, *Salvia miltiorrhiza* has been gradually applied in various clinical fields. It is believed that tanshinones will play a more important role in clinical application with the deepening of basic pharmacological and metabolic studies and clinical studies of tanshinones.

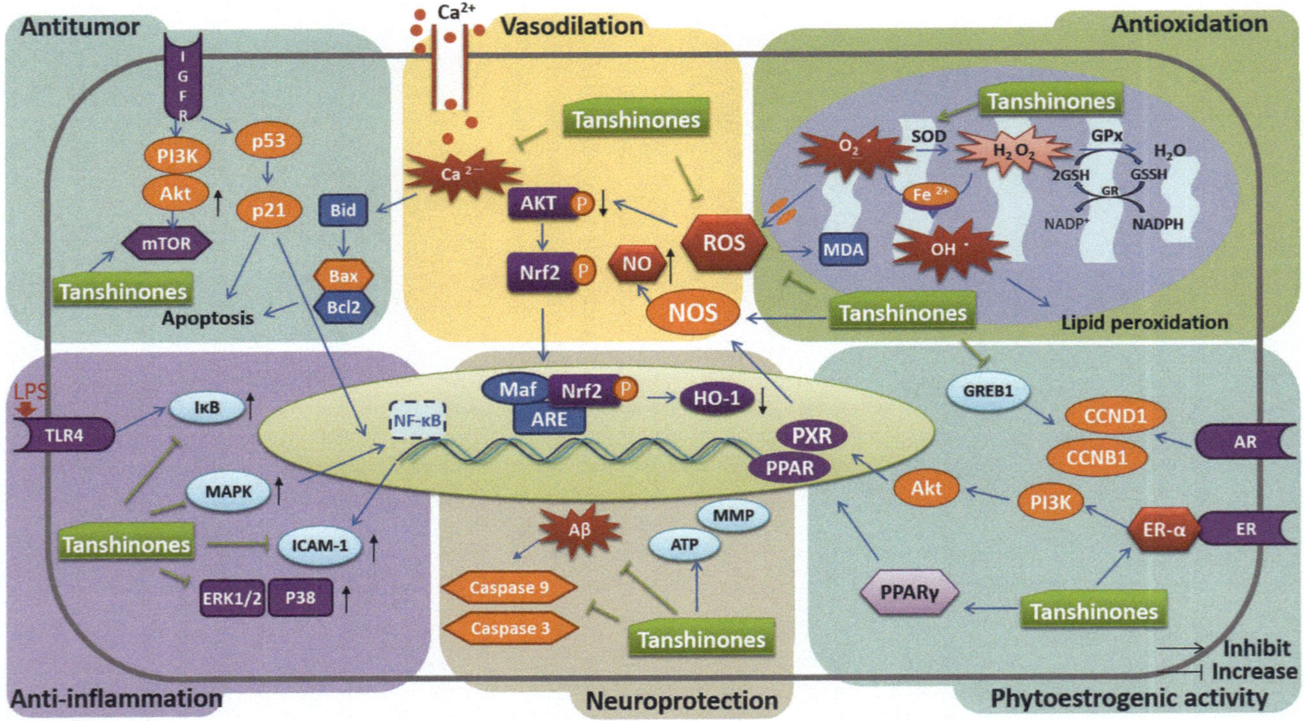

Fig. 2 Pharmacological activities of tanshinones mostly related to antioxidation, anti-inflammation, antitumor, phytoestrogenic activity, vasodilation and neuroprotection. Note: *Aβ*, amyloid β-protein; *AKT*, protein kinase B; *AR*, androgen receptor; *ARE*, antioxidant response element; *ATP*, adenosine triphosphate; *Bax*, B-cell lymphoma-2 associated X protein; *Bcl2*, B-cell lymphoma-2; *Bid*, B-cell lymphoma-2 homology 3 interacting domain death agonist; *Caspase 3*, cysteine aspartic protease 3; *Caspase 9*, cysteine aspartic protease 3; *CCNB1*, cyclin B1; *CCND1*, cyclin D1; *ERK*, extracellular signal regulated kinase; *ER-α*, estrogen receptor α; *FAS*, fatty acid synthase; *GPx*, glutathione peroxidase; *GREB1*, growth regulation by estrogen in breast cancer 1; *GSH*, glutathione; *GSSH*, oxidized glutathione; *HO-1*, heme oxygenase 1; H_2O_2, hydrogen peroxide; *IGFR*, insulin-like growth factor 1 receptor; *IkB*, I kappa-B; *LRR*, leucine-rich repeat; *Maf*, transcription factor belonging to the AP-1 family (MAF or c-MAF); *MAPK*, mitogen-activated protein kinase; *MMP*, matrix metalloproteinase; *mTOR*, mammalian target of rapamycin; *NADP+*, oxidized form of nicotinamide adenine dinucleotide phosphate; *NADPH*, nicotinamide adenine dinucleotide phosphate; *NF-kB*, nuclear factor-kappa B; *NO*, nitric oxide; *NOS*, nitric oxide synthase; *Nrf2*, nuclear factor erythroid 2-related factor 2; *PI3K*, phosphoinositide 3-kinase; *PPARγ*, peroxisome proliferator-activated receptor gamma; *PXR*, pregnane X receptor; *ROS*, reactive oxygen species; *SOD*, super oxide dismutase, *TLR4*, toll like receptor 4.

Acknowledgments

National Key R&D Program of China (SQ2018YFC170023) and the National Science Fund for Distinguished Young Scholars (81125024) supported this work.

Conflict of interest

The authors declare no other competing interests.

References

Banerji, B., Killi, S. K., Katarkar, A., Chatterjee, S., Tangella, Y., Prodhan, C., et al. (2017). Neo-tanshinlactone D-ring modified novel analogues induce apoptosis in human breast cancer cell via DNA damage. *Bioorganic & Medicinal Chemistry*, *25*(1), 202–212. https://doi.org/10.1016/j.bmc.2016.10.026.

Cai, H.-D., Su, S.-L., Li, Y., Zhu, Z., Guo, J., Zhu, Y., et al. (2016). Simultaneous determination of four tanshinones by UPLC-TQ/MS and their pharmacokinetic application after administration of single ethanol extract of danshen combined with water extract in normal and adenine-induced chronic renal failure rats. *Molecules (Basel, Switzerland)*, *21*(12), 1630. https://doi.org/10.3390/molecules21121630.

Cao, L., Huang, B., Fu, X., Yang, J., Lin, Y., & Lin, F. (2017). Effects of tanshinone IIA on the regulation of renal proximal tubular fibrosis. *Molecular Medicine Reports*, *15*(6), 4247–4252. https://doi.org/10.3892/mmr.2017.6498.

Cao, E. H., Liu, X. Q., Wang, J. J., & Xu, N. F. (1996). Effect of natural antioxidant tanshinone II-A on DNA damage by lipid peroxidation in liver cells. *Free Radical Biology & Medicine*, *20*(6), 801–806.

Chen, J., Bi, Y., Chen, L., Zhang, Q., & Xu, L. (2018). Tanshinone IIA exerts neuroprotective effects on hippocampus-dependent cognitive impairments in diabetic rats by attenuating ER stress-induced apoptosis. *Biomedicine & Pharmacotherapy*, *104*, 530–536. https://doi.org/10.1016/j.biopha.2018.05.040.

Chen, Y. H., Lin, S. J., Ku, H. H., Shiao, M. S., Lin, F. Y., Chen, J. W., et al. (2001). Salvianolic acid B attenuates VCAM-1 and ICAM-1 expression in TNF-alpha-treated human aortic endothelial cells. *Journal of Cellular Biochemistry*, *82*(3), 512–521.

Chen, X., Wu, R., Kong, Y., Yang, Y., Gao, Y., Sun, D., et al. (2017). Tanshinone IIA attenuates renal damage in STZ-induced diabetic rats via inhibiting oxidative stress and inflammation. *Oncotarget*, *8*(19), 31915–31922. https://doi.org/10.18632/oncotarget.16651.

Cheng, T. O. (2006). Danshen: A popular chinese cardiac herbal drug. *Journal of the American College of Cardiology*, *47*(7), 1498. author reply 1499-1500. https://doi.org/10.1016/j.jacc.2006.01.001.

Commission, C. P. (2015). *Pharmacopoeia of the People's Republic of China* (2015th ed.). Beijing: Chemical Industry Press.

Dai, C., Liu, Y., & Dong, Z. (2017). Tanshinone I alleviates motor and cognitive impairments via suppressing oxidative stress in the neonatal rats after hypoxic-ischemic brain damage. *Molecular Brain*, *10*(1), 52. https://doi.org/10.1186/s13041-017-0332-9.

Dai, H., Wang, M., Li, X., Li, Y., Wang, L., & Xue, M. (2009). *LC-DAD-MS identification of metabolites of tanshinone drugs in vivo. 4* (pp. 9–10). Information of the Chinese Pharmacological Society.

Dasgupta, S., Lonard, D. M., & O'Malley, B. W. (2014). Nuclear receptor coactivators: Master regulators of human health and disease. *Annual Review of Medicine*, *65*, 279–292. https://doi.org/10.1146/annurev-med-051812-145316.

Di Cesare Mannelli, L., Piccolo, M., Maione, F., Ferraro, M. G., Irace, C., De Feo, V., et al. (2018). Tanshinones from *Salvia miltiorrhiza* Bunge revert chemotherapy-induced neuropathic pain and reduce glioblastoma cells malignancy. *Biomedicine & Pharmacotherapy, 105*, 1042–1049. https://doi.org/10.1016/j.biopha.2018.06.047.

Dianat, M., Sadeghi, N., Badavi, M., Panahi, M., & Taheri Moghadam, M. (2014). Protective effects of co-administration of gallic acid and cyclosporine on rat myocardial morphology against ischemia/reperfusion. *Jundishapur Journal of Natural Pharmaceutical Products, 9*(4), e17186.

Dong, H., Mao, S., Wei, J., Liu, B., Zhang, Z., Zhang, Q., et al. (2012). Erratum to: Tanshinone IIA protects PC12 cells fromβ-amyloid25–35-induced apoptosis via PI3. *Molecular Biology Reports, 39*(6), 7213.

Du, G.-H. (2018). *Natural small molecule drugs from plants*. Springer Nature America, Inc.

Elmore, S. (2007). Apoptosis: A review of programmed cell death. *Toxicologic Pathology, 35*(4), 495–516. https://doi.org/10.1080/01926230701320337.

Fan, G.-W., Gao, X.-M., Wang, H., Zhu, Y., Zhang, J., Hu, L.-M., et al. (2009). The anti-inflammatory activities of Tanshinone IIA, an active component of TCM, are mediated by estrogen receptor activation and inhibition of iNOS. *The Journal of Steroid Biochemistry and Molecular Biology, 113*(3–5), 275–280. https://doi.org/10.1016/j.jsbmb.2009.01.011.

Fan, G., Jiang, X., Wu, X., Fordjour, P. A., Miao, L., Zhang, H., et al. (2016). Anti-inflammatory activity of tanshinone IIA in LPS-stimulated RAW264.7 macrophages via miRNAs and TLR4-NF-kappaB pathway. *Inflammation, 39*(1), 375–384. https://doi.org/10.1007/s10753-015-0259-1.

Fan, G., Zhu, Y., Guo, H., Wang, X., Wang, H., & Gao, X. (2011). Direct vasorelaxation by a novel phytoestrogen tanshinone IIA is mediated by nongenomic action of estrogen receptor through endothelial nitric oxide synthase activation and calcium mobilization. *Journal of Cardiovascular Pharmacology, 57*(3), 340–347.

Fang, Z. Y., Lin, R., Yuan, B. X., Yang, G. D., Liu, Y., & Zhang, H. (2008). Tanshinone IIA downregulates the CD40 expression and decreases MMP-2 activity on atherosclerosis induced by high fatty diet in rabbit. *Journal of Ethnopharmacology, 115*(2), 217–222. https://doi.org/10.1016/j.jep.2007.09.025.

Fitzwalter, B. E., & Thorburn, A. (2017). A caspase-independent way to kill cancer cells. *Nature Cell Biology, 19*(9), 1014–1015. https://doi.org/10.1038/ncb3604.

Gao, S., Liu, Z., Li, H., Little, P. J., Liu, P., & Xu, S. (2012). Cardiovascular actions and therapeutic potential of tanshinone IIA. *Atherosclerosis, 220*(1), 3–10. https://doi.org/10.1016/j.atherosclerosis.2011.06.041.

Guasch, L., Sala, E., Mulero, M., Valls, C., Salvado, M. J., Pujadas, G., et al. (2013). Identification of PPARgamma partial agonists of natural origin (II): In silico prediction in natural extracts with known antidiabetic activity. *PLoS One, 8*(2). e55889. https://doi.org/10.1371/journal.pone.0055889.

Guo, Z., Yan, M., Chen, L., Fang, P., Li, Z., Wan, Z., et al. (2018). Nrf2-dependent antioxidant response mediated the protective effect of tanshinone IIA on doxorubicin-induced cardiotoxicity. *Experimental and Therapeutic Medicine, 16*(4), 3333–3344. https://doi.org/10.3892/etm.2018.6614.

Han, D. (2011). Study the effect of tanshinoneIIA on apoptosis of myocardial cells of inchemia-reperfusion rats. *Modern Preventive Medicine, 38*(13), 2572–2574.

Hao, W., Chen, L., Wu, L. F., Yang, F., Niu, J. X., Kaye, A. D., et al. (2016). Tanshinone IIA exerts an antinociceptive effect in rats with cancer-induced bone pain. *Pain Physician, 19*(7), 465–476.

Hu, H., Zhai, C., Qian, G., Gu, A., Liu, J., Ying, F., et al. (2015). Protective effects of tanshinone IIA on myocardial ischemia reperfusion injury by reducing oxidative stress, HMGB1 expression, and inflammatory reaction. *Pharmaceutical Biology, 53*(12), 1752–1758. https://doi.org/10.3109/13880209.2015.1005753.

Huang, K.-H., Fang, W.-L., Li, A. F.-Y., Liang, P.-H., Wu, C.-W., Shyr, Y.-M., et al. (2018). Caspase-3, a key apoptotic protein, as a prognostic marker in gastric cancer after curative surgery. *International Journal of Surgery*, *52*, 258–263.

Huang, N., Li, Y., Zhou, Y., Zhou, Y., Feng, F., Shi, S., et al. (2019). Neuroprotective effect of tanshinone IIA-incubated mesenchymal stem cells on Abeta25-35-induced neuroinflammation. *Behavioural Brain Research*, *365*, 48–55. https://doi.org/10.1016/j.bbr.2019.03.001.

Jia, L. Q., Zhang, N., Xu, Y., Chen, W. N., Zhu, M. L., Song, N., et al. (2016). Tanshinone IIA affects the HDL subfractions distribution not serum lipid levels: Involving in intake and efflux of cholesterol. *Archives of Biochemistry and Biophysics*, *592*, 50–59. https://doi.org/10.1016/j.abb.2016.01.001.

Jiang, L., Zeng, H., Ni, L., Qi, L., Xu, Y., Xia, L., et al. (2019). HIF-1α preconditioning potentiates antioxidant activity in ischemic injury: The role of sequential administration of dihydrotanshinone I and protocatechuic aldehyde in cardioprotection. *Antioxidants & Redox Signaling*, *31*(3), 227–242. https://doi.org/10.1089/ars.2018.7624. Epub 2019 Apr 3.

Jieensinue, S., Zhu, H., Li, G., Dong, K., Liang, M., & Li, Y. (2018). Tanshinone IIA reduces SW837 colorectal cancer cell viability via the promotion of mitochondrial fission by activating JNK-Mff signaling pathways. *BMC Cell Biology*, *19*(1), 21. https://doi.org/10.1186/s12860-018-0174-z.

Jin, Y. C., Kim, C. W., Kim, Y. M., Nizamutdinova, I. T., Ha, Y. M., Kim, H. J., et al. (2009). Cryptotanshinone, a lipophilic compound of salvia miltiorrriza root, inhibits TNF-alpha-induced expression of adhesion molecules in HUVEC and attenuates rat myocardial ischemia/reperfusion injury in vivo. *European Journal of Pharmacology*, *614*(1–3), 91–97. https://doi.org/10.1016/j.ejphar.2009.04.038.

Kakisawa, H., Hayashi, T., Okazaki, I., & Ohashi, M. (1968). Isolation and structures of new tanshinones. *Tetrahedron Letters*, *9*(28), 2331–3234.

Kim, S. K., Jung, K. H., & Lee, B. C. (2009). Protective effect of Tanshinone IIA on the early stage of experimental diabetic nephropathy. *Biological & Pharmaceutical Bulletin*, *32*(2), 220–224.

Kiraz, Y., Adan, A., Yandim, M. K., & Baran, Y. (2016). Major apoptotic mechanisms and genes involved in apoptosis. *Tumor Biology*, *37*(7), 8471–8486.

Koushki, D., Latifi, S., Norouzi Javidan, A., & Matin, M. (2015). Efficacy of some non-conventional herbal medications (sulforaphane, tanshinone IIA, and tetramethylpyrazine) in inducing neuroprotection in comparison with interleukin-10 after spinal cord injury: A meta-analysis. *The Journal of Spinal Cord Medicine*, *38*(1), 13–22. https://doi.org/10.1179/2045772314Y.0000000215.

Kubli, D., Zhang, X., Lee, Y., Hanna, R., Quinsay, M., Nguyen, C., et al. (2013). Parkin protein deficiency exacerbates cardiac injury and reduces survival following myocardial infarction. *The Journal of Biological Chemistry*, *288*(2), 915–926.

Lam, F. F., Yeung, J. H., Chan, K. M., & Or, P. M. (2008). Dihydrotanshinone, a lipophilic component of *Salvia miltiorrhiza* (danshen), relaxes rat coronary artery by inhibition of calcium channels. *Journal of Ethnopharmacology*, *119*(2), 318–321. https://doi.org/10.1016/j.jep.2008.07.011.

Li, J., Bai, Y., Bai, Y., Zhu, R., Liu, W., Cao, J., et al. (2017). Pharmacokinetics of caffeic acid, ferulic acid, formononetin, cryptotanshinone, and tanshinone IIA after oral administration of naoxintong capsule in rat by HPLC-MS/MS. *Evidence-based Complementary and Alternative Medicine: eCAM*, *2017*, 9057238. https://doi.org/10.1155/2017/9057238.

Li, L., Bonneton, F., Chen, X. Y., & Laudet, V. (2015). Botanical compounds and their regulation of nuclear receptor action: The case of traditional Chinese medicine. *Molecular and Cellular Endocrinology*, *401*, 221–237. https://doi.org/10.1016/j.mce.2014.10.028.

Li, Y., Fan, Y., Su, H., Wang, Q., Li, G. F., Hu, Y., et al. (2019). Metabolic characteristics of tanshinone I in human liver microsomes and S9 subcellular fractions. *Xenobiotica*, *49*(2), 152–160. https://doi.org/10.1080/00498254.2018.1432087.

Li, Y., Guo, Y., Chen, Y., Wang, Y., You, Y., Yang, Q., et al. (2015). Establishment of an interleukin-1beta-induced inflammation-activated endothelial cell-smooth muscle cell-mononuclear cell co-culture model and evaluation of the anti-inflammatory effects of tanshinone IIA on atherosclerosis. *Molecular Medicine Reports*, *12*(2), 1665–1676. https://doi.org/10.3892/mmr.2015.3668.

Li, H., Kong, D., Dou, Z., & Zheng, K. (2019). Study on apoptosis of breast Cancer cell MCF-7 induced by total tanshinone through mitochondrial pathway. *Journal of Chinese Medicinal Materials*, *42*(1), 184–188.

Li, P., Wang, G. J., Li, J., Hao, H. P., & Zheng, C. N. (2006). Identification of tanshinone IIA metabolites in rat liver microsomes by liquid chromatography-tandem mass spectrometry. *Journal of Chromatography A*, *1104*(1–2), 366–369. https://doi.org/10.1016/j.chroma.2005.12.047.

Li, Y., Wang, J., Wang, Z., Feng, J., Liang, Q., & Zheng, Z. (2007). Effect of tanshinone II A on endothelial nitric oxide synthase gene expression and intracellular Ca2+ level induced by angiotensin II in cultured porcine arotic endothelial cells. *Chinese Journal of Critical Care Medicine*, *27*(8), 720–723.

Li, Y., & Zhou, Y. (2018). The therapeutic effect of tanshinone IIA on propionibacterium acnes-induced inflammation in vitro. *Dermatologic Therapy*, *31*(6). e12716. https://doi.org/10.1111/dth.12716.

Lin, H. H., Chung, Y., Cheng, C. T., Ouyang, C., Fu, Y., Kuo, C. Y., et al. (2018). Autophagic reliance promotes metabolic reprogramming in oncogenic KRAS-driven tumorigenesis. *Autophagy*, *14*(9), 1481–1498. https://doi.org/10.1080/15548627.2018.1450708.

Lin, W.-J., & Kuang, H.-Y. (2014). Oxidative stress induces autophagy in response to multiple noxious stimuli in retinal ganglion cells. *Autophagy*, *10*(10), 1692–1701.

Lin, T. Y., Lu, C. W., Huang, S. K., & Wang, S. J. (2013). Tanshinone IIA, a constituent of danshen, inhibits the release of glutamate in rat cerebrocortical nerve terminals. *Journal of Ethnopharmacology*, *147*(2), 488–496. https://doi.org/10.1016/j.jep.2013.03.045.

Lin, R., Wang, W. R., Liu, J. T., Yang, G. D., & Han, C. J. (2006). Protective effect of tanshinone IIA on human umbilical vein endothelial cell injured by hydrogen peroxide and its mechanism. *Journal of Ethnopharmacology*, *108*(2), 217–222. https://doi.org/10.1016/j.jep.2006.05.004.

Liu, F., Huang, Z. Z., Sun, Y. H., Li, T., Yang, D. H., Xu, G., et al. (2017). Four main active ingredients derived from a traditional chinese medicine guanxin shutong capsule cause cardioprotection during myocardial ischemia injury calcium overload suppression. *Phytotherapy Research*, *31*(3), 507–515. https://doi.org/10.1002/ptr.5787.

Liu, Y., Liu, J., Wu, X., & Chai, C. (2007). The study of the strain rate imaging to evaluate the local ischemia myocardial systolic and diastolic function. *Journal of Ultrasound in Clinical Medicine*, *2007*(07), 418–420.

Liu, J., Wu, J., Wang, X., & Cai, Z. (2007). Study of the phase I and phase II metabolism of a mixture containing multiple tanshinones using liquid chromatography/tandem mass spectrometry. *Rapid Communications in Mass Spectrometry*, *21*(18), 2992–2998. https://doi.org/10.1002/rcm.3182.

Liu, X., Ye, M., An, C., Pan, L., & Ji, L. (2013). The effect of cationic albumin-conjugated PEGylated tanshinone IIA nanoparticles on neuronal signal pathways and neuroprotection in cerebral ischemia. *Biomaterials*, *34*(28), 6893–6905. https://doi.org/10.1016/j.biomaterials.2013.05.021.

Lu, L., Li, C., Li, D., Wang, Y., Zhou, C., Shao, W., et al. (2013). Cryptotanshinone inhibits human glioma cell proliferation by suppressing STAT3 signaling. *Molecular and Cellular Biochemistry*, *381*(1–2), 273–282. https://doi.org/10.1007/s11010-013-1711-x.

Luo, H., Sheng, L., Zhang, S., Xu, L., & Wei, P. (1983). Bile excretion and intrahepatic transformation of tanshinone, an active component of anti-mycobacterium. *Acta Pharmaceutica Sinica*, *1*, 1–6.

Lusis, A. (2000). Atherosclerosis. *Nature*, *407*(6801), 233–241.

Mao, S., Wang, Y., Zhang, M., & Hinek, A. (2014). Phytoestrogen, tanshinone IIA diminishes collagen deposition and stimulates new elastogenesis in cultures of human cardiac fibroblasts. *Experimental Cell Research*, *323*(1), 189–197. https://doi.org/10.1016/j.yexcr.2014.02.001.

Nambiar, J., Vijayakumar, G., Drishya, G., Shaji, S. K., Pandurangan, N., Kumar, G. B., et al. (2019). (I-3,II-3)-biacacetin-mediated cell death involves mitochondria. *Molecular and Cellular Biochemistry*, *451*(1–2), 79–90. https://doi.org/10.1007/s11010-018-3395-8.

Pan, Y., & Kupper, T. S. (2018). Metabolic reprogramming and longevity of tissue-resident memory T cells. *Frontiers in Immunology*, *9*, 1347. https://doi.org/10.3389/fimmu.2018.01347.

Pang, H., Wu, L., Tang, Y., Zhou, G., Qu, C., & Duan, J. (2016). Chemical analysis of the herbal medicine *Salviae miltiorrhizae* radix et rhizoma (Danshen). *Molecules (Basel, Switzerland)*, *21*(1), 51.

Park, O. K., Choi, J. H., Park, J. H., Kim, I. H., Yan, B. C., Ahn, J. H., et al. (2012). Comparison of neuroprotective effects of five major lipophilic diterpenoids from Danshen extract against experimentally induced transient cerebral ischemic damage. *Fitoterapia*, *83*(8), 1666–1674. https://doi.org/10.1016/j.fitote.2012.09.020.

Park, J. H., Park, O., Cho, J. H., Chen, B. H., Kim, I. H., Ahn, J. H., et al. (2014). Anti-inflammatory effect of tanshinone I in neuroprotection against cerebral ischemia-reperfusion injury in the gerbil hippocampus. *Neurochemical Research*, *39*(7), 1300–1312. https://doi.org/10.1007/s11064-014-1312-4.

Ren, C., & Du, S. (2018). Tanshinone IIA protects hippocampal neuronal cells from radiation injury. *Guangdong Medical Journal*, *39*(6), 807–810.

Sashidhara, K. V., Rosaiah, J. N., Kumar, M., Gara, R. K., Nayak, L. V., Srivastava, K., et al. (2010). Neo-tanshinlactone inspired synthesis, in vitro evaluation of novel substituted benzocoumarin derivatives as potent anti-breast cancer agents. *Bioorganic & Medicinal Chemistry Letters*, *20*(23), 7127–7131. https://doi.org/10.1016/j.bmcl.2010.09.040.

Shu, M., Hu, X., Huang, Z., Huang, D., & Zhang, S. (2016). Effects of tanshinone IIA on fibrosis in a rat model of cirrhosis through heme oxygenase-1, inflammation, oxidative stress and apoptosis. *Molecular Medicine Reports*, *13*(4), 3036–3042.

Song, M., Hang, T. J., Zhang Zh, X., Du, R., & Chen, J. (2005). Determination of cryptotanshinone and its metabolite in rat plasma by liquid chromatography-tandem mass spectrometry. *Journal of Chromatography B, Analytical Technologies in the Biomedical and Life Sciences*, *827*(2), 205–209. https://doi.org/10.1016/j.jchromb.2005.09.014.

Sun, J., Yang, M., Han, J., Wang, B., Ma, X., Xu, M., et al. (2007). Profiling the metabolic difference of seven tanshinones using high-performance liquid chromatography/multi-stage mass spectrometry with data-dependent acquisition. *Rapid Communications in Mass Spectrometry*, *21*(14), 2211–2226. https://doi.org/10.1002/rcm.3080.

Tan, Y. L., Ou, H. X., Zhang, M., Gong, D., Zhao, Z. W., Chen, L. Y., et al. (2019). Tanshinone IIA promotes macrophage cholesterol efflux and attenuates atherosclerosis of apoE-/- mice by Omentin-1/ABCA1 pathway. *Current Pharmaceutical Biotechnology*, *20*, 422–432. https://doi.org/10.2174/1389201020666190404125213.

Tang, S., Shen, X. Y., Huang, H. Q., Xu, S. W., Yu, Y., Zhou, C. H., et al. (2011). Cryptotanshinone suppressed inflammatory cytokines secretion in RAW264.7 macrophages through inhibition of the NF-kappaB and MAPK signaling pathways. *Inflammation*, *34*(2), 111–118. https://doi.org/10.1007/s10753-010-9214-3.

Tang, F., Wu, X., Wang, T., Wang, P., Li, R., Zhang, H., et al. (2007). Tanshinone II A attenuates atherosclerotic calcification in rat model by inhibition of oxidative stress. *Vascular Pharmacology*, *46*(6), 427–438. https://doi.org/10.1016/j.vph.2007.01.001.

Tao, J., Wang, Z., Liu, Q., & Fang, G. (1996). Study of tanshinone on myocardial reperfusion injury. *Chinese Journal of Anesthesiology*, *5*, 202–204.

Wang, X., Bastow, K. F., Sun, C. M., Lin, Y. L., Yu, H. J., Don, M. J., et al. (2004). Antitumor agents. 239. Isolation, structure elucidation, total synthesis, and anti-breast cancer activity of neo-tanshinlactone from *Salvia miltiorrhiza*. *Journal of Medicinal Chemistry*, *47*(23), 5816–5819. https://doi.org/10.1021/jm040112r.

Wang, L., Cheng, L., Zhang, B., Wang, N., & Wang, F. (2019). Tanshinone prevents alveolar bone loss in ovariectomized osteoporosis rats by up-regulating phosphoglycerate dehydrogenase. *Toxicology and Applied Pharmacology*, *376*, 9–16. https://doi.org/10.1016/j.taap.2019.05.014.

Wang, M., Dai, H., Li, X., Li, Y., Wang, L., & Xue, M. (2010). Structural elucidation of metabolites of tanshinone I and its analogue dihydrotanshinone I in rats by HPLC-ESI-MSn. *Journal of Chromatography B, Analytical Technologies in the Biomedical and Life Sciences*, *878*(13–14), 915–924. https://doi.org/10.1016/j.jchromb.2010.02.014.

Wang, C., Du, X., Yang, R., Liu, J., Xu, D., Shi, J., et al. (2015). The prevention and treatment effects of tanshinone IIA on oestrogen/androgen-induced benign prostatic hyperplasia in rats. *The Journal of Steroid Biochemistry and Molecular Biology*, *145*, 28–37. https://doi.org/10.1016/j.jsbmb.2014.09.026.

Wang, B., Ge, Z., Cheng, Z., & Zhao, Z. (2017). Tanshinone IIA suppresses the progression of atherosclerosis by inhibiting the apoptosis of vascular smooth muscle cells and the proliferation and migration of macrophages induced by ox-LDL. *Biology Open*, *6*(4), 489–495. https://doi.org/10.1242/bio.024133.

Wang, Q., Jiang, C., Zheng, X., Zhu, X., Yan, S., Wang, H., et al. (2017). Insight into the pharmacokinetic behavior of tanshinone IIA in the treatment of Crohn's disease: Comparative data for tanshinone IIA and its two glucuronidated metabolites in normal and recurrent colitis models after oral administration. *Xenobiotica*, *47*(1), 66–76. https://doi.org/10.3109/00498254.2016.1160158.

Wang, J., Liu, J., & Du, M. (2019). Effects of tanshinone IIA on cardiac function and mitophagy of myocardial infraction rats. *Chinese Journal of Immunology*, *35*(4), 40–45.

Wang, Z., Sun, D., Guo, F., Huang, D., Zhang, W., Yang, E. D., et al. (2019). Study on extraction technology and activity of tanshinone from *Salvia miltiorrhiza*. *Journal of Anhui Agricultural University*, *46*(1), 90–97.

Wang, X., Wang, Y., Jiang, M., Zhu, Y., Hu, L., Fan, G., et al. (2011). Differential cardioprotective effects of salvianolic acid and tanshinone on acute myocardial infarction are mediated by unique signaling pathways. *Journal of Ethnopharmacology*, *135*(3), 662–671. https://doi.org/10.1016/j.jep.2011.03.070.

Wang, Y., Yan, J., Li, S., Cai, X., Wang, W., Luo, K., et al. (2014). Pharmacokinetics and tissue distribution study of tanshinone IIA after oral administration of Bushen Huoxue Qubi granules to rats with blood stasis syndrome. *Pharmacognosy Magazine*, *10*(39), 285–291. https://doi.org/10.4103/0973-1296.137369.

Wang, R., Zhang, H., Wang, Y., Yu, X., & Yuan, Y. (2016). Effects of salvianolic acid B and tanshinone IIA on the pharmacokinetics of losartan in rats by regulating the activities and expression of CYP3A4 and CYP2C9. *Journal of Ethnopharmacology*, *180*, 87–96. https://doi.org/10.1016/j.jep.2016.01.021.

Wei, B., Li, W. W., Ji, J., Hu, Q. H., & Ji, H. (2014). The cardioprotective effect of sodium tanshinone IIA sulfonate and the optimizing of therapeutic time window in myocardial ischemia/reperfusion injury in rats. *Atherosclerosis*, *235*(2), 318–327. https://doi.org/10.1016/j.atherosclerosis.2014.05.924.

Wei, Y., Li, P., Wang, C., Peng, Y., Shu, L., Jia, X., et al. (2012). Metabolism of tanshinone IIA, cryptotanshinone and tanshinone I from radix *Salvia miltiorrhiza* in zebrafish. *Molecules (Basel, Switzerland)*, *17*(7), 8617–8632. https://doi.org/10.3390/molecules17078617.

Weng, Y.-S., Kuo, W.-W., Lin, Y.-M., Kuo, C.-H., Tzang, B.-S., Tsai, F.-J., et al. (2013). Danshen mediates through estrogen receptors to activate Akt and inhibit apoptosis effect of Leu27IGF-II-induced IGF-II receptor signaling activation in cardiomyoblasts. *Food and Chemical Toxicology*, *56*, 28–39. https://doi.org/10.1016/j.fct.2013.01.008.

Xie, M., & Shen, Z. (1983). Absorption, distribution, excretion and metabolism of cryptotanshinone. *Acta Pharmaceutica Sinica*, *18*(2), 90–96.

Xu, Z., Chen, L., Xiao, Z., Zhu, Y., Jiang, H., Jin, Y., et al. (2018). Potentiation of the anticancer effect of doxorubicinin drug-resistant gastric cancer cells by tanshinone IIA. *Phytomedicine*, *51*, 58–67. https://doi.org/10.1016/j.phymed.2018.05.012.

Xu, J., Li, F., Zhang, B., Song, K., Wang, Z., Liu, D., et al. (2009). Estimation of chlorophyll-a concentration using field spectral data: A case study in inland case-II waters, North China. *Environmental Monitoring and Assessment*, *158*(1–4), 105–116. https://doi.org/10.1007/s10661-008-0568-z.

Xu, S., Liu, Z., Huang, Y., Chen, J., Chen, S., Shen, X., et al. (2014). Effectiveness of combination therapy of atorvastatin and non lipid-modifying tanshinone IIA from Danshen in a mouse model of atherosclerosis. *International Journal of Cardiology*, *174*(3), 878–880. https://doi.org/10.1016/j.ijcard.2014.04.226.

Xue, M., Cui, Y., Wang, H., Luo, Y., Zhang, B., & Zhou, Z. (1999). Pharmacokinetics of cryptotanshinone and its metabolite on pigs. *Acta Pharmaceutica Sinica*, *34*(2), 81–84.

Yang, J. X., Pan, Y. Y., Ge, J. H., Chen, B., Mao, W., Qiu, Y. G., et al. (2016). Tanshinone II A attenuates TNF-alpha-induced expression of VCAM-1 and ICAM-1 in endothelial progenitor cells by blocking activation of NF-kappaB. *Cellular Physiology and Biochemistry*, *40*(1–2), 195–206. https://doi.org/10.1159/000452537.

Yang, W., Zhang, J., Shi, L., Ji, S., Yang, X., Zhai, W., et al. (2019). Protective effects of tanshinone IIA on SH-SY5Y cells against oAβ1–42-induced apoptosis due to prevention of endoplasmic reticulum stress. *The International Journal of Biochemistry & Cell Biology*, *107*, 82–91. https://doi.org/10.1016/j.biocel.2018.12.011.

Ye, Y., Xu, W., & Zhong, W. (2010). Effects of cryptotanshinone on proliferation and apoptosis of Helacell line of cervical cancer. *China Journal of Chinese Materia Medica*, *35*(1), 118–121.

Yu, T., Zhou, Z., Mu, Y., de Lima Lopes, G., & Luo, K. Q. (2014). A novel anti-cancer agent, acetyltanshinone IIA, inhibits oestrogen receptor positive breast cancer cell growth by down-regulating the oestrogen receptor. *Cancer Letters*, *346*(1), 94–103. https://doi.org/10.1016/j.canlet.2013.12.023.

Zeng, J., Wang, M., Shen, S., Zhang, Z., Jiang, J., & Qiu, F. (2015). Pharmacokinetics of cryptotanshinone with single and multiple doses in rats. *Journal of Human University of Chinese medicine*, *35*(4), 1–5.

Zhang, X., Cao, Y., Wang, L., Yuan, X., & Fang, Z. (2017). Inhibitory effects of tanshinones towards the catalytic activity of UDP-glucuronosyltransferases (UGTs). *Pharmaceutical Biology*, *55*(1), 1703–1709. https://doi.org/10.3109/13880209.2015.1045621.

Zhang, X. S., Ha, S., Wang, X. L., Shi, Y. L., Duan, S. S., & Li, Z. A. (2015). Tanshinone IIA protects dopaminergic neurons against 6-hydroxydopamine-induced neurotoxicity through miR-153/NF-E2-related factor 2/antioxidant response element signaling pathway. *Neuroscience*, *303*, 489–502. https://doi.org/10.1016/j.neuroscience.2015.06.030.

Zhang, Z., He, H., Qiao, Y., Huang, J., Wu, Z., Xu, P., et al. (2018). Tanshinone IIA pretreatment protects H9c2 cells against anoxia/reoxygenation injury: Involvement of the translocation of Bcl-2 to mitochondria mediated by 14-3-3η. *Oxidative Medicine and Cellular Longevity*, *2018*, 3583921. https://doi.org/10.1155/2018/3583921.

Zhang, H. S., & Wang, S. Q. (2007). Nrf2 is involved in the effect of tanshinone IIA on intracellular redox status in human aortic smooth muscle cells. *Biochemical Pharmacology*, *73*(9), 1358–1366. https://doi.org/10.1016/j.bcp.2007.01.004.

Zhang, Y., Wei, L., Sun, D., Cao, F., Gao, H., Zhao, L., et al. (2010). Tanshinone IIA pretreatment protects myocardium against ischaemia/reperfusion injury through the phosphatidylinositol 3-kinase/Akt-dependent pathway in diabetic rats. *Diabetes, Obesity & Metabolism*, *12*(4), 316–322. https://doi.org/10.1111/j.1463-1326.2009.01166.x.

Zhang, T., Zhong, S., Wang, Y., Dong, S., Guan, T., Hou, L., et al. (2019). In vitro and in silico perspectives on estrogenicity of tanshinones from *Salvia miltiorrhiza*. *Food Chemistry*, *270*, 281–286. https://doi.org/10.1016/j.foodchem.2018.07.098.

Zhao, Y. P., Wang, F., Jiang, W., Liu, J., Liu, B. L., Qi, L. W., et al. (2019). A mitochondrion-targeting tanshinone IIA derivative attenuates myocardial hypoxia reoxygenation injury through a SDH-dependent antioxidant mechanism. *Journal of Drug Targeting*, *27*, 896–902. https://doi.org/10.1080/1061186X.2019.1566338.

Zheng, X., Wang, S., Zhao, X., Zhao, X., Liu, Q., & Zheng, J. (2007). Analysis on danshen-related metabolites induced by compound danshen dripping pills in human serum. *Negative*, *28*(5), 435–437.

Zhu, Z., Liu, Z., Zhou, L., Tian, C., Tao, L., Wei, Z., et al. (2014). Effect of cryptotanshinone on metastasis of human breast cancer cell line MDA-MB-231 and its molecular mechanism. *Chinese Journal of Experimental Traditional Medical Formulae*, *20*(11), 160–165.

Zhu, Y., Tang, Q., Wang, G., & Han, R. (2017). Tanshinone IIA protects hippocampal neuronal cells from reactive oxygen species through changes in autophagy and activation of phosphatidylinositol 3-kinase, protein kinas B, and mechanistic target of rapamycin pathways. *Current Neurovascular Research*, *14*(2), 132–140.

Zhu, J., Xu, Y., Ren, G., Hu, X., Wang, C., Yang, Z., et al. (2017). Tanshinone IIA sodium sulfonate regulates antioxidant system, inflammation, and endothelial dysfunction in atherosclerosis by downregulation of CLIC1. *European Journal of Pharmacology*, *815*, 427–436. https://doi.org/10.1016/j.ejphar.2017.09.047.

Zong, W. X., Rabinowitz, J. D., & White, E. (2016). Mitochondria and cancer. *Molecular Cell*, *61*(5), 667–676. https://doi.org/10.1016/j.molcel.2016.02.011.

Further reading

Liu, A. H., Guo, H., Ye, M., Lin, Y. H., Sun, J. H., Xu, M., et al. (2007). Detection, characterization and identification of phenolic acids in Danshen using high-performance liquid chromatography with diode array detection and electrospray ionization mass spectrometry. *Journal of Chromatography A*, *1161*(1–2), 170–182. https://doi.org/10.1016/j.chroma.2007.05.081.

Xijun, W. (2015). Methodology for systematic analysis of in vivo efficacy material base of traditional Chinese medicine—Chinmedomics. *China Journal Chinese Materia Médica*, *40*(1), 13–17.

CHAPTER THREE

Pharmacological action and potential targets of chlorogenic acid

Mingsan Miao*, Liling Xiang
Department of Medicine, Henan University of Chinese Medicine, Zhengzhou, China
*Corresponding author: e-mail address: miaomingsan@163.com

Contents

Abstract

Chlorogenic acid is a widely distributed natural compound with many important pharmacological effects, which are found in a variety of plants. It is also an important secondary metabolite in plants. As a natural plant extract from a wide range of sources, in vitro and in vivo studies have found that the main pharmacological effects of chlorogenic acid are antioxidant, antiinflammatory, antibacterial, antiviral, hypoglycemic, lipid lowering, anticardiovascular, antimutagenic, anticancer, immunomodulatory, etc. Therefore it may play an important role in promoting human health. For example, it can provide new ideas and new ways for the prevention and treatment of cardiovascular disease, cancer, diabetes, and other chronic diseases, but the specific mechanism of action is unclear. Due to the difficulty of extraction and purification, poor stability, poor solubility, low absolute bioavailability of oral administration, the possibility of

Advances in Pharmacology, Volume 87
ISSN 1054-3589
https://doi.org/10.1016/bs.apha.2019.12.002

allergies caused by injection, and so on, there are difficulties in its medicinal research and development. The further study of chlorogenic acid will provide an important theoretical basis for its rational use.

Abbreviation

CGA chlorogenic acid

1. Introduction

Chlorogenic acid has the molecular formula $C_{16}H_{18}O_9$ and molecular weight 354.30. The structure is shown in Fig. 1. When heated and exposed to light, its biological activity can be lost. It is widely found in higher dicotyledonous plants and ferns. Chlorogenic acid (CGA) is a kind of phenylalanine compound produced by the shikimic acid pathway during aerobic respiration. Because CGA has many important biological activities, it has been widely used in many fields, such as medicine, food, health care, and the chemical industry. It is the main active ingredient of many traditional Chinese herbal compound preparations for antibacterial and antiinflammatory purposes, for example, clearing away heat and detoxifying. The content of CGA in honeysuckle and *Eucommia ulmoides* Oliv. is high. It is reported that CGA is absorbed in the stomach of rats by prototype (Lafay et al., 2006). Most CGAs are hydrolyzed to caffeic acid and quinic acid in the intestine through the action of special esterase and then absorbed. After absorption, it is metabolized into glucuronic acid glycosides and sulfate metabolites. The oral absorption rate of CGA is low. It exists mainly in the form of metabolites in plasma and is excreted through the kidneys. In recent years, CGA as has been internationally regarded as plant gold. It has attracted increasing attention, and there are many reports

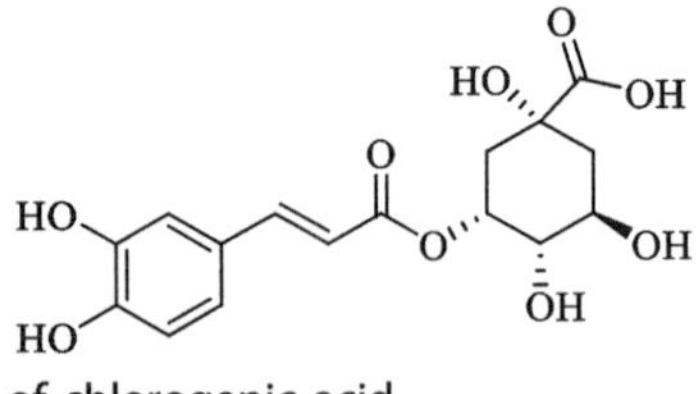

Fig. 1 Structure diagram of chlorogenic acid.

on various aspects of its research. CGA is an important bioactive substance. It has antioxidant, antiinflammatory, antibacterial, antiviral, hypoglycemic, lipid-lowering, anticardiovascular, antimutagenic, anticancer, immune regulation, and other biological functions. However, the specific mechanism of action is unclear.

2. Antioxidant effect of chlorogenic acid

CGA is a new and efficient natural phenolic antioxidant. Its natural antioxidant properties depend on its special molecular structure. It contains five active hydroxyl groups and one carboxyl group. The phenolic hydroxyl group structure reacts easily with free radicals and can form hydrogen radicals with an antioxidant effect to eliminate the activity of hydroxyl radicals and superoxide anions, therefore playing a strong antioxidant role. Antioxidant activity is one of the important activities of CGA, research shows (Hu, Yu, & Zhao, 2006) that CGA has a scavenging effect on three kinds of reactive oxygen species ($^{-}O_2$,·OH and H_2O_2). The scavenging effect and concentration is dose dependent. When the concentration is high, the scavenging effect on these three reactive oxygen species is obvious and stable. When the concentration is low, the scavenging effect on $^{-}O_2$· and ·OH deteriorates, even producing an oxidation-promoting effect.

Under normal conditions of the body, the generation and elimination of free radicals are in equilibrium. When the free radicals are out of balance, various functional obstacles and diseases can occur in the body. For example, when peroxidation is particularly serious, the lipid structure of the cell membrane will be destroyed, and damage to membrane enzymes may lead to cell dysfunction (Bagdas et al., 2015). A recent study has found that CGA has a very strong antioxidant effect and can accelerate wound repair in diabetic rats without affecting the levels of superoxide dismutase and catalase in wounds (Kim, Pan, Kim, Lee, & Park, 2018). A recent research has studied the protective effect of CGA on alcoholic liver injury. It was found that CGA alleviated liver injury by reducing the accumulation of oxidative products such as superoxide, hydrogen peroxide, and hydroxyl radicals, and inhibiting oxidative stress (Zhou et al., 2016). Some researchers studied that CGA ameliorated intestinal mitochondrial injury by increasing antioxidant effects and activity of respiratory complexes. CGA can improve the intestinal mitochondria induced by hydrogen peroxide, increasing the activity of respiratory chain complexes I, IV, and V, and also changing the ultrastructure of mitochondria and mitochondrial damage in rats with colitis induced by trinitrobenzene sulfonic acid. Therefore it is proved that CGA may be useful for prevention of intestinal diseases, which can lessen and treat mitochondria damage with trinitrobenzene sulfonic acid. It was also found (Luo et al., 2013) that CGA can reduce the apoptotic rate of nucleus pulposus cells induced by hydrogen peroxide, and its mechanism might be related to promoting the expression of Bcl-2 and inhibiting the expression of caspase-3.

CGA can inhibit the activity of xanthine oxidase, reduce the production of oxygen free radicals in the body, and reduce the level of lipid peroxidation in the body by upregulating the activity of antioxidant enzymes (Lou et al., 2016). The possible mechanisms for CGA to exert its antioxidant activity are as follows. It can (1) promote the metabolism of amino acids and glutathione, and improve the level of lipid metabolism; (2) upregulate the signal pathway of nuclear factor E2-related factor 2/antioxidant response element (Nrf2-ARE), inhibiting the degradation of Nrf2 protein mediated by ubiquitin, stabilizing the concentration of Nrf2 protein in cytoplasm, enhancing the transcriptional activity of Nrf2 protein under stress conditions, and protecting and promoting the expression of protective genes such as antioxidant proteins and phase II detoxifying enzymes (Boettler et al., 2011), thereby improving the antioxidant capacity in the body; (3) promote the phosphorylation of protein kinase B and the expression of fork protein transcription factor, antioncogene p53, and antiapoptotic protein B-cell lymphoma-2 by upregulating the signal pathway of phosphatidylinositol-3 kinase/protein kinase B (PI3K-Akt) to inhibit cell apoptosis (Lou et al., 2016); and (4) relate the antioxidant activity of CGA to the mitogen-activated protein kinase (MAPK) signaling pathway. Studies have shown (Ji et al., 2013) that CGA can inhibit phosphorylation of extracellular signal-regulated kinase, c-Jun amino-terminal kinase, and p38 MAPK in the MAPK pathway (Tosovic, Markovic, Dimitric Markovic, Mojovic, & Milenkovic, 2017). A study has found that CGA can produce an antioxidant effect by hydrogen atom transfer or free radical adduct in acidic and neutral media. When in a basic environment (such as physiological pH), sequential proton loss electron transfer has a very high rate, which may be the antioxidant mechanism of CGA.

3. Antiinflammatory effect of chlorogenic acid

Its antiinflammatory effect is another important biological property of CGA. Ohkawara, Takeda, and Nishihira (2017) studied CGA on inflammatory injury of pancreatic and lung tissues in mice with pancreatitis caused by L-arginine. CGA can reduce pancreatic-related tissues and inhibit the activity of the pancreatic enzyme. At the same time, it can significantly reduce the level of macrophage migration inhibitory factor in the pancreas and serum of mice, indicating that CGA has a strong antiinflammatory effect. Yun, Kang, and Lee (2012) studied the protective effect of CGA on liver ischemia/reperfusion injury. It was found that CGA could significantly improve liver function and pathological injury, and inhibit oxidative stress and tumor necrosis factor-α (TNF-α). The protective effect of CGA protects liver tissue by inhibiting inflammatory reaction and strengthening the antioxidant defense system. When Yu, Zhang, and Wang (2016) studied the effect of CGA on human periodontal ligament cells (hHDLCs), they found that CGA can significantly increase the activity of alkaline phosphatase, promote the proliferation of hHDLCs, promote the formation of mineralized nodules of hHDLCs, inhibit the expression of interleukin (IL)-6, and then inhibit the inflammatory response of human periodontal ligament cells. CGA has a strong antiinflammatory effect on arachidonic acid metabolism by inhibiting the activation of inflammatory factors such as HIF-1a, ICAM-1, VCAM-1, TNF-α, IL-6, and nuclear factor-kappa B (NK-κB) p65, thus protecting cerebral ischemia/reperfusion injury (Miao, Cao, Li, Fang, & Miao, 2017).

Inflammation is the defense response of the body to damaged local tissues. CGA can be involved in the signal pathway of tyrosine kinase/signal transducer and transcriptional activator 3, and inhibit the expression of IL-6 receptor β subunit, tyrosine kinase 1 phosphorylation signal transducer, and transcriptional activator 3 under oxidative stress. It can also reverse regulate the expression and secretion of inflammatory factors (Lou et al., 2016). The inflammatory response is a physiological response to tissue damage caused by exogenous or endogenous factors, and is an important manifestation of autoimmunity. The NK-κB pathway is closely related to the body's autoimmunity, and plays a key regulatory role in the secretion of proinflammatory cytokines, chemokines, and adhesion molecules. The Toll-like receptor (TLR) signaling pathway is an important CGA regulation pathway, and plays the role of an antiinflammatory. CGA inhibits TLR4 signaling pathway activation, downregulates myeloid differentiation factor 88 type, induces nitric oxide synthase (NOS) and an enzyme called cyclooxygenase 2, raises the BMP activin membrane-bound inhibitory factor, thereby inhibiting the TNF-αβ, IL-6 and IL-1 secretion, and relieve inflammation of the liver injury and fibrosis (Ruifeng et al., 2014).

Subsequent studies have found that CGA can also improve the body's inflammatory response by inhibiting TLR2, TLR3, and TLR9 signaling pathways (Lou et al., 2016). A recent research has demonstrated that induced inflammation of fibroblast-like synovial cells (RSC-364) through white cell medium, and found that CGA can inhibit the expression of key molecules in JAK/STAT and the NK-κB signaling pathway and inhibit the activation of these signaling pathways in inflammatory response, thus inhibiting the proliferation of synovial cells. It was found by flow cytometry and Western blot that CGA shows good therapeutic potential in the treatment of rheumatoid arthritis. After pretreatment of diabetic nephropathy model with CGA, the results showed that the expression of nuclear factor red blood cell-derived factor 2, nuclear translocation, and heme oxygenase-1 (HO-1) were significantly increased. The phosphorylation of I and B and NK-κB were significantly decreased. CGA played an antiinflammatory effect by regulating Nrf2/HO-1 and the NK-κB pathway (Bao et al., 2018).

4. Antibacterial and antiviral effects of chlorogenic acid

In terms of antibacterial activity, CGA has broad-spectrum antibacterial activity, and has certain inhibitory on *Escherichia coli*, *Staphylococcus aureus*, yeast, *Aspergillus niger*, and *Bacillus subtilis*, as well as good resistance activity against *Staphylococcus aureus* and *Escherichia coli*. CGA has a stronger effect on fungi than bacteria, accompanied by a certain dose effect (Zhu, Zhang, & Lo, 2004). It is clinically used for treating acute bacterial infection. Studies have found that CGA can destroy the biofilm of *Pseudomonas aeruginosa* and *Aspergillus fumigatus* and affect the normal growth of these strains to achieve a bacteriostatic effect (Yan, Xiao, Zhou, & Yang, 2017). The bacteriostatic effect of CGA is mainly affected by temperature and increases with the increases in temperature, but when the temperature exceeds 60 °C, the bacteriostatic effect obviously decreases (Karunanidhi, Thomas, van Belkum, & Neela, 2013). The early research has found that CGA has a significant inhibitory effect on the envelope synthesis of *Stenotrophomonas maltophilia* organisms. It is believed that CGA can be used as a safety antibacterial drug or a combination of antibacterial drugs to treat *Stenotrophomonas maltophilia* infection.

At present, the antibacterial mechanism of CGA is unclear. According to existing literature, the antibacterial mechanism of CGA may be related to the following aspects: (1) The bacteriostatic mechanism of CGA to *E. coli* may be caused by destroying the structure of the bacterial cell wall and membrane, which leads to an increase in cell permeability, thus causing cell electrolyte, enzymes, DNA, and RNA to leak out, thus affecting cell structure stability and gradually causing cell death (Zhou, Luo, Xiong, & Tang, 2014). (2) CGA contains a phenolic hydroxyl group, which is the most suitable reaction substrate for phenolic enzyme catalysis. It can affect the activity of related metabolic enzymes, reduce the level of substance and energy metabolism, and cause the metabolic process to be blocked, thus inhibiting the activity of bacteria (Feng et al., 2005). Studies have found that the antibacterial mechanism of CGA may be related to noncompetitive inhibition of arylamine acetyltransferase in bacteria. CGA can change the permeability of cell membranes by inhibiting a change in β-galactosidase to affect a content change in protein. It does so by reducing sugar and acetone in the metabolic process of bacteria and hindering the material and energy metabolism and protein synthesis of the strain. It can also inhibit the metabolism of sugar by bacteria, resulting in insufficient energy of bacteria and further affecting their growth and reproduction (Luo et al., 2016). (3) CGA has strong polarity and high affinity for macromolecular substances such as lipids. It can bind to the surface of bacteria and change their membrane structure, increasing the permeability of the bacterial membrane, causing partial leakage of DNA, RNA, electrolyte, enzymes, and nutrients in bacteria, and affecting protein synthesis (Francisco et al., 2013). (4) CGA may reduce the number of bacterial flagella by inhibiting their synthesis, thus reducing the colony effect of bacteria, which is another possible mechanism for CGA to play an antibacterial role (Ren et al., 2015).

Regarding antivirus, there are few related studies, and its mechanism of action is unclear. Studies have found that CGA has significant blocking and inhibiting effects on influenza A virus FM1 strain, herpes simplex virus, porcine parvovirus in vitro, and porcine reproductive and respiratory syndrome virus (Ojha et al., 2013). CGA has obvious inhibitory effects on respiratory syncytial virus, a synergistic effect when combined with licorice, and enhances an in vitro antirespiratory syncytial virus effect (Liao et al., 2017). CGA is the main antiviral active ingredient of honeysuckle flower. After purification, CGA has certain therapeutic effects on influenza virus, respiratory syncytial virus, viral myocarditis, herpes virus, and adenovirus. The mechanism of action of CGA possibly plays an effective antiviral role by appropriately downregulating interferon (IFN)-β and regulating the TLR3 signaling pathway through the key signaling molecules TLR3, TBK1, and IRF3 (Du, 2017). Some enzyme inhibition experiments proved that CGA and its derivatives can inhibit ceramidase activity and thus have antiviral activity (Gamaleldin Elsadig Karar, Matei, Jaiswal, Illenberger, & Kuhnert, 2016; Ma, Bolraa, Ji, He, & Ma, 2016).

5. Hypoglycemic and lipid-lowering effects of chlorogenic acid

CGA can maintain blood glucose concentration and prevent diabetes to a certain extent. Peng et al. used a high-fat diet to cause small intestinal glucose metabolism disorder and disrupted blood glucose balance in rats (Peng, Zhu, Zhong, Xu, & Wang, 2015). By adding CGA to a high-fat diet, the expression of glucagon proglucagon mRNA in different intestinal segments (duodenum, jejunum, ileum, and colon) was analyzed by real-time quantitative polymerase chain reaction. It was concluded that CGA could affect glucose metabolism by regulating the expression of glucagon transporter and glucagon in the intestine. Thus CGA controls blood glucose and insulin to maintain blood glucose balance. Ma et al. performed mouse experiments and found that CGA could prevent obesity and obesity-related metabolic syndrome in mice induced by diet. CGA increases the sensitivity of fatty liver and insulin and reduces chronic inflammation in obese mice (Ma, Gao, & Liu, 2015). These findings suggest that CGA has potential health benefits in managing obesity and obesity-related metabolic disorders.

The hypoglycemic mechanism of CGA may be related to the inhibition of the glucose-6-phosphate-shifting enzyme and glucose absorption. CGA has been identified as a novel specific inhibitor of glucose-6-phosphate-shifting enzyme in rat liver microsomes. Because glucose-6-phosphate-shifting enzyme plays an important role in the regulation of blood glucose balance in vivo, it is essential to produce endogenous glucose from glycogen isogenesis and glycogen decomposition. Intake of CGA will help to reduce hepatic glycogen excretion in type 2 diabetes mellitus. As a result, CGA has become a potential choice for the treatment of diabetes. It was also found that CGA could stimulate insulin secretion mediated by glucagon-like peptide 1 and affect blood glucose content. Studies have shown that CGA can activate AMP-activated protein kinase (AMPK), upregulate the gene expression of glucose transporter 4 (GLUT4) to stimulate the absorption of glucose in skeletal muscle, downregulate the gene expression of glucose-6-phosphate-shifting enzyme, inhibit gluconeogenesis, and reduce the synthesis of fatty acids. CGA promotes GLUT4 migration to cell membranes by activating

AMPK, thus promoting glucose uptake (Jung, Lee, Park, Jeon, & Choi, 2006; Ong, Hsu, & Tan, 2012). Beam and others believe that CGA can regulate the transport mechanism of glucose to skeletal muscle by influencing insulin content to a certain extent (Beam et al., 2015).

In terms of lipid lowering, Ma et al. showed that CGA can effectively prevent dietary obesity and related metabolic syndrome (Ma et al., 2015). Balzan et al. pointed out that an extract of Paraguay tea could significantly reduce the contents of triacylglycerol and cholesterol in rat plasma, and CGA played an important role in this process (Balzan et al., 2013). Previous study also pointed out that CGA can regulate cholesterol metabolism by inhibiting the activity of hydroxymethyl glutaric coenzyme A reductase (Hao et al., 2016). Liu and other studies proved that a long-term high-fat diet can produce a large accumulation of fat in liver cells, and CGA has a significant effect on reducing the accumulation of fat in liver caused by high-sugar and high-fat diets (Liu et al., 2015).

Rodriguez de Sotillo found that intravenous administration to rats of CGA at 5 mg/mL for 3 weeks reduced plasma cholesterol and triglyceride by 44% and 58%, respectively, and also significantly reduced liver triglyceride levels (Rodriguez de Sotillo & Hadley, 2002). Frank et al. also showed that the contents of vitamin E and cholesterol in the lung and liver of Sprague–Dawley rats decreased when CGA and caffeic acid were added to their food (Frank, Kamal-Eldin, Razdan, Lundh, & Vessby, 2003).

CGA has also been shown to reduce fatty acid synthesis and fat deposition by downregulating the gene expression of aconitase catalase, fatty acid synthetase, and nuclear transcription factor peroxisome proliferator-activated receptor-gamma 2 (Zheng, Qiu, Zhang, & Li, 2014). Pancreatic lipase is a kind of lipase synthesized and secreted by the pancreas, which is responsible for the decomposition of 50–70% dietary fat. It is reported that plant extracts such as CGA are natural inhibitors of pancreatic lipase and can be used in the intervention of obesity and diabetes (De la Garza, Milagro, Boque, Campion, & Martinez, 2011).

6. Anticardiovascular effects of chlorogenic acid

Oxygen free radicals are one of the important factors causing endothelial injury. Vascular endothelial cell injury is the basis of pathological conditions such as platelet aggregation, coagulation, apoptosis and proliferation of vascular smooth muscle cells, and disorder of vascular tension regulation. As a free radical scavenger and antioxidant, CGA has been widely recognized. By scavenging oxygen free radicals and antilipid peroxidation, it can increase the concentration of potassium ions in blood, reduce the levels of triacylglycerol and cholesterol in blood, protect vascular endothelial cells, and thus have an effective protective effect on the cardiovascular system. Isochlorogenic acid B has a strong inhibitory effect on the biosynthesis of thrombin and damage to endothelin cells induced by hydrogen peroxide, and it can promote the release of prostaglandin and antiplatelet agglutination in rats.

It has been found that CGA can reduce cerebral infarction and blood–brain barrier and brain edema by inhibiting lipid peroxidation and matrix metalloproteinase activity, and significantly inhibiting brain injury (Lee et al., 2012). Kim et al. showed that the apoptotic nucleus agglutination of neurons induced by hydrogen peroxide was strongly inhibited and the activity of antioxidant enzymes was increased after treatment with CGA (Kim et al., 2012). Inflammatory factors such as IL-1, IL-6, and TNF-α can lead to cardiomyocyte hypertrophy, abnormal myocardial contractility, and cardiomyocyte apoptosis. It has been found that CGA can protect myocardium by inhibiting the expression of inflammatory factors in myocardial cells. The MEK/ERK signaling pathway is the main pathway for many cytokines to regulate apoptosis and proliferation. During the process of cardiomyocyte injury, the MEK1/ERK1/2 signaling pathway can be abnormally activated by G-protein-coupled receptors, receptor encephaline kinase, cardiotrophin-1, and stress stimulation, which play an important regulatory role in the growth, proliferation, and apoptosis of cardiomyocytes. Restoration of perfusion of myocardial tissue after ischemia can induce and accelerate cell apoptosis. Geng et al. confirmed that CGA can inhibit the activation of the MEK/ERK signaling pathway and reduce myocardial ischemia/reperfusion injury in rats (Geng, Zhang, & Li, 2019). Anchor protein-B is expressed in many tissues and cells, and plays an important role in the correct localization of membrane proteins and intracellular proteins. Deficiency of anchor protein-B leads to arrhythmia, and its level is significantly decreased in myocardial tissue with failure. The decrease in expression is related to the increase in reactive oxygen species (Kashef et al., 2012). He conducted experiments in suckling mice to prove that CGA can regulate the expression of anchoring protein-B in myocardial cells after hypoxia-reoxygenation through the reactive oxygen species pathway, thus playing a protective role in myocardial cells (He, Shen, Liu, Cao, & Hong, 2014).

7. Antimutagenic and anticancer effects of chlorogenic acid

CGA has a strong ability to inhibit mutation. It can inhibit the mutation induced by aflatoxin B and nitrosation, and effectively reduce the mutation of bone marrow red blood cells caused by radiation. The study found that CGA has radiation protection. The results of comet assay show that CGA can significantly reduce DNA damage caused by X-rays in human lymphocytes, and the damage is reduced by 5.99–53.57% (Cinkilic et al., 2013). Li et al. irradiated human skin fibroblast ESF-1 with 40 J/cm^2 ultraviolet A and 70 mJ/cm^2 ultraviolet B, then treated it with different concentrations of CGA. After 24 h, it was found that CGA could significantly enhance the photoaging cell activity induced by ultraviolet A and damaged cell activity induced by ultraviolet B. In addition, CGA can increase the activity of superoxide dismutase and decrease the content of malondialdehyde and the activity of lactate dehydrogenase in cell culture medium (Li, Song, Chen, & Xu, 2013).

In terms of anticancer, CGA has significant inhibitory effects on colorectal cancer, liver cancer, laryngeal cancer, lung cancer, colon cancer, etc., and is considered to be an effective chemical protective agent for cancer. CGA can also reduce the utilization rate of carcinogens and transport in the liver to achieve anticancer effects. Because of invasion, infinite proliferation and metastasis of tumor hepatocytes are the most critical steps in the formation and diffusion of malignant tumor cells, and CGA has a certain inhibitory effect on tumor hepatocytes. CGA can inhibit the proliferation of human lung cancer A549 cells to some extent. The effect of CGA on the proliferation of lung cancer cells was detected by the tetrazolium method. The apoptotic rate was observed by flow cytometry. The results showed that CGA can inhibit the proliferation and metastasis of A549 cells and promote cell apoptosis (Tian et al., 2016). CT26 colon cancer cells in logarithmic growth phase were inoculated into mice, and CGA was used for intervention. From the tumor inhibition rate and pathological sections, it was found that CGA significantly inhibited CT26 colon cancer xenografts (Xiao et al., 2012). In addition, CGA inhibited the growth of HCT116 and HT29 colon cancer cells in vitro in a dose-dependent manner, induced cell cycle arrest in the S phase, and inhibited the activation of extracellular signal-related kinases in both cell types (Hou, Liu, Han, Yan, & Li, 2017).

Excessive growth of human acute promyelocytic cells can trigger leukemia. Liu et al. divided human acute promyelocytic cells into an experimental group and a control group, and treated the experimental group with 1.0, 5.0, and 10.0 μmol/L CGA, respectively. After 48 h, the growth of human acute promyelocytes was significantly inhibited in a dose-dependent manner; after 72 h, the growth inhibition rate and apoptosis rate of human acute promyelocytic cells were significantly increased in a dose-dependent manner compared with the control group. Its mechanism of action is to inhibit the growth of the G_0 and G_1 phases of the cell cycle, thereby inhibiting the growth of human acute promyelocytic cells and inducing apoptosis (Liu, Zhou, Qiu, Lu, & Wang, 2013). In the study of the effect of CGA on the retinoblastoma cell line HXO-RB44, we found that CGA may inhibit the proliferation of the retinoblastoma cell line by increasing the expression of HXO-RB44 oncogene and reducing the expression of cyclin to inhibit the proliferation of this cell line (Zhao, He, Yao, Liu, & Zheng, 2016).

CGA can produce anticancer effects by blocking the cell growth cycle, inducing apoptosis, and inhibiting the proliferation of cancer cells. The main molecular mechanisms may be related to the following aspects: (1) Induction of tumor cell apoptosis may be related to increased intracellular reactive oxygen species associated with decreased aminopeptidase N, epidermal growth factor receptor tyrosine kinase, and matrix metalloproteinase activity (Tian et al., 2016). (2) The intensity of signal factors in signal transduction pathway of cell growth and reproduction should be reduced, as should the viability of cancer cells. (3) The activity of quinone oxidoreductase-glutathione transferase and nicotinamide adenine dinucleotide phosphate should be increased, and the induction of the carcinogenic effect of oxidants resisted. (4) The activity of carcinogenic kinases such as MAPK to prevent cell carcinogenesis should be reduced. (5) The expression of tumor suppressor genes such as Nrf2 should be stimulated and the growth of cancer cells inhibited. CGA can also regulate the expression of cholesterol metabolism-related genes and proteins by inhibiting lipid accumulation in hepatocellular carcinoma cells, thus promoting the metabolic disorder of hepatocellular carcinoma cells and inhibiting their growth (Lai et al., 2017).

8. Immunomodulatory effects of chlorogenic acid

CGA has certain immunomodulatory ability, but there is little research on its immunomodulatory effect at home and abroad. The activation of immune cells is the first link of the inflammatory response. CGA plays an immunomodulatory role by inhibiting the production of antiinflammatory cytokines by macrophages. In vitro studies showed that CGA could significantly enhance the proliferation of T-cells induced by influenza virus antigen and induce the production of IFN-γ and IFN-α from human lymphocytes and human peripheral blood leukocytes (Jin et al., 2006). In addition, Dai Yi found that CGA can improve the metabolism and phagocytosis of peritoneal macrophages in mice, promote the release of NO, proinflammatory cytokines, IL-1β, and TNF-α, and inhibit the release of antiinflammatory cytokines IL-10 in a dose-dependent manner, playing an immunomodulatory role under normal and lipolipid-stimulated conditions (Dai, Xu, Shangguan, & Zhao, 2015). Studies have shown that for allergic rhinitis in mice, CGA can significantly reduce the spleen index of mice, increase the thymus index and the content of IFN-γ in mouse nasal lavage, and reduce the IL-4 of mouse nasal lavage fluid. CGA significantly reduced the levels of histamine, IgE, IL-4, IL-5, and IL-10 in the serum of allergic rhinitis mice, increased the content of IFN-γ, and increased the value of IFN-γ/IL-4. It also downregulated the expression of IL-4, IL-5, and IL-10 mRNA in nasal mucosa of allergic rhinitis mice, upregulated the expression of IFN-γ mRNA, and exerted immunomodulatory effects through various immune cytokines to slow down allergic rhinitis in mice (Li, Jiang, Liu, Di, & Hong, 2015).

In addition, CGA can induce autoimmunity to remove malignant tumor cells. Normally, the body can recognize tumor cells by autoimmune reaction and remove them by cellular immunity. However, malignant tumors can inhibit cellular immunity and escape the recognition of immune cells, thus multiplying in large numbers in the body. Studies by Yang and others have shown that CGA can induce the expression of NOS, TNF-α, and macrophage inflammatory protein-2, regulate the immune system to recognize cancer cells correctly, and eliminate them through its own cellular immune function to prevent further canceration of cells (Yang, Zhang, Wang, Li, & Lv, 2018). Kang et al. studied the effect of CGA on BALB/cEMT-6 female mice by expression microarray. It was found that CaN and NFAT genes related to the immune system regulatory pathway were activated, and the CaN/NFAT signaling pathway was widely used. This can increase the expression of Th1 cytokines (IFN-γ and IL-2), inhibit the expression of Th2 cytokines (IL-4 and IL-10), and activate T-cells, macrophages, natural killer cells and B-cells to regulate the immune function (Kang et al., 2015). Recent studies have shown that CGA can inhibit the growth of glioma cells by promoting STAT1 activation, increasing lipopolysaccharide/IFN-λ-mediated M1 macrophage-related markers such as inducible NOS, major histocompatibility complex II, and CD11c, and reducing the expression of IL-4-mediated M2 macrophage markers Arg and CD206 by inhibiting STAT6 (Yang, Yang, Kang, Kang, & Li, 2018). In addition, the proportion of CD11c-positive macrophages in G422 mice treated with CGA increased and M2-positive macrophages decreased, which was consistent with the weight loss of tumors in G422 mice (Xue et al., 2017).

9. Conclusion

CGA is a kind of natural compound that is widely distributed and has many pharmacological activities: it has antioxidant, antiinflammatory, antibacterial, antiviral, hypoglycemic, lipid lowering, anticardiovascular, antimutagenic, antitumor effects, and can regulate the immune system. It has high clinical application value too. Its biological activity and function have been given increased attention and its application is now becoming more and more extensive. At present, research into CGA is gradually improving, for example, the production efficiency of CGA is showing signs of progress. However, the biosynthesis and regulation, pharmacological activity and development, and utilization of CGA are not systematic and are far from perfect. Its pharmacological activity, action mechanism, structure–activity relationship, toxicology, and clinical research still need further study to fully tap into its potential medicinal value, and make it play a greater role in medicine and the chemical, cosmetics, and food industries.

Acknowledgments

This work was supported by the National "Major New Drug Creation" Science and Technology Major Project (2009ZX09103-324), Central Plains Scholars (162101510003).

Conflict of interest

The authors declare that there are no conflicts of interest.

References

Bagdas, D., Etoz, B. C., Gul, Z., Ziyanok, S., Inan, S., Turacozen, O., et al. (2015). In vivo systemic chlorogenic acid therapy under diabetic conditions: Wound healing effects and cytotoxicity/genotoxicity profile. *Food and Chemical Toxicology*, *81*, 54–61.

Balzan, S., Hernandes, A., Reichert, C. L., Donaduzzi, C., Pires, V. A., Gasparotto, A., Jr., et al. (2013). Lipid-lowering effects of standardized extracts of Ilex paraguariensis in high-fat-diet rats. *Fitoterapia*, *86*, 115–122.

Bao, L., Li, J., Zha, D., Zhang, L., Gao, P., Yao, T., et al. (2018). Chlorogenic acid prevents diabetic nephropathy by inhibiting oxidative stress and inflammation through modulation of the Nrf2/HO-1 and NF-kB pathways. *International Immunopharmacology, 54*, 245–253.

Beam, J. R., Gibson, A. L., Kerksick, C. M., Conn, C. A., White, A. C., & Mermier, C. M. (2015). Effect of post-exercise caffeine and green coffee bean extract consumption on blood glucose and insulin concentrations. *Nutrition, 31*(2), 292–297.

Boettler, U., Volz, N., Pahlke, G., Teller, N., Kotyczka, C., Somoza, V., et al. (2011). Coffees rich in chlorogenic acid or N-methylpyridinium induce chemopreventive phase II-enzymes via the Nrf2/ARE pathway in vitro and in vivo. *Molecular Nutrition & Food Research, 55*(5), 798–802.

Cinkilic, N., Cetintas, S. K., Zorlu, T., Vatan, O., Yilmaz, D., Cavas, T., et al. (2013). Radioprotection by two phenolic compounds: Chlorogenic and quinic acid, on X-ray induced DNA damage in human blood lymphocytes in vitro. *Food and Chemical Toxicology, 53*, 359–363.

Dai, Y., Xu, M. S., Shangguan, X. C., & Zhao, M. Y. (2015). Immunoregulation effect of chlorogenic acid on mouse peritoneal macrophages. *Natural Product Research and Development, 27*(12), 2128–2133.

De la Garza, A. L., Milagro, F. I., Boque, N., Campion, J., & Martinez, J. A. (2011). Natural inhibitors of pancreatic lipase as new players in obesity treatment. *Planta Medica, 77*(8), 773–785.

Du, J. (2017). Regulation effect of chlorogenic acid on TLR3 signal transduction pathway in RAW264.7 cells infected with RSV. *Journal of Qiqihar University of Medicine, 38*(6), 626–628.

Feng, R., Lu, Y., Bowman, L. L., Qian, Y., Castranova, V., & Ding, M. (2005). Inhibition of activator protein-1, NF-kappaB, and MAPKs and induction of phase 2 detoxifying enzyme activity by chlorogenic acid. *The Journal of Biological Chemistry, 280*(30), 27888–27895.

Francisco, V., Costa, G., Figueirinha, A., Marques, C., Pereira, P., Miguel Neves, B., et al. (2013). Anti-inflammatory activity of Cymbopogon citratus leaves infusion via proteasome and nuclear factor-kappaB pathway inhibition: Contribution of chlorogenic acid. *Journal of Ethnopharmacology, 148*(1), 126–134.

Frank, J., Kamal-Eldin, A., Razdan, A., Lundh, T., & Vessby, B. (2003). The dietary hydroxycinnamate caffeic acid and its conjugate chlorogenic acid increase vitamin e and cholesterol concentrations in Sprague-Dawley rats. *Journal of Agricultural and Food Chemistry, 51*(9), 2526–2531.

Gamaleldin Elsadig Karar, M., Matei, M. F., Jaiswal, R., Illenberger, S., & Kuhnert, N. (2016). Neuraminidase inhibition of dietary chlorogenic acids and derivatives—Potential antivirals from dietary sources. *Food & Function, 7*(4), 2052–2059.

Geng, J., Zhang, Z., & Li, W. (2019). Protective effect of chlorogenic acid preconditioning on myocardial ischemia-reperfusion injury in rats. *Chinese Journal of Modern Applied Pharmacy, 36*(06), 682–685.

Hao, S., Xiao, Y., Lin, Y., Mo, Z., Chen, Y., Peng, X., et al. (2016). Chlorogenic acid-enriched extract from Eucommia ulmoides leaves inhibits hepatic lipid accumulation through regulation of cholesterol metabolism in HepG2 cells. *Pharmaceutical Biology, 54*(2), 251–259.

He, W. F., Shen, Y., Liu, X., Cao, Q., & Hong, K. (2014). Effect and mechanism of chlorogenic acid on ankyrin-B of cardiomyocytes under hypoxia reoxygenation. *Journal of Clinical Cardiology, 30*(8), 725–726.

Hou, N., Liu, N., Han, J., Yan, Y., & Li, J. (2017). Chlorogenic acid induces reactive oxygen species generation and inhibits the viability of human colon cancer cells. *Anti-Cancer Drugs, 28*(1), 59–65.

Hu, Z. F., Yu, W. L., & Zhao, Y. P. (2006). Study on the scavenging of ROS and anti-lipid peroxidation by chlorogenic acid. *Food Science*, *2*, 128–130.

Ji, L., Jiang, P., Lu, B., Sheng, Y., Wang, X., & Wang, Z. (2013). Chlorogenic acid, a dietary polyphenol, protects acetaminophen-induced liver injury and its mechanism. *The Journal of Nutritional Biochemistry*, *24*(11), 1911–1919.

Jin, X. H., Ohgami, K., Shiratori, K., Suzuki, Y., Koyama, Y., Yoshida, K., et al. (2006). Effects of blue honeysuckle (*Lonicera caerulea* L.) extract on lipopolysaccharide-induced inflammation in vitro and in vivo. *Experimental Eye Research*, *82*(5), 860–867.

Jung, U. J., Lee, M. K., Park, Y. B., Jeon, S. M., & Choi, M. S. (2006). Antihyperglycemic and antioxidant properties of caffeic acid in db/db mice. *The Journal of Pharmacology and Experimental Therapeutics*, *318*(2), 476–483.

Kang, T. Y., Yang, H. R., Zhang, J., Li, D., Lin, J., Wang, L., et al. (2015). Corrigendum to "the studies of chlorogenic acid antitumor mechanism by gene chip detection: The immune pathway gene expression" *Journal of Analytical Methods in Chemistry*, *2015*, 538–539.

Karunanidhi, A., Thomas, R., van Belkum, A., & Neela, V. (2013). In vitro antibacterial and antibiofilm activities of chlorogenic acid against clinical isolates of *Stenotrophomonas maltophilia* including the trimethoprim/sulfamethoxazole resistant strain. *BioMed Research International*, *2013*, 3920–3958.

Kashef, F., Li, J., Wright, P., Snyder, J., Suliman, F., Kilic, A., et al. (2012). Ankyrin-B protein in heart failure: Identification of a new component of metazoan cardioprotection. *The Journal of Biological Chemistry*, *287*(36), 30268–30281.

Kim, J., Lee, S., Shim, J., Kim, H. W., Kim, J., Jang, Y. J., et al. (2012). Caffeinated coffee, decaffeinated coffee, and the phenolic phytochemical chlorogenic acid up-regulate NQO1 expression and prevent H(2)O(2)-induced apoptosis in primary cortical neurons. *Neurochemistry International*, *60*(5), 466–474.

Kim, H., Pan, J. H., Kim, S. H., Lee, J. H., & Park, J. W. (2018). Chlorogenic acid ameliorates alcohol-induced liver injuries through scavenging reactive oxygen species. *Biochimie*, *150*, 131–138.

Lafay, S., Gil-Izquierdo, A., Manach, C., Morand, C., Besson, C., & Scalbert, A. (2006). Chlorogenic acid is absorbed in its intact form in the stomach of rats. *The Journal of Nutrition*, *136*(5), 1192–1197.

Lai, L. L., Xiao, Y., Peng, X. F., Leng, E. N., Mo, Z. T., Li, W. N., et al. (2017). Influence of chlorogenic acid extracted from Folium eucommiae and crocin on cholesterol metabolism of hepatoma carcinoma cells. *Shandong Medical Journal*, *57*(8), 17.

Lee, K., Lee, J. S., Jang, H. J., Kim, S. M., Chang, M. S., Park, S. H., et al. (2012). Chlorogenic acid ameliorates brain damage and edema by inhibiting matrix metalloproteinase-2 and 9 in a rat model of focal cerebral ischemia. *European Journal of Pharmacology*, *689*(1–3), 89–95.

Li, H. X., Jiang, H. B., Liu, S. N., Di, L. J., & Hong, T. (2015). Effect and mechanism of chlorogenic acid in allergic rhinitis mice. *Chinese Journal of Biochemical Drugs*, *35*(6), 1–5.

Li, J. M., Song, L. Y., Chen, Q. Y., & Xu, Y. M. (2013). Protective effects of ultraviolet radiation induced photoaging in ESF-1 cell by chlorogenic acid. *Information on Traditional Chinese Medicine*, *30*(4), 25–27.

Liao, W. B., Shen, B. D., Shen, C. Y., Zheng, J., Xu, P. H., Sun, J., et al. (2017). Combined antiviral effect of chlorogenic acid and glycyrrhizin against respiratory syncytial virus infection in vitro. *Pharmaceutical Journal of Chinese People's Liberation Army*, *33*(1), 12–16.

Liu, Y. L., Song, Z., Peng, B. J., Xu, S. H., Zhu, Q., & Wang, Z. (2015). Effects of chlorogenic acid on apoptosis-related gene expressions in rats with non-alcoholic fatty liver disease caused by high-fat diet. *Chinese Journal of Animal Nutrition*, *27*(7), 2140–2149.

Liu, Y. J., Zhou, C. Y., Qiu, C. H., Lu, X. M., & Wang, Y. T. (2013). Chlorogenic acid induced apoptosis and inhibition of proliferation in human acute promyelocytic leukemia HL60 cells. *Molecular Medicine Reports*, *8*(4), 1106–1110.

Lou, L., Zhou, J., Liu, Y., Wei, Y. I., Zhao, J., Deng, J., et al. (2016). Chlorogenic acid induces apoptosis to inhibit inflammatory proliferation of IL-6-induced fibroblast-like synoviocytes through modulating the activation of JAK/STAT and NF-kappaB signaling pathways. *Experimental and Therapeutic Medicine*, *11*(5), 2054–2060.

Luo, Y. C., Huang, L. M., Yang, Y., Zhu, M., Wen, Y. L., Liu, Y., et al. (2016). Study on the mechanism of chlorogenic acid inhibiting *Staphylococcus aureus*. *Journal of Southwest University (Natural Science Edition)*, *38*(3), 15–19.

Luo, Y. Y., Yin, M., Wu, Y. H., He, D. W., Wei, Q. Q., & Yin, C. C. (2013). Protective effects of chlorogenic acid against hydrogen peroxide induced rat nucleus pulposus cells. *Apoptosis*, *35*(4), 656–660.

Ma, J. N., Bolraa, S., Ji, M., He, Q. Q., & Ma, C. M. (2016). Quantification and antioxidant and anti-HCV activities of the constituents from the inflorescences of *Scabiosa comosa* and *S. tschilliensis*. *Natural Product Research*, *30*(5), 590–594.

Ma, Y., Gao, M., & Liu, D. (2015). Chlorogenic acid improves high fat diet-induced hepatic steatosis and insulin resistance in mice. *Pharmaceutical Research*, *32*(4), 1200–1209.

Miao, M., Cao, L., Li, R., Fang, X., & Miao, Y. (2017). Protective effect of chlorogenic acid on the focal cerebral ischemia reperfusion rat models. *Saudi Pharmaceutical Journal*, *25*(4), 556–563.

Ohkawara, T., Takeda, H., & Nishihira, J. (2017). Protective effect of chlorogenic acid on the inflammatory damage of pancreas and lung in mice with l-arginine-induced pancreatitis. *Life Sciences*, *190*, 91–96.

Ojha, D., Mukherjee, H., Ghosh, S., Bag, P., Mondal, S., Chandra, N. S., et al. (2013). Evaluation of anti-infective potential of a tribal folklore Odina wodier Roxb against some selected microbes and herpes simplex virus associated with skin infection. *Journal of Applied Microbiology*, *115*(6), 1317–1328.

Ong, K. W., Hsu, A., & Tan, B. K. (2012). Chlorogenic acid stimulates glucose transport in skeletal muscle via AMPK activation: A contributor to the beneficial effects of coffee on diabetes. *PLoS One*, 7(3), e32718.

Peng, B. J., Zhu, Q., Zhong, Y. L., Xu, S. H., & Wang, Z. (2015). Chlorogenic acid maintains glucose homeostasis through modulating the expression of SGLT-1, GLUT-2, and PLG in different intestinal segments of Sprague-Dawley rats fed a high-fat diet. *Biomedical and Environmental Sciences*, *28*(12), 894–903.

Ren, S., Wu, M., Guo, J., Zhang, W., Liu, X., Sun, L., et al. (2015). Sterilization of polydimethylsiloxane surface with Chinese herb extract: A new antibiotic mechanism of chlorogenic acid. *Scientific Reports*, *5*, 10464.

Rodriguez de Sotillo, D. V., & Hadley, M. (2002). Chlorogenic acid modifies plasma and liver concentrations of: Cholesterol, triacylglycerol, and minerals in (fa/fa) Zucker rats. *The Journal of Nutritional Biochemistry*, *13*(12), 717–726.

Ruifeng, G., Yunhe, F., Zhengkai, W., Ershun, Z., Yimeng, L., Minjun, Y., et al. (2014). Chlorogenic acid attenuates lipopolysaccharide-induced mice mastitis by suppressing TLR4-mediated NF-kappaB signaling pathway. *European Journal of Pharmacology*, *729*, 54–58.

Tian, W., Dou, Y. W., Wang, H. T., Zhu, J. F., Dai, Y. L., & Xiang, H. (2016). Effect of chlorogenic acid on lung cancer A549 cell apoptosis and mechanism. *Journal of Preventive Medicine of Chinese People's Liberation Army*, *34*(6), 854.

Tosovic, J., Markovic, S., Dimitric Markovic, J. M., Mojovic, M., & Milenkovic, D. (2017). Antioxidative mechanisms in chlorogenic acid. *Food Chemistry*, *237*, 390–398.

Xiao, H. R., Liu, Y., Sun, Q. Y., He, M. J., Yang, Y., & Bao, X. (2012). Study on the inhibitory effects of chlorogenic acid on CT26 colon cancer. *West China Journal of Pharmaceutical Sciences*, *27*(3), 269–271.

Xue, N., Zhou, Q., Ji, M., Jin, J., Lai, F., Chen, J., et al. (2017). Chlorogenic acid inhibits glioblastoma growth through repolarizating macrophage from M2 to M1 phenotype. *Scientific Reports*, 7, 39011.

Yan, Y. W., Xiao, L., Zhou, X., & Yang, H. Q. (2017). Pharmacological effect of chlorogenic acid and countermeasures for medicinal research and development. *China Pharmacy*, *28*(19), 2729–2732.

Yang, J. Y., Yang, S. B., Kang, Z., Kang, X., & Li, W. B. (2018). The prospect of chlorogenic acid in the treatment of glioma. *Chinese Journal of Clinical Oncology*, *45*(5), 256–259.

Yang, X. L., Zhang, J. L., Wang, J. F., Li, X. Q., & Lv, J. T. (2018). Research progress in anti-tumor and mechanism of chlorogenic acid. *Chinese Journal of Experimental Traditional Medical Formulae*, *24*(19), 229–234.

Yu, G. X., Zhang, F., & Wang, L. (2016). The effect of chlorogenic acid on the bioactivity of lipopolysaccharide treated human periodontal ligament cells. *Chinese Journal of Conservative Dentistry*, *26*(6), 343–347.

Yun, N., Kang, J. W., & Lee, S. M. (2012). Protective effects of chlorogenic acid against ischemia/reperfusion injury in rat liver: Molecular evidence of its antioxidant and anti-inflammatory properties. *The Journal of Nutritional Biochemistry*, *23*(10), 1249–1255.

Zhao, J. B., He, X. W., Yao, S. Y., Liu, J. S., & Zheng, D. Y. (2016). Inhibitory effect of chlorogenic acid on the growth of retinoblastoma cell line HXO-Rb44. *Journal of Xi'an Jiaotong University (Medical Sciences)*, *37*(5), 734.

Zheng, G., Qiu, Y., Zhang, Q. F., & Li, D. (2014). Chlorogenic acid and caffeine in combination inhibit fat accumulation by regulating hepatic lipid metabolism-related enzymes in mice. *The British Journal of Nutrition*, *112*(6), 1034–1040.

Zhou, Z. E., Luo, Q. S., Xiong, J. H., & Tang, K. J. (2014). Antimicrobial mechanisms of 3-O-caffeoyl quinic acid and 3,5-di-O-caffeoyl quinic acid against *Escherichia coli*. *Food Science and Technology*, *39*(3), 228–232.

Zhou, Y., Zhou, L. L., Ruan, Z., Mi, S. M., Jiang, M., Li, X. L., et al. (2016). Chlorogenic acid ameliorates intestinal mitochondrial injury by increasing antioxidant effects and activity of respiratory complexes. *Bioscience, Biotechnology, and Biochemistry*, *80*(5), 962–971.

Zhu, X., Zhang, H., & Lo, R. (2004). Phenolic compounds from the leaf extract of artichoke (*Cynara scolymus* L.) and their antimicrobial activities. *Journal of Agricultural and Food Chemistry*, *52*(24), 7272–7278.

Further reading

Kang, T. Y., Yang, H. R., Zhang, J., Li, D., Lin, J., Wang, L., et al. (2013). The studies of chlorogenic acid antitumor mechanism by gene chip detection: The immune pathway gene expression. *Journal of Analytical Methods in Chemistry*, *2013*, 617243.

CHAPTER FOUR

Astragaloside IV derived from *Astragalus membranaceus*: A research review on the pharmacological effects

Jianqin Zhang[a], Chuxuan Wu[a], Li Gao[a], Guanhua Du[b], Xuemei Qin[a,*]
[a]Modern Research Center for Traditional Chinese Medicine, Shanxi University, Taiyuan, China
[b]Institute of Materia Medica, Chinese Academy of Medical Science and Peking Union Medical College, Beijing, P. R. China
*Corresponding author: e-mail address: qinxm@sxu.edu.cn

Contents

Abstract

Decoctions prepared from the roots of *Astragali Radix* are known as "Huangqi" and are widely used in traditional Chinese medicine for treatment of viral and bacterial infections, inflammation, as well as cancer. Astragaloside IV (AS-IV), one of the major compounds from the aqueous extract of *Astragalus membranaceus*, is a cycloartane-type triterpene glycoside chemical. To date, many studies in cellular and animal models have demonstrated that AS-IV possesses potent protective effects in cardiovascular, lung, kidney and brain. Based on studies over the past several decades, this review systematically summarizes the pharmacological effects, pharmacokinetics and the toxicity of AS-IV. We analyze in detail the pharmacological effects of AS-IV on neuroprotection, liver

Advances in Pharmacology, Volume 87
ISSN 1054-3589
https://doi.org/10.1016/bs.apha.2019.08.002

protection, anti-cancer and anti-diabetes, attributable to its antioxidant, anti-inflammatory, anti-apoptotic properties, and the roles in enhancement of immunity, attenuation of the migration and invasion of cancer cells and improvement of chemosensitivity of chemotherapy drugs. In addition, the latest developments in the combination of AS-IV and other active ingredients of traditional Chinese medicine or chemical drugs are detailed. These pharmacological effects are associated with multiple signaling pathways, including the Raf-MEK-ERK pathway, EGFR-Nrf2 signaling pathway, Akt/PDE3B signaling pathway, AMPK signaling pathway, NF-κB signaling pathway, Nrf2 antioxidant signaling pathways, PI3K/Akt/mTOR signaling pathway, PKC-α-ERK1/2-NF-κB pathway, IL-11/STAT3 signaling pathway, Akt/GSK-3β/β-catenin pathway, JNK/c-Jun/AP-1 signaling pathway, PI3K/Akt/NF-κB pathway, miRNA-34a/LDHA pathway, Nox4/Smad2 pathway, JNK pathway and NF-kB/PPARγ pathway. This review will provide an overall understanding of the pharmacological functions of astragaloside IV on neuroprotection, liver protection, anti-cancer and anti-diabetes. In light of this, AS-IV will be a potent alternative therapeutic agent for treatment of the above mentioned diseases.

Abbreviations

AAA	abdominal aortic aneurysm
Akt	serine/threonine-specific protein kinase
AMPKα	AMP-activated protein kinase α
AR	retina aldose reductase
AS-IV	astragaloside IV
ATF4	activating transcription factor-4
Bax	B-cell lymphoma 2-associated X protein
BCL2	B-cell lymphoma 2
B7-H3	a member of the B7 family of immunoregulatory proteins
CAG	cycloastragenol
CHOP	C/EBP homologous protein
CRC	colorectal cancer
CREB1	CAMP responsive element binding protein 1
CNS	central nervous system
DRG	dorsal root ganglia
Drp-1	dynamin-related protein 1
EGFR	epidermal growth factor receptor
eIF2α	eukaryotic translation initiation factor-α
EMT	the epithelial-mesenchymal transition
eNOS	endothelial nitric oxide synthase
ERG	electroretinogram
ERK1/2	extracellular signal-regulated protein kinases 1 and 2
Fis-1	mitochondrial fission protein 1
GA	glycated albumin
GLUT4	glucose transporter
G6Pase	glucose-6-phosphatase
GRP78	glucose-regulated protein 78
HBeAg	hepatitis B e antigen

HBsAg	hepatitis B surface antigen
HCC	hepatocellular carcinoma
HFD	high-fat diet
HK-2	proximal renal tubular epithelial cells
ICAM-1	intercellular adhesion molecule-1
IDO	indoleamine 2,3-dioxygenase
IKK	inhibitory κB kinase
IL-1β	interleukin-1β
ILK	integrin-linked kinase
IR	insulin resistance
iNOS	inducible nitric oxide synthase
JNK	c-Jun N-terminal kinases
MCP-1	monocyte chemoattractant protein-1
MEK1/2	mitogen-activated protein kinase
MFF	mitochondrial fission factor
mTOR	mammalian target of rapamycin
MNNG	*N*-methyl-N′-nitro-*N*-nitrosoguanidine
NAFLD	non-alcoholic fatty liver disease
NAG	*N*-acetyl-β-D-glucosaminidase
NFAT2	nuclear factor of activated T cells
NF-κB	nuclear factor kappa-light-chain-enhancer of activated B cells
NGAL	neutrophil gelatinase-associated lipocalin
NO	nitric oxide
NOTCH3	eurogenic locus notch homolog protein 3
Nox4	NADPH oxidase 4
Nrf2	NF-E2-related factor 2
OGD/R	oxygen and glucose deprivation/re-oxygenation
ORP150	150 kDa oxygen-regulated protein
Ox-LDL	low density lipoproteins
PDE3B	the predominant isoform of phosphodiesterase
PERK	protein kinase RNA (PKR)-like ER kinase
PI3K	phosphoinositide 3-kinases
PINK1	PTEN-induced putative kinase 1/Parkin
PKC-α	protein kinase C alpha type
PLGC	precancerous lesions of gastric carcinoma
P2X3	anti-P2X purinoceptor 3
RCECs	capillary endothelial cells
RGCs	retinal ganglion cell
RSK2	ribosomal S6 kinase 2
SERCA2b	sarcoendoplasmic reticulum Ca^{2+} ATPase 2b
SOD	superoxide dismutase
TGF-β1	transforming growth factor-beta 1
TLR4	toll-like receptor 4
TM	tunicamycin
TNF-α	tumor-necrosis factor-α
TRAF5	tumor-necrosis factor (TNF) receptor (TNFR)-associated factor 5
TRPA1	transient receptor potential ankyrin 1

TRPC6 transient receptor potential channel 6
TRPV1 transient receptor potential cation channel subfamily V member 1
VSMC vascular smooth muscle cell

1. Introduction

Astragalus was formally described in 1753 by Carl Linnaeus in his Species Plantarum. *Astragalus membranaceus* was initially recorded in one of the most famous ancient Chinese medical book, *Shen Nong Ben Cao Jing*, in 200 AD with a wide range of therapeutical effects and no toxicity (Sun & Sun, 2010). In the Chinese Pharmacopeia (ISBN 978-7-5067-8929-5) 2015 edition, Astragali Radix, also known as Huangqi, is defined as the dried roots of *A. membranaceus* (Fisch.) Bge. var. *mongholicus* (Bge.) Hsiao or *A. membranaceus* (Fisch.) Bge. *Astragali Radix* is considered to be a high-grade traditional Chinese medicine, which nourishes *Qi* and blood, and has multiple protective effects on immune system, cardiovascular system, nervous system, liver and kidney (Auyeung, Han, & Ko, 2016; Liu, Bao, & Liu, 2014).

As reported , three main chemical compounds are contained in *Astragali Radix* (Huangqi), including polysaccharides (heteropolysaccharide and dextran), saponins and flavonoids. With the development of extraction and separation technologies, more than 40 constituents of astragalus saponins have been identified from the dried astragalus roots by using HPLC and GC-MS (Liu et al., 2014).

Astragaloside IV (AS-IV, also known as astragalus saponin IV, Fig. 1) is one of the main active ingredients of *A. membranaceus* and is used as a quality control marker of Huangqi in the Chinese Pharmacopeia (2015 version). AS-IV is 3-*O*-beta-D-xylopyranosyl-6-*O*-beta-D-glucopyranosyl-cycloastragenol and its molecular formula is $C_{14}H_{68}O_{14}$. AS-IV has various pharmacological activities, including protective effects on cerebral injury and CNS, cardiovascular disease, respiratory system, kidney, endocrine system, organic immune system, liver and cancer due to its wide range of pharmacological actions, such as antioxidant, cardioprotective effects, anti-inflammatory, antiviral, antibacterial, antifibrosis, anti-diabetes and immunoregulation effects (Li, Hou, Xu, Liu, & Tu, 2017; Ren, Zhang, Mu, Sun, & Liu, 2013).

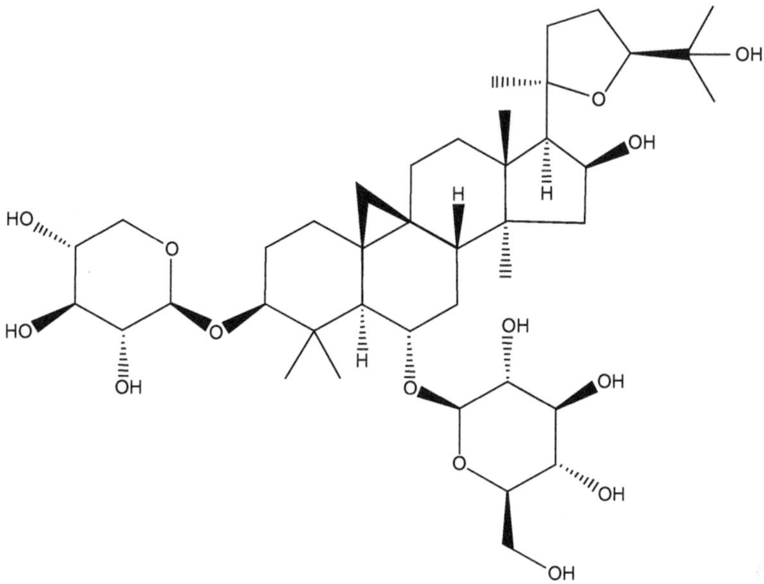

Fig. 1 Chemical structure of astragaloside IV.

In this study, we summarize the pharmacological effects of AS-IV on neuroprotection, liver protection, anti-cancer and anti-diabetes and the latest research on other diseases.

2. The protective effect of AS-IV on nervous system

At present, millions of people around the world are affected by neurological disorders such as stroke, dementia, epilepsy, Alzheimer's disease (AD), and Parkinson's disease (PD). Huge treatment costs have put enormous economic pressure on society for amelioration of these afflictions. Environmental, genetic factors and functional and sensory loss occurs due to neuronal cell damage can contribute to the neurological diseases (Costa et al., 2018). Oxidative stress, defined as the increased generation of reactive oxygen species and its oxidative products of biomacromolecules (Li et al., 2016), is an important component of neurodegenerative diseases (An, Wei, Qian, Li, & Wang, 2018; Zhang et al., 2012).

The pharmacological mechanism of AS-IV in Alzheimer's disease (AD), Parkinson's disease (PD), cerebral ischemia and autoimmune encephalomyelitis has been thoroughly and systematically summarized by Costa et al. in 2018 (Costa et al., 2018). Based on 16 articles published between 2007 and

2017, the authors concluded that AS-IV can attenuate behavioral and neurochemical deficits due to its antioxidant, anti-apoptotic and anti-inflammatory properties, which point to new strategies in drug development (Costa et al., 2018). In addition, other experiments revealed the function of neuroprotective effect by using different cell models, damage models in murine cortical neurons and mouse models of sciatic nerve injury.

The spontaneous discharge of cultured primary hippocampal neurons is regarded as a good model for physiological and pathological neuronal networks in vitro. Zhu et al. (2008) investigated the changes in the spontaneous neuronal excitability induced by AS-IV with the cultured hippocampal network. A dose of 40 mg/L AS-IV (dissolved in DMSO) could inhibit the frequencies of synchronized spontaneous Ca^{2+} oscillations to 59.39% ± 3.25% (mean ± SEM). The application of 40 mg/L AS-IV could significantly decrease the frequency of the spontaneous postsynaptic currents to 43.78% ± 7.72% (mean ± SEM) and the spontaneous excitatory postsynaptic currents to 49.25% ± 7.06% (mean ± SEM), while there was no difference in the frequency in the DMSO group, respectively. Also, AS-IV repressed voltage-gated K^+ and Na^+ currents of cultured rat hippocampal neurons. These data suggest that AS-IV may depress the spontaneous neuronal excitability, which provides a new insight for AS-IV as a neuroprotector , although these findings lack information relevant for interpretation of the data, including dose/concentration dependency data as well as a comparison to other active moieties (Zhu et al., 2008).

Nowadays, the proteomic is considered to be a powerful tool in the development of novel biomarker candidates for early detection of disease and identification of new targets for therapeutics, based on the protein expression changes under the organism's different physiological states and the stages of disease progress (Hanash, 2003). A comprehensive shotgun proteomic profiling procedure, based on an online 2D-nano-LC-MS/MS system, was used to investigate proteomic variations after treatment with 100 μM AS-IV in PC12 cells, which exposed to 5 mM glutamate at 24 h. The findings of this work demonstrated that proteins related to signal transduction, immune system, signaling molecules and interaction, and energy metabolism play key roles in the neuroprotective effect of AS-IV. The Raf-MEK-ERK pathway was involved in the neuroprotective effect of AS-IV against glutamate-induced neurotoxicity in PC12 cells (Yue et al., 2015).

AS-IV may exert a therapeutic effect on ischemia stroke. Studies have shown that pretreatment of AS-IV (10–50 μM, for 6 h) significantly inhibited oxygen and glucose deprivation/re-oxygenation (OGD/R) induced neuron viability loss. Importantly, the activation of EGFR-Nrf2 signaling pathway is responsible for the neuroprotection of AS-IV on cortical neurons against OGD/R damages (Gu et al., 2015).

In addition to its neuroprotective effects, AS-IV also exhibits pharmacological effects in refractory neuropathic pain. Shi et al. (2015) systematically investigated the antinociceptive activity of AS-IV in an animal model of chronic constriction injury (CCI) in neuropathic pain. AS-IV could alleviate neuropathic pain by two ways: (a) down-regulation of the expressions of important molecules associated with neuropathic pain in the DRG, such as P2X3, TRPA1, and TRPV1, and (b) restoration of the histological structure of the damaged sciatic nerve by accumulating GFRα1 in the debris of myelin between the Schwann cells and the damaged axon (Shi et al., 2015).

In the peripheral nervous system, AS-IV also can protect and promote peripheral nerve regeneration (Cheng et al., 2006). Growth-associated protein 43, as a specific molecular marker during nerve injury plays a vital role in nerve growth, development and regeneration (Shen & Meiri, 2013). AS-IV (10 or 5 mg/kg per day) may contribute to sciatic nerve regeneration and functional recovery in mouse model of sciatic nerve injury with the underlying mechanism of the up-regulation of growth-associated protein-43 expression (Zhang & Chen, 2013).

3. The protective effect of AS-IV on liver

As the largest solid organ, the liver carries out many vital roles in the human body, such as detoxification, the production of chemicals and drug metabolism, which are the main causes of oxidative stress, drug-induced liver injury, and insulin resistance (IR) injury. Recent studies have shown that AS-IV offers protection of the liver through various pharmacological effects, such as antioxidation (Han, Li, Lin, Ma, & Huang, 2014), anti-infection (Wang et al., 2009) and anti-inflammation (Wei, Liu, Chen, Sheng, & Liu, 2019).

In general, high-fat diet feeding can result in adipose dysfunction with inducing endogenous glucose production in mice. Du et al. noted that pretreatment with AS-IV contributed to the limitation of hepatic lipid deposition and the depression of excessive hepatic glucose through reduction of cAMP accumulation via regulation of Akt/PDE3B (Du et al., 2017). IR is a crucial factor for non-alcoholic fatty liver disease, with the characterization of lipid accumulation in hepatocytes. AS-IV exerts the potential to be developed as a drug for treatment of hepatic steatosis due to its strong activities in inhibiting IR and lipid accumulation in HepG2 cells via regulating AMPK-dependent phosphorylation of SREBP-1c at Ser372 (Wang, Li, Hao, & Li, 2018).

4. The anti-cancer effect of AS-IV

Many recent studies have shown that AS-IV exerted beneficial anti-cancer effects against various tumor types based on immune-enhancement activity (Li, Ye, & Chen, 2018), inhibition of tumor growth (Zhang et al., 2014) and inhibition of tumor migration and invasion (Zhu & Wen, 2018).

Lung cancer is the most frequently occurring cancer and the leading cause of death (18.4%) among all cancer deaths worldwide (Bray et al., 2018). It was reported that AS-IV had certain protective and adjuvant therapeutic effects on lung-related diseases and lung cancer (Zhang et al., 2014; Zhang, Chen, Xu, & Tian, 2018; Zhou, Zhuo, & Cai, 2018). In an orthotopic lung cancer model induced by IDO-overexpression in C57BL/6 mice, AS-IV remarkably suppressed the growth of tumor in vivo. AS-IV can improve the immune response by inhibiting the expression of Tregs and inducing the activity of CTLs (Zhang et al., 2014). AS-IV attenuates the migration and invasion of A549 cells by regulating PKC-α-ERK1/2-NF-κB pathway (Cheng et al., 2014). In addition, AS-IV enhances chemosensitivity to cisplatin in human non-small cell lung cancer cells via inhibition of B7-H3, which can be used as a potential therapeutic approach for lung cancer patients (He et al., 2016).

Hepatocellular carcinoma (HCC) is the seventh most prevalent malignancy in both sexes (Bray et al., 2018). At present, some progress has been made with AS-IV in the treatment of liver cancer. AS-IV successfully inhibited migration ability, cell viability and invasiveness of HCC cells through blocking IL-11/STAT3 signaling pathway via significantly down-regulating the expression of lncRNA-ATB in a dose- and time-dependent manner (Li, Ye, & Chen, 2018), and suppressing epithelial-mesenchymal transition by targeting the Akt/GSK-3β/β-catenin pathway (Qin et al., 2017). Multidrug resistance has become a major obstacle in cancer chemotherapy, which is considered to be mediated by P glycoprotein (P-gp) encoded by the multidrug resistance (mdr1) gene (Chen et al., 2016). Wang et al. found that AS-IV (0.1 mM) reversed the drug resistance of Bel-7402/FU human hepatic cancer cells by depressing the expression of mdr1 and blocking the JNK/c-Jun/AP-1 signaling pathway, although authors did not examine the effects of down-regulation of mdr1 gene expression on oral bioavailability and clearance of other drugs (Wang et al., 2017).

Gastric cancer (including cardia and noncardia gastric cancer) is an important cancer worldwide and considered to be the fifth most frequently diagnosed cancer and the third leading cause of cancer death (Bray et al., 2018). It has been reported that AS-IV possesses anti-metastasis activity of gastric cancer cells through inhibition of the PI3K/Akt/NF-κB pathway (Zhu & Wen, 2018). Because the diagnosis of gastric carcinoma tends to be at an advanced stage, in-depth research of precancerous lesions of gastric carcinoma (PLGC) is becoming important in preventing the formation and development of gastric carcinoma (Yoon & Kim, 2015). Recent research demonstrates that AS-IV protects the gastric mucosal injury, prevents and cures gastric mucosal atrophy in MNNG-induced precancerous lesions of gastric carcinoma in rats (Cai et al., 2018), and it could reverse PLGC via regulation on glycolysis through the miRNA-34a/LDHA pathway (Zhang et al., 2018).

According to the statistics, colorectal cancer (CRC), is another frequent cancer and the second leading cause of cancer death (9.2%) with a poor prognosis in both males and females (Bray et al., 2018). Similar to previous reports in lung cancer, AS-IV also enhances cisplatin chemosensitivity in human colorectal cancer through inhibition of NOTCH3 (Xie, Li, Li, & Luo, 2016), and AS-IV inhibits cell proliferation of CRC cells by down-regulating the expression of B7-H3 (Wang, Mou, Cui, Wang, & Zhang, 2018). Ye, Su, Chen, Zheng, & Liu (2017) found that AS-IV could suppress EMT and reduce chemotherapy-resistant by inducing miR-134 expression which significantly down-regulated the CREB1 signaling in colorectal cancer cell Line SW-480 (Ye et al., 2017).

5. The protective effect of AS-IV on diabetes

Diabetes is a metabolic disorder characterized by elevated blood glucose. Insulin can uptake glucose by the cells, when the body does not make sufficient insulin or does not use insulin well, glucose will stay in the blood (Zhu, Zheng, Chen, Gu, & Huang, 2016). Without treatment, the high level of glucose can damage the eyes, kidneys, heart, gastric mucosa, and can also lead to coma and death (Chen et al., 2008; Ding et al., 2014; Ju et al., 2019; Liu et al., 2017; Mai, Li, Yin, & Li, 2015; Wang, Siu, &

Zhang, 2017). Accumulating evidence suggests that AS-IV exhibits a hypoglycemic effect in diabetic mice (Lu, Li, Guo, Chen, & Li, 2015; Lv et al., 2010) and can alleviate the above mentioned complications of diabetes through a variety of underlying molecular mechanisms (Table 1).

5.1 Pharmacological effects of AS-IV on diabetic nephropathy

Diabetic nephropathy (DN) is the chronic loss of kidney function occurring in conjunction with diabetes mellitus (Song et al., 2018; Sun et al., 2016). Proteinuria (Gui, et al., 2013; Wang et al., 2015), hypertension, podocyte apoptosis (Yao et al., 2016) and increased reactive oxygen species (He et al., 2018) are pathological features of DN. Recently, several in vitro and in vivo studies indicated that AS-IV could attenuate DN through the following mechanisms:

5.1.1 AS-IV protects against kidney injury by inhibiting oxidative stress and NF-κB-mediated inflammatory pathway

The findings of a recent study demonstrated that AS-IV can prevent rat kidney injury induced by iatrogenic hyperinsulinemia through inhibiting oxidative stress, IL-1β and TNF-α overproduction, repressing ERK1/2 activation, and improving TRPC6 expression (He et al., 2018). Likewise, Qi et al. found that AS-IV can ameliorate EMT induced by glycated albumin in NRK-52E cell line by regulation of the impaired redox balance (Qi, Niu, Qin, Qiao, & Gu, 2014). AS-IV attenuates DN by ameliorating oxidative stress (Chen et al., 2018; Gui et al., 2012), inhibiting NF-κB mediated inflammatory genes expression in streptozotocin (STZ)-induced diabetic rats (Gui et al., 2013) and in human mesangial cells (Sun et al., 2014).

5.1.2 AS-IV protects against kidney injury through ameliorating albuminuria

Albuminuria is an important hallmark feature in the development of DN. The mechanisms in the renoprotective function of AS-IV in the pathogenesis of DN through reducing albuminuria via decreasing ER-stress (Wang et al., 2015), inhibiting NF-κB mediated inflammatory genes expression (Gui et al., 2013), and restoring the balance of Bax and Bcl-2 expression and inhibiting caspase-3 activation (Gui et al., 2012).

Table 1 Astragaloside IV prevention mechanism of diabetes complications.

Diabetes complications	Model class	Modeling method	Pharmacological effect	Molecular mechanism	References
Diabetic nephropathy	The immortalized mouse podocyte cell	HG	Improves HG-induced podocyte adhesion dysfunction	α3β1 integrin↑, ILK↓	Chen et al. (2008)
	Mouse podocytes	HG	Prevents HG-induced podocyte apoptosis	Bax↓, Bcl-2↑, caspase-3↓	Gui et al. (2012)
	Sprague-Dawley rats	STZ			
	Sprague-Dawley rats	STZ	Inhibits NF-κB mediated inflammatory genes expression	TNF-α↓, MCP-1↓, ICAM-1↓, α1-chain type IV collagen↓	Gui et al. (2013)
	Sprague-Dawley rats	STZ	Inhibits of endoplasmic reticulum stress-induced podocyte apoptosis	PERK↓, ATF4↓, CHOP↓, TRB3↓, Bcl-2↑, Bax↓, eIF2α↓, GRP78↓	Chen et al. (2014)
	Mouse podocytes	HG			
	Human glomerular mesangial cell line	HG	Prevents damage to human mesangial cells	ROS↓, NF-κB↓, Nox4↑, Akt↓, Nox4↓, IκBα↓	Sun et al. (2014)
	The rat proximal tubular epithelial cell line NRK-52E	glycated albumin	Induces NRK-52E cell line EMT through oxidative stress	SOD↓, NADPH oxidase↓, E-cadherin↑, α-smooth muscle actin↓	Qi, Niu, Qin, Qiao, and Gu (2014)
	Sprague-Dawley rats	STZ	Attenuates proteinuria	GRP78↓, ORP150↓, caspase-3↓, eIF2α↓, PERK↓, JNK↓	Wang et al. (2015)
	Human podocytes	TM			

Continued

Table 1 Astragaloside IV prevention mechanism of diabetes complications.—cont'd

Diabetes complications	Model class	Modeling method	Pharmacological effect	Molecular mechanism	References
	Sprague-Dawley rats	STZ	Decreases blood glucose levels	Integrin β1↑, ILK↓, α-actinin-4↓	Lu, Li, Guo, Chen, and Li (2015)
	Sprague-Dawley rats	STZ	Inhibits oxidative stress	TRPC6↑, IL-1β↓, TNF-α, Erk1/2↓	He et al. (2018)
	Mouse podocytes	HG	Prevents HG-induced podocyte apoptosis	Bax↓, NFAT2↓, TRPC6↓, intracellular Ca^{2+}↓	Yao et al. (2016)
	db/db mice	STZ	Reduces albuminuria	Akt/mTOR↓, NF-κB↓, Erk1/2↓	Sun et al. (2016)
	db/db mice	STZ	Modulates the mitochondrial	Drp-1↓, Fis-1↓, MFF↓, PINK1/Parkin-mediated mitophagy↓	Liu et al. (2017)
	C57BL/6J mice	STZ, HG	Inhibits podocyte apoptosis and ER-stress	SERCA2b↑, AMPKα↑, Angiotensinogen↓,mTOR↓	Guo et al. (2017)
	Proximal renal tubular epithelial cells	palmitic acid	Alleviates PA-induced apoptosis of HK-2 cells	Bax↓, cleaved-caspase3↓, Nrf2↑, Bcl-2↑	Chen et al. (2018)
	C57BL/6J mice	STZ	Reduces albuminuria and serum creatinine levels, ameliorates mesangial matrix expansion and greater foot process width	ERK1/E2↓, MEK1/2↓, RSK2↓, NAG↓, NGAL↓, TGF-β1↓	Song et al. (2018)

	Sprague-Dawley rats	STZ	Attenuates albuminuria and decreases podocyte apoptosis	TRAF5↓, lncRNA -TUG1↑	Lei, Zhang, Li, and Ren (2018) and Lei, Zhang, Ren, and Luo (2018)
	mouse podocytes (MPC5)	HG			
	Sprague-Dawley rats	STZ	Suppresses podocyte apoptosis	MIR-378↑, TRAF5↓	Lei, Zhang, Li, and Ren (2018) and Lei, Zhang, Ren, and Luo (2018)
Diabetic retinopathy	Sprague-Dawley rats	HFD, STZ	Inhibits ER-stress-induced renal tubular epithelial cells apoptosis	GRP78↓, p-PERK↓, ATF4↓, CHOP↓, caspase-3↓, Bax/Bcl-2↓	Ju et al. (2019)
	db/db mice	STZ	Improves the amplitude in pattern ERG and reduces the apoptosis of RGCs	AR↓, ERK1/2↓, NF-κB↓	Ding et al. (2014)
	Sprague-Dawley rats RCECs	HG	Antioxidative function	Nox4↓, SOD↑, GSH↑, GSH-peroxidase↑, CAT↑	Qiao, Fan, and Tang (2017)
Diabetic gastropathy	Sprague-Dawley rats	STZ	Antioxidative function	iNOS↓, COX-2↓, mucin1↑	Wang, Siu, and Zhang (2017)
Diabetes vascular complications	Vascular smooth muscle cell	HG	Inhibits proliferation and promotes apoptosis in HG-induced rat vascular smooth muscle cells	α-smooth muscle actin↑, $\Delta\Psi m$↓	Yuan et al. (2008)

Continued

Table 1 Astragaloside IV prevention mechanism of diabetes complications.—cont'd

Diabetes complications	Model class	Modeling method	Pharmacological effect	Molecular mechanism	References
Diabetes vascular complications	Human umbilical vein endothelial cells	STZ	Inhibits H_2O_2-induced human umbilical vein endothelial cell apoptosis	Transforming growth factor-β 1↓, Nox4↓, Smad2↓, Bax↓, Caspase-3↓, Bcl-2↑	Mai, Li, Yin, and Li (2015)
	Human umbilical vein endothelial cell	HG	Promotes cell proliferation, reduces cell apoptosis	TNF-α↓, IL-1β↓, JNK↓, Bax↓, cytochrome c↓, cleaved-caspase-9↓, cleaved-caspase-3↓, Bcl-2↑	You et al. (2019)
Type 2 diabetic	C57BL/6J mice	STZ, HFD	Decreases the blood glucose, TG and insulin levels	Glycogen phosphorylase↓, G6Pase↓	Lv et al. (2010)
Diabetes	The mouse myoblast cell line C2C12	Palmitate	Facilitates glucose transport	Insulin-stimulated translocation of GLUT4↑, TLR4↓, IKK↓, IκBα ↓, NF-κB↓, MCP-1↓, IL-6↓, TNF-α↓	Zhu, Zheng, Chen, Gu, and Huang (2016)

5.1.3 AS-IV protects against kidney injury through attenuating podocytes apoptosis

Podocytes apoptosis has been considered a key factor contributing to the development of diabetic nephropathy and albuminuria. It is well-documented that AS-IV suppresses podocytes apoptosis through different underlying molecular mechanisms, such as modulating TRAF5 expression through enhancing the expression of miR-378 (Lei, Zhang, Ren, & Luo, 2018) and regulating TUG1 (Lei, Zhang, Li, & Ren, 2018), down-regulating TRPC6 (He et al., 2018; Yao et al., 2016), inhibiting endoplasmic reticulum stress and oxidative stress (Chen et al., 2014; Gui et al., 2012; Guo et al., 2017) and improving HG-induced podocyte adhesion dysfunction by $\alpha_3\beta_1$ integrin up-regulation and ILK inhibition (Chen et al., 2008).

5.2 Pharmacological effects of AS-IV on vascular complications

Vascular complications are a main cause of morbidity and mortality in diabetic patients. AS-IV prevents human umbilical vein endothelial cell apoptosis by inhibiting Nox4 expression through the Nox4/Smad2 pathway (H_2O_2-induced cell apoptosis) (Mai et al., 2015) and suppressing the JNK pathway (HG-induced cell apoptosis) (You et al., 2019). Yuan et al., also found that AS-IV protects VSMC against HG-induced cell proliferation by promoting apoptosis and regulating phenotypic modulation of VSMC (Yuan et al., 2008).

5.3 Pharmacological effects of AS-IV on diabetic retinopathy

Diabetic retinopathy, one of the most common microvascular complications of diabetes, is considered to be the major cause of blindness in adults (Ding et al., 2014). Administration of AS-IV significantly down-regulates AR activity, depresses the activation of ERK1/2 phosphorylation and NF-kB, and reduces the apoptosis of RGCs in db/db mice with DR (Ding et al., 2014). Qiao et al. found that AS-IV exerts protective effects in HG-injured RCECs by its anti-oxidative function (Qiao, Fan, & Tang, 2017).

6. The latest research progress of AS-IV

As an important active compound from Chinese herbal medicine, AS-IV has been used for therapeutic purposes in cardiovascular disease in China (Wang et al., 2018). Previous studies have demonstrated that AS-IV possesses cardioprotective action through antioxidant, anti-inflammatory and anti-apoptosis effects (Li et al., 2017; Zheng et al., 2018). Abdominal aortic aneurysm (AAA), characterized by macrophage infiltration-mediated inflammation and oxidative stress, is a potentially life-threatening cardiovascular disease. Recent research noted that the protective action of AS-IV against 3,4-Benzopyrene-induced abdominal aortic aneurysm is due to the abrogation of oxidative stress and the improvement of phosphorylation of PI3K/AKT. These results indicated that AS-IV provides potential interference in the formation of AAA (Wang, Zhou, et al., 2018).

Based on literature research, it appears that most pharmacological studies of AS-IV concentrated on the individual compounds. Compound medicine is one of the main features of traditional Chinese medicine (Sun & Sun, 2010). Recent studies have shown that AS-IV, as one of the key active components of *A. membranaceus*, has promising efficacy in combination with other compounds in many cells or animal disease models (Chu et al., 2017; Wang et al., 2013). For cerebral ischemia injury, studies demonstrated that AS-IV combined with Ginsenoside Rg1, Ginsenoside Rb1, and Notoginsenoside R1 (the active ingredients of *Panax notoginseng*) could enhance the protective effects on cerebral ischemia injury by anti-inflammation and anti-apoptosis (Huang et al., 2015). Meanwhile, Chu et al. noted that combined administration of paeoniflorin and AS-IV could relieve ischemic brain edema through depression of connexin43 expression via activation of JNK and ERK pathways (Chu et al., 2017). Similarly, compared with the control group, combined administration of AS-IV and atorvastatin significantly inhibited the development of atherosclerotic lesions via the NF-kB/PPARg pathway (Sun, Rui, Pan, Zhang, & Wang, 2018).

Endothelium dysfunction is considered to be a crucial factor in the development of vascular disease in diabetes mellitus. Recent experimentation indicated that AS-IV combined with ferulic acid protects against vascular endothelial dysfunction in diabetic rats, related to NF-κB pathway involving down-regulation of Ox-LDL, up-regulation of NO and eNOS, and activation of NF-κB P65, MCP-1 and TNF-α (Yin, Qi, Song, Zhang, & Teng, 2014). Moreover, combined administration of AS-IV and ferulic acid has significant effects on synergistic promotion of blood vessel regeneration from electrospun fibrous scaffolds (Wang et al., 2013).

7. Pharmacokinetics and toxicity of AS-IV

The bioavailability of AS-IV after p.o. administration is only 7.4% in beagle dogs and 3.66% in rats (Zhang, Zhu, Chen, & Du, 2007), such low absolute bioavailability will restrict its application in oral administration. Meanwhile, Huang et al. found that the low absorption in Caco-2 cells mainly due to its poor intestinal permeability, high molecular weight, low lipophilicity and its paracellular transport (Huang et al., 2006).

Following i.v. injection of AS-IV (1.5 mg/kg), AS-IV can be detected in the selected tissues, including skin, adipose tissue, heart, muscle, duodenum, brain, kidney, lung, spleen, liver, stomach and ovary in rats (Zhang et al., 2006). After i.v. administration, the highest concentration of AS-IV is observed in liver, lung and kidney (Chang et al., 2012; Zhang et al., 2006). AS-IV have linear pharmacokinetic characteristics in both rats and dogs. The rate of AS-IV combining with plasma protein is about 83–90% (Zhang et al., 2006, 2007). AS-IV can be slowly eliminated by hepatic clearance (0.0041/kg/min) (Zhang et al., 2006).

In order to ensure the clinical safety of AS-IV, its preclinical toxicity was conducted. Zhu et al. found that AS-IV has maternal toxic after intravenous administration (1.0 mg/kg) in rats and fetal toxicity at a dose higher than 0.5 mg/kg, while it is devoid of teratogenic effects in rats and rabbits (Zhu et al., 2009). The research of further reproductive toxicity test in Sprague-Dawley rats showed that AS-IV causes the delay for fur development, eye opening, and cliff parry reflex of pups after maternal under 1.0 mg/kg AS-IV exposure for 4 weeks, while no influence over the memory and learning of F1 pups (Wan et al., 2010). Based on these findings, AS-IV should be used with caution to women during peripartum.

8. Conclusion

Over the last few decades, an increasing number of literatures have provided abundant evidence that AS-IV, as one of the important chemical extracted from *A. membranaceus*, exerts various pharmacological effects on neuroprotection, liver protection, anti-cancer and anti-diabetes, which are mainly due to its antioxidant, anti-inflammatory, anti-apoptotic properties, and the roles of enhancement of immunity, attenuation of the migration and invasion of cancer cell and improvement of chemosensitivity to chemotherapy drugs. Numerous studies have shown that the multi-level, multi-target pharmacological effects of AS-IV are in line with the complex pathogenesis of diseases, and may be a potential candidate clinical drug for the treatment of diseases and disease-related complications.

There are still many problems in the development and utilization of AS-IV as a new clinical drug:

(1) Direct target and specific molecular mechanism of AS-IV in the treatment of diseases is still uncertain. As part of the research process of AS-IV for treatment of diseases, bioinformatics methods should be introduced to predict the target of drugs or to verify the interaction between drugs and targets in vitro and in vivo to determine the targets of AS-IV for treatment of specific disease.

(2) Combining AS-IV with other agents may be an effective to treat diseases. In the theory of Chinese medicine, *Astragali Radix*, known as the "ten medicine and eight *Astragali Radix*," is a commonly used as a "*bu Qi*" Chinese herbal medicine, emphasizing the importance of AS-IV combinations. The combination of astragaloside IV with other active ingredients of traditional Chinese medicine or chemical drugs may be an effective way to achieve complementary advantages, reduce toxicity and increase efficiency.

(3) AS-IV, as an important bioactive chemicals derived from *A. membranaceus* has poor clinical application due to its low water-soluble and oral bioavailability. It is a feasible and effective method to develop new water-soluble derivatives of AS-IV. LS-102, a novel water-soluble derivative of AS-IV, showed a pharmacokinetic profile different from AS-IV with higher bioavailability. No acute toxicity effect was detected in mice treated with LS-102 even at the high dose of 5000 mg/kg body weight (Qing et al., 2019). Thus, it is reasonable to speculate that LS-102 might provide better clinical efficacy and be a potential candidate for the new drug (Sun et al., 2019).

(4) At present, few studies have been done on the toxicity and the potential adverse effects of AS-IV in vivo and in vitro. For more safe clinical application, research on toxicity and side effects of AS-IV should be given attention. Cycloastragenol (CAG), the main metabolite of AS-IV, can inhibit the UGT1A8 and UGT2B7 activity in vivo (Ran et al., 2016). This result indicates that an in vivo herb–drug interaction between AST/CAG and drugs mainly undergoing UGT1A8- or UGT2B7-catalyzed metabolism might occur.

Acknowledgments

The Applied Basic Research of Shanxi Province (No. 201601D202058), 2016 Provincial Support National Research Foundation of Shanxi Province (No. 226546001), Key laboratory of Effective Substances Research and Utilization in TCM of Shanxi province (201605D111004).

Conflict of interest

The authors report no conflicts of interest.

References

An, H. T., Wei, D. F., Qian, Y. J., Li, N., & Wang, X. M. (2018). SQYZ granules, a traditional Chinese herbal, attenuate cognitive deficits in AD transgenic mice by modulating on multiple pathogenesis processes. *American Journal of Translational Research*, *10*(11), 3857–3875.

Auyeung, K. K., Han, Q. B., & Ko, J. K. (2016). *Astragalus membranaceus*: A review of its protection against inflammation and gastrointestinal cancers. *The American Journal of Chinese Medicine*, *44*(1), 1–22.

Bray, F., Ferlay, J., Soerjomataram, I., Siegel, R. L., Torre, L. A., & Jemal, A. (2018). Global cancer statistics 2018: GLOBOCAN estimates of incidence and mortality worldwide for 36 cancers in 185 countries. *CA: A Cancer Journal for Clinicians*, *68*, 394–424.

Cai, T. T., Zhang, C. Z., Zhao, Z. M., Li, S. Y., Cai, H. B., & Chen, X. D. (2018). The gastric mucosal protective effects of astragaloside IV in mnng-induced GPL rats. *Biomedicine & Pharmacotherapy*, *104*, 291–299.

Chang, Y. X., Sun, Y. G., Li, J., Zhang, Q. H., Guo, X. R., Zhang, B. L., et al. (2012). The experimental study of Astragalus membranaceus on meridian tropsim: The distribution study of astragaloside IV in rat tissues. *Journal of Chromatography B*, *911*, 71–75.

Chen, Y. F., Gui, D. K., Chen, J. G., He, D. Y., Luo, Y. L., & Wang, N. S. (2014). Down-regulation of PERK-ATF4-CHOP pathway by Astragaloside IV is associated with the inhibition of endoplasmic reticulum stress-induced podocyte apoptosis in diabetic rats. *Cellular Physiology and Biochemistry*, *33*(6), 1975–1987.

Chen, J. G., Gui, D. K., Chen, Y. F., Mou, L. J., Liu, Y., & Huang, J. H. (2008). Astragaloside IV improves high glucose-induced podocyte adhesion dysfunction via α3β1 integrin upregulation and integrin-linked kinase inhibition. *Biochemical Pharmacology*, *76*(6), 796–804.

Chen, C. Y., Liu, N. Y., Lin, H. C., Lee, C. Y., Hung, C. C., & Chang, C. S. (2016). Synthesis and bioevaluation of novel benzodipyranone derivatives as P-glycoprotein inhibitors for multidrug resistance reversal agents. *European Journal of Medicinal Chemistry*, *118*, 219–229.

Chen, Q. Q., Su, Y., Ju, Y. H., Ma, K. K., Li, W. Z., & Li, W. P. (2018). Astragalosides IV protected the renal tubular epithelial cells from free fatty acids-induced injury by reducing oxidative stress and apoptosis. *Biomedicine & Pharmacotherapy*, *108*, 679–686.

Cheng, X. D., Gu, J. F., Zhang, M. H., Yuan, J. R., Zhao, B. J., Jiang, J., et al. (2014). Astragaloside IV inhibits migration and invasion in human lung cancer A549 cells via regulating PKC-α-ERK1/2-NF-κB pathway. *International Immunopharmacology*, *23*, 304–313.

Cheng, C. Y., Yao, C. H., Liu, B. S., Liu, C. J., Chen, G. W., & Chen, Y. S. (2006). The role of astragaloside in regeneration of the peripheral nerve system. *Journal of Biomedical Materials Research Part A*, *76*(3), 463–469.

Chu, H. I., Huang, C. Y., Gao, Z. D., Dong, J., Tang, Y. P., & Dong, Q. (2017). Reduction of ischemic brain edema by combined use of paeoniflorin and astragaloside IV via down-regulating connexin 43. *Phytotherapy Research*, *31*(9), 1410–1418.

Costa, I. M., Lima, F. O. V., Fernandes, L. C. B., Norrara, B., Neta, F. I., Alves, R. D., et al. (2018). Astragaloside IV supplementation promotes a neuroprotective effect in experimental models of neurological disorders: A systematic review. *Current Neuropharmacology*, *16*, 1–18.

Ding, Y. Z., Yuan, S. T., Liu, X. Y., Mao, P. A., Zhao, C., Huang, Q., et al. (2014). Protective effects of astragaloside IV on db/db mice with diabetic retinopathy. *PLoS One*, *9*(11) e112207.

Du, Q., Zhang, S. H., Li, A. Y., Mohammad, I. S., Liu, B. L., & Li, Y. W. (2017). Astragaloside IV inhibits adipose lipolysis and reduces hepatic glucose production via Akt dependent PDE3B expression in HFD-fed mice. *Frontiers in Physiology*, *9*, 15.

Gu, D. M., Lu, P. H., Zhang, K., Wang, X., Sun, M., Chen, G. Q., et al. (2015). EGFR mediates astragaloside IV-induced Nrf2 activation to protect cortical neurons against in vitro ischemia/reperfusion damages. *Biochemical and Biophysical Research Communications*, *457*, 391–397.

Gui, D. K., Guo, Y. P., Wang, F., Liu, W., Chen, J. G., Chen, Y. F., et al. (2012). Astragaloside IV, a novel antioxidant, prevents glucose-induced podocyte apoptosis in vitro and in vivo. *PLoS One*, 7(6) e39824.

Gui, D. K., Huang, J. H., Guo, Y. P., Chen, J. G., Chen, Y. F., & Xiao, W. Z. (2013). Astragaloside IV ameliorates renal injury in streptozotocin-induced diabetic rats through inhibiting NF-κB-mediated inflammatory genes expression. *Cytokine*, *61*(2013), 970–977.

Guo, H. J., Wang, Y., Zhang, X. M., Zang, Y. J., Zhang, Y., Wang, L., et al. (2017). Astragaloside IV protects against podocyte injury via SERCA2-dependent ER stress reduction and AMPKα-regulated autophagy induction in streptozotocin-induced diabetic nephropathy. *Scientific Reports*, 7(1), 6852.

Han, L., Li, J., Lin, X., Ma, Y. F., & Huang, Y. F. (2014). Protective effect of astragaloside IV on oxidative damages of chang liver cell induced by ethanol and H_2O_2. *China Journal of Chinese Materia Medica*, *39*(22), 4430–4435, [in Chinese].

Hanash, S. (2003). Disease proteomics. *Nature*, *422*, 226–232.

He, K. Q., Li, W. Z., Chai, X. Q., Yin, Y. Y., Jiang, Y., & Li, W. P. (2018). Astragaloside IV prevents kidney injury caused by iatrogenic hyperinsulinemia in a streptozotocin-induced diabetic rat model. *International Journal of Molecular Medicine*, *41*(2), 1078–1088.

He, C. S., Liu, Y. C., Xu, Z. P., Dai, P. C., Chen, X. W., & Jin, D. H. (2016). Astragaloside IV enhances cisplatin chemosensitivity in non-small cell lung cancer cells through inhibition of B7-H3. *Cellular Physiology and Biochemistry*, *40*, 1221–1229.

Huang, X. P., Ding, H., Lu, J. D., Tang, Y. H., Deng, B. X., & Deng, C. Q. (2015). Effects of the combination of the main active components of Astragalus and Panax notoginseng on inflammation and apoptosis of nerve cell after cerebral ischemia-reperfusion. *The American Journal of Chinese Medicine*, *43*(7), 1–20.

Huang, C. R., Wang, G. J., Wu, X. L., Li, H., Xie, H. T., LV, H., et al. (2006). Absorption enhancement study of astragaloside IV based on its transport mechanism in caco-2 cells. *European Journal of Drug Metabolism and Pharmacokinetics*, *31*(1), 5–10.

Ju, Y. H., Su, Y., Chen, Q. Q., Ma, K. K., Ji, T. J., Wang, Z. Y., et al. (2019). Protective effects of Astragaloside IV on endoplasmic reticulum stress-induced renal tubular epithelial cells apoptosis in type 2 diabetic nephropathy rats. *Biomedicine & Pharmacotherapy*, *109*, 84–92.

Lei, X., Zhang, L. M., Li, Z. L., & Ren, J. G. (2018). Astragaloside IV/lncRNA-TUG1/TRAF5 signaling pathway participates in podocyte apoptosis of diabetic nephropathy rats. *Drug Design, Development and Therapy*, *12*, 2785–2793.

Lei, X., Zhang, B. d., Ren, J. G., & Luo, F. L. (2018). Astragaloside suppresses apoptosis of the podocytes in rats with diabetic nephropathy via miR-378/TRAF5 signaling pathway. *Life Sciences*, *206*, 77–83.

Li, T., Chen, S., Feng, T., Dong, J., Li, Y., & Li, H. (2016). Rutin protects against aging-related metabolic dysfunction. *Food & Function*, 7(2), 1147–1154.

Li, X. Z., Ding, Y. Z., Wu, H. F., Bian, Z. P., Xu, J. D., Gu, C. R., et al. (2017). Astragaloside IV prevents cardiac remodeling in the apolipoprotein E-deficient mice by regulating cardiac homeostasis and oxidative stress. *Cellular Physiology and Biochemistry, 44*, 2422–2438.

Li, L., Hou, X. J., Xu, R. F., Liu, C., & Tu, M. (2017). Research review on the pharmacological effects of astragaloside IV. *Fundamental and Clinical Pharmacology, 31*, 17–36.

Li, Y. L., Ye, Y., & Chen, H. Y. (2018). Astragaloside IV inhibits cell migration and viability of hepatocellular carcinoma cells via suppressing long noncoding RNA ATB. *Biomedicine & Pharmacotherapy, 99*(2018), 134–141.

Liu, D. L., Bao, H. Y., & Liu, Y. (2014). Progress on chemical constituents and pharmacological effects of Astragali Radix in recent five years. *Food and Drug, 16*, 68–70, [in Chinese].

Liu, X. H., Wang, W. J., Song, G. F., Wei, X., Zeng, Y. J., Han, P. X., et al. (2017). Astragaloside IV ameliorates diabetic nephropathy by modulating the mitochondrial quality control network. *PLoS One, 12*(8) e0182558.

Lu, W. S., Li, S., Guo, W. W., Chen, L. L., & Li, Y. S. (2015). Effects of Astragaloside IV on diabetic nephropathy in rats. *Genetics and Molecular Research, 14*(2), 5427–5434.

Lv, L., Wu, S. Y., Wang, G. F., Zhang, J. J., Pang, J. X., Liu, Z. Q., et al. (2010). Effect of astragaloside IV on hepatic glucose-regulating enzymes in diabetic mice induced by a high-fat diet and streptozotocin. *Phytotherapy Research, 24*(2), 219–224.

Mai, Y. h., Li, W. Z., Yin, Y. Y., & Li, W. P. (2015). AST IV inhibits H2O2-induced human umbilical vein endothelial cell apoptosis by suppressing Nox4 expression through the TGF-β1/Smad2 pathway. *International Journal of Molecular Medicine, 35*, 1667–1674.

Qi, W. W., Niu, J. Y., Qin, Q. J., Qiao, Z. D., & Gu, Y. (2014). Astragaloside IV attenuates glycated albumin-induced epithelial-to-mesenchymal transition by inhibiting oxidative stress in renal proximal tubular cells. *Cell Stress & Chaperones, 19*(1), 105–114.

Qiao, Y., Fan, C. L., & Tang, M. K. (2017). Astragaloside IV protects rat retinal capillary endothelial cells against high glucose-induced oxidative injury. *Drug Design, Development and Therapy, 11*, 3567–3577.

Qin, C. G., Ma, D. N., Ren, Z. G., Zhu, X. D., Wang, C. H., Wang, Y. C., et al. (2017). Astragaloside IV inhibits metastasis in hepatoma cells through the suppression of epithelial-mesenchymal transition via the Akt/GSK-3β/β-catenin pathway. *Oncology Reports, 37*, 1725–1735.

Qing, L. S., Chen, T. B., Sun, W. X., Chen, L., Luo, P., Zhang, Z. F., et al. (2019). Pharmacokinetics comparison, intestinal absorption and acute toxicity assessment of a novel water-soluble astragaloside IV derivative (astragalosidic acid, LS-102). *European Journal of Drug Metabolism and Pharmacokinetics, 44*(2), 251–259.

Ran, R. X., Zhang, C. Z., Li, R. S., Chen, B. W., Zhang, W. H., Zhao, Z. Y., et al. (2016). Evaluation and comparison of the inhibition effect of astragaloside IV and aglycone cycloastragenol on various UDP-glucuronosyl transferase (UGT) isoforms. *Molecules, 21*, 1616.

Ren, S., Zhang, H., Mu, Y. P., Sun, M. Y., & Liu, P. (2013). Pharmacological effects of Astragaloside IV: A literature review. *Journal of Traditional Chinese Medicine, 33*(3), 413–416.

Shen, Y., & Meiri, K. (2013). GAP-43 dependency defines distinct effects of netrin-1 on cortical and spinal neurite outgrowth and directional guidance. *International Journal of Developmental Neuroscience, 31*(1), 11–20.

Shi, G. B., Fan, R., Zhang, W., Yang, C., Wang, Q., Song, J., et al. (2015). Antinociceptive activity of astragaloside IV in the animal model of chronic constriction injury. *Behavioural Pharmacology, 26*(5), 436–446.

Song, G. F., Han, P. X., Sun, H. L., Shao, M. M., Yu, X. W., Wang, W. J., et al. (2018). Astragaloside IV ameliorates early diabetic nephropathy by inhibition of MEK1/2-ERK1/2-RSK2 signaling in streptozotocin-induced diabetic mice. *Journal of International Medical Research, 46*(7), 2883–2897.

State Pharmacopoeia Commission. (2015). *Pharmacopoeia of the People's Republic of China* (1st ed.) (p. 301). . Beijing: Chemical Industry Press. in Chinese.
Sun, L., Li, W. P., Li, W. Z., Xiong, L., Li, G. P., & Ma, R. (2014). Astragaloside IV prevents damage to human mesangial cells through the inhibition of the NADPH oxidase/ROS/Akt/N-κB pathway under high glucose conditions. *International Journal of Molecular Medicine, 34*(1), 167–176.
Sun, B., Rui, R. P., Pan, H. Y., Zhang, L. C., & Wang, X. L. (2018). Effect of combined use of astragaloside IV (AsIV) and atorvastatin (AV) on expression of PPAR-g and inflammation-associated cytokines in atherosclerosis rats. *Medical Science Monitor, 24*, 6229–6236.
Sun, X. Y., & Sun, F. Y. (2010). *Shen Nong Ben Cao Jing*. Taiyuan: Shanxi Science and Technology Press, pp. 112–113. in Chinese.
Sun, H. L., Wang, W. J., Han, P. X., Shao, M. M., Song, G. F., Du, H., et al. (2016). Astragaloside IV ameliorates renal injury in db/db mice. *Scientific Reports, 6*, 32545.
Sun, W. X., Zhang, Z. F., Xie, J., He, Y., Cheng, Y., Ding, L. S., et al. (2019). Determination of a astragaloside IV derivative LS-102 in plasma by ultra-performance liquid chromatography-tandem mass spectrometry in dog plasma and its application in a pharmacokinetic study. *Phytomedicine, 53*, 243–251.
Wan, X. Y., Zhu, J. B., Zhu, Y. P., Ma, X. L., Zheng, Y. W., Zhang, T. B., et al. (2010). Effect of astragaloside IV on the general and peripartum reproductive toxicity in Sprague-Dawley rats. *International Journal of Toxicology, 29*, 505–516.
Wang, C. Y., Li, Y., Hao, M. J., & Li, W. M. (2018). Astragaloside IV inhibits triglyceride accumulation in insulin-resistant HepG2 cells via AMPK-induced SREBP-1c phosphorylation. *Frontiers in Physiology, 9*, 345.
Wang, S. G., Li, J. Y., Huang, H., Gao, W., Zhuang, C. l., Li, B., et al. (2009). Anti-hepatitis B virus activities of astragaloside IV isolated from radix astragali. *Biological and Pharmaceutical Bulletin, 32*(1), 132–135.
Wang, P. P., Luan, J. J., Xu, W. K., Wang, L., Xu, D. J., Yang, C. Y., et al. (2017). Astragaloside IV downregulates the expression of MDR1 in Bel-7402/FU human hepatic cancer cells by inhibiting the JNK/c-Jun/AP-1 signaling pathway. *Molecular Medicine Reports, 16*, 2761–2766.
Wang, S. X., Mou, J. G., Cui, L. S., Wang, X. G., & Zhang, Z. Q. (2018). Astragaloside IV inhibits cell proliferation of colorectal cancer cell lines through down-regulation of B7-H3. *Biomedicine & Pharmacotherapy, 102*, 1037–1044.
Wang, N. D., Siu, F., & Zhang, Y. B. (2017). Effect of astragaloside IV on diabetic gastric mucosa in vivo and in vitro. *American Journal of Translational Research, 9*(11), 4902–4913.
Wang, Z. S., Xiong, F., Xie, X. H., Chen, D., Pan, J. H., & Cheng, L. (2015). Astragaloside IV attenuates proteinuria in streptozotocin-induced diabetic nephropathy via the inhibition of endoplasmic reticulum stress. *BMC Nephrology, 16*, 44.
Wang, H., Zhang, Y., Xia, T., Wei, W., Chen, F., Guo, X. Q., et al. (2013). Synergistic promotion of blood vessel regeneration by astragaloside IV and ferulic acid from electrospun fibrous mats. *Molecular Pharmaceutics, 10*, 2394–2403.
Wang, J. N., Zhou, Y. Y., Wu, S. Z., Huang, K. Y., Thapa, S., Tao, L. Y., et al. (2018). Astragaloside IV attenuated 3,4-benzopyrene-induced abdominal aortic aneurysm by ameliorating macrophage-mediated inflammation. *Frontiers in Pharmacology, 9*, 496.
Wei, R. D., Liu, H., Chen, R., Sheng, Y. J., & Liu, T. (2019). Astragaloside IV combating liver cirrhosis through the PI3K/Akt/mTOR signaling pathway. *Experimental and Therapeutic Medicine, 17*, 393–397.
Xie, T., Li, Y., Li, S. L., & Luo, H. F. (2016). Astragaloside IV enhances cisplatin chemosensitivity in human colorectal cancer via regulating NOTCH3. *Oncology Research, 24*, 447–453.

Yao, X. M., Liu, Y. J., Wang, Y. M., Wang, H., Zhu, B. B., Liang, Y. P., et al. (2016). Astragaloside IV prevents high glucose-induced podocyte apoptosis via downregulation of TRPC6. *Molecular Medicine Reports*, *13*(6), 5149–5156.

Ye, Q., Su, L., Chen, D. G., Zheng, W. Y., & Liu, Y. (2017). Astragaloside IV induced miR-134 expression reduces EMT and increases chemotherapeutic sensitivity by suppressing CREB1 signaling in colorectal cancer cell line SW-480. *Cellular Physiology and Biochemistry*, *43*, 1617–1626.

Yin, Y. H., Qi, F. H., Song, Z. H., Zhang, B., & Teng, J. L. (2014). Ferulic acid combined with astragaloside IV protects against vascular endothelial dysfunction in diabetic rats. *Bioscience Trends*, *8*(4), 217–226.

Yoon, H., & Kim, N. (2015). Diagnosis and management of high risk group for gastric cancer. *Gut and Liver*, *9*(1), 5–17.

You, L. Z., Fang, Z. H., Shen, G. M., Wang, Q., He, Y., Ye, S., et al. (2019). Astragaloside IV prevents high glucos-induced cell apoptosis and inflammatory reactions through inhibition of the JNK pathway in human umbilical vein endothelial cells. *Molecular Medicine Reports*, *19*(3), 1603–1612.

Yuan, W., Zhang, Y., Ge, Y. K., Yan, M., Kuang, R., & Zheng, X. X. (2008). Astragaloside IV inhibits proliferation and promotes apoptosis in rat vascular smooth muscle cells under high glucose concentration in vitro. *Planta Medica*, *74*(10), 1259–1264.

Yue, R. C., Li, X., Chen, B. Y., Zhao, J., He, W. W., Yuan, H., et al. (2015). Astragaloside IV attenuates glutamate-induced neurotoxicity in PC12 cells through Raf-MEK-ERK pathway. *PLoS One*, *10*(5), e0126603.

Zhang, C. Z., Cai, T. T., Zeng, X. H., Cai, D. K., Chen, Y. X., Huang, X. J., et al. (2018). Astragaloside IV reverses MNNG-induced precancerous lesions of gastric carcinoma in rats: Regulation on glycolysis through miRNA-34a/LDHA pathway. *Phytotherapy Research*, *32*, 1364–1372.

Zhang, X. H., & Chen, J. J. (2013). The mechanism of astragaloside IV promoting sciatic nerve regeneration. *Neural Regeneration Research*, *8*(24), 2256–2265.

Zhang, X. Z., Chen, J., Xu, P., & Tian, X. (2018). Protective effects of astragaloside IV against hypoxic pulmonary hypertension. *Medicinal Chemistry Communications*, *9*, 1715.

Zhang, Z. G., Wu, L., Wang, J. L., Yang, J. D., Zhang, J., Zhang, J., et al. (2012). Astragaloside IV prevents MPP+-induced SH-SY5Y cell death via the inhibition of Bax-mediated pathways and ROS production. *Molecular and Cellular Biochemistry*, *364*, 209–216.

Zhang, W. D., Zhang, C., Liu, R. H., Li, H. L., Zhang, J. T., Mao, C., et al. (2006). Preclinical pharmacokinetics and tissue distribution of a natural cardioprotective agent astragaloside IV in rats and dogs. *Life Sciences*, *79*, 808–815.

Zhang, A. l., Zheng, Y. H., Que, Z. J., Zhang, L. L., Lin, S. C., Le, V., et al. (2014). Astragaloside IV inhibits progression of lung cancer by mediating immune function of Tregs and CTLs by interfering with IDO. *Journal of Cancer Research and Clinical Oncology*, *140*(11), 1883–1890.

Zhang, Q., Zhu, L. L., Chen, G. G., & Du, Y. U. (2007). Pharmacokinetics of stragaloside iv in beagle dogs. *European Journal of Drug Metabolism and Pharmacokinetics*, *32*(2), 75–79.

Zheng, Q., Zhu, J. Z., Bao, X. Y., Zhu, P. C., Tong, Q., Huang, Y. Y., et al. (2018). A preclinical systematic review and meta-analysis of astragaloside IV for myocardial ischemia/reperfusion injury. *Frontiers in Physiology*, *9*, 795.

Zhou, M. Q., Zhuo, L. Y., & Cai, C. (2018). Astragaloside IV inhibits cigarette smoke-induced pulmonary inflammation in mice. *Inflammation*, *41*(5), 1671–1680.

Zhu, S. Q., Qi, L., Rui, Y. F., Li, R. X., He, X. P., & Xie, Z. P. (2008). Astragaloside IV inhibits spontaneous synaptic transmission and synchronized Ca^{2+} oscillations on hippocampal neurons. *Acta Pharmacologica Sinica*, *29*(1), 57–64.

Zhu, J. B., Wan, X. Y., Zhu, Y. P., Ma, X. L., Zheng, Y. W., & Zhang, T. B. (2009). Effect of astragaloside IV on the embryo-fetal development of Sprague-Dawley rats and New Zealand White rabbits. *Journal of Applied Toxicology*, *29*, 381–385.

Zhu, J. H., & Wen, K. (2018). Astragaloside IV inhibits TGF-β1-induced epithelial mesenchymal transition through inhibition of the PI3K/Akt/NF-κB pathway in gastric cancer cells. *Phytotherapy Research*, *2018*, 1–8.

Zhu, R. F., Zheng, J. J., Chen, L. H., Gu, B., & Huang, S. G. (2016). Astragaloside IV facilitates glucose transport in C2C12 myotubes through the IRS1/AKT pathway and suppresses the palmitate-induced activation of the IKK/IκBα pathway. *Internatonal Journal of Molecular Medicine*, *37*(6), 1697–1705.

Further reading

Cheng, M. X., Chen, Z. Z., Cai, Y. L., Liu, C. A., & Tu, B. (2011). Astragaloside IV protects against ischemia reperfusion in a murine model of orthotopic liver transplantation. *Transplantation Proceedings*, *43*, 1456–1461.

Li, L., Huang, W. X., Wang, S. K., Sun, K. C., Zhang, W. X., Ding, Y. M., et al. (2018). Astragaloside IV attenuates acetaminophen-induced liver injuries in mice by activating the Nrf2 signaling pathway. *Molecules*, *23*, 2032.

CHAPTER FIVE

Modern traditional Chinese medicine: Identifying, defining and usage of TCM components

David J. Newman*
Newman Consulting LLC, Wayne, PA, United States
*Corresponding author: e-mail address: djnewman664@verizon.net

Contents

Abstract

TCM-based medications have been used for millennia in China and have always been "different" from current Western-based medicines in that they frequently are still mixtures of predominately plant products. From the early 20th Century, there has been a move to identify both the actual compounds in these mixes, and then over the past approximately 50 years, to utilize early information for current diseases, with an example

Advances in Pharmacology, Volume 87
ISSN 1054-3589
https://doi.org/10.1016/bs.apha.2019.07.001

being artemisinin for treatment of malaria. Since that discovery, Western scientists, together with their Chinese counterparts, have begun to investigate how TCM compositions can be utilized to discover new agents, sometimes the actual TCM-based compound(s) but also by utilizing the pharmacophores from such preparations that have utility in human diseases. The examples in this review include artemisinin derivatives and their manifold bioactivities, indirubins and derivatives as antitumor agents, arsenicals predominately as treatment for leukemia, though extending into other cancer types. Finally, there are sections discussing the use of current computerized techniques that combine metabolomics, mass spectroscopy/HPLC, and network pharmacology with the aim of identifying the "active principles" in relevant TCM preparations and finally how high content screening can be utilized in conjunction with the other analytical techniques.

Abbreviations

Abl1	tyrosine-protein kinase *ABL1*
Abl T315I	amino acid substitutions in Abl, threonine to isoleucine
AML	acute myeloid leukemia
APL	acute promyelocytic leukemia
ART	artemisinin
Aur A	aurora kinase A, also known as serine/threonine-protein kinase 6
BAD	Bcl2 antagonist of cell death
Bcl-xL	antiapoptotic member of the Bcl-2 family at outer mitochondrial membrane
BH3	B-cell lymphoma 2 (Bcl-2) homology 3
c-Kit	receptor tyrosine kinase
c-Src	proto-oncogene tyrosine-protein kinase
CDK1-cyclin B	cyclin B has to bind to cyclin-dependent kinase 1 for activation of the complex
CDK2	cyclin-dependent kinase 2
CDK5/p25	cyclin-dependent kinase 5 plus protein P25 is an activator of GSK
CLK1	dual specificity kinase acting on both serine/threonine and tyrosine-containing substrates
CML	chronic myelogenous leukemia
DHA	dihydroartemisinin
ds-DNA	double-stranded DNA
DYRK1A	dual specificity tyrosine phosphorylation regulated kinase 1A
DYRK2	*cf* DYRK1A; member of the same gene family
EphB4	ephrin type-B receptor 4
GSK-3	glycogen synthase kinase 3 is a serine/threonine-protein kinase
HCC	hepatocellular carcinoma
HCS	high content screening
HPLC	high pressure (or performance) liquid chromatography
IPA	ingenuity pathway analysis (Qiagen Bioinformatics, USA)
JAK2	Janus kinase 2 involved in cytokine signaling
Mcl-1	myeloid cell leukemia-1

MS^n	mass Spectroscopy involving multiple MS collection/analysis systems
NF-κB	nuclear factor kappa light chain enhancer of activated B cells
PARP	poly ADP ribose polymerase
PDE5	phosphodiesterase 5 (GDP)
PDGF	platelet-derived growth factor
PDGFR	platelet-derived growth factor receptor
PTK	phosphotyrosine kinase
Rho	Rho GTPases a family of molecular switches controlling signal-transduction pathways
ROS	reactive oxygen species
TACE	transarterial chemoembolization may be offered as a main treatment for liver cancer
SCF	stem cell factor
siBAD	small interfering RNAs directed against BAD
TCM	traditional Chinese medicine
TNF-α	tumor necrosis factor alpha
TUNEL	terminal deoxynucleotidyl transferase (TdT) dUTP nick-end labeling

1. Introduction

TCM (Traditional Chinese Medicine) is what can be described today as an example of the use of a polypharmacologic approach. As such the mixture(s) of medicinal plants and/or metallic components (an example being arsenious trioxide [As_2O_3]), is not directed at a single target in the Western sense but effects changes in a number of related but as yet, ill-defined, or often unknown pharmacological targets. In contrast, Western drug searchers for at least the last 30 years, were usually "wedded" to the concept of one target, one drug and assumed that such a compound, once identified, would be specific for that target. The difference could also be expressed in a simpler statement. TCM started with a mixture that was efficacious in Man, and today what can be called "SCM" or "Scientific Chinese Medicine," would aim to identify the active agent(s), whereas the Western concept started with a "defined" assay *in vitro* and proceeded through a long process to identify an active *in vivo* entity, even though until approximately the early 1940s, the West still relied on single materials isolated from medicinal plants without significant efficacy or even toxicity testing.

This lack of testing in the modern sense was due to a relatively simple fact, the discipline now known as pharmacology did not exist in a formalized manner until the late 1940s, early 1950s, and its scientific underpinnings can be traced back to the compilation and publication of what has become the major handbook of drug interactions with the human body, Goodman and Gilman's treatise first published in 1941 (Goodman & Gilman, 1941). This textbook of over 1800 pages, relied upon published and peer reviewed data, with the underpinning of the novel science of pharmacodynamics. Currently this treatise is in its 13th edition (2017), and further discussion of the problems that surrounded drug discovery before its publication, and afterward, is well covered in a recent book by Kirsch and Ogas which covers the problems involved in drug discovery today (Kirsch & Ogas, 2017). Although many pharmacopeias had been published in the previous 2000 years in the West, they were effectively compilations of what had been reported as useful, but aside from the "Al-Canon of Avicenna" (Moosavi, 2009) until roughly the 17th Century, these were not what could be considered formal medical texts in the pattern of those published from roughly 300 BCE in China, with an excellent example being the Yellow Emperor's Classic of Medicine, though the actual dates might have been much earlier (Curran, 2008).

There is one area, microbial infections, where although the effects could be seen, the possible causative agents both eukaryotic and prokaryotic microbes, were unknown prior to the work of van Leeuwenhoek (Dobell, 1932) in the middle 1600s and even then, it took another 250 years for the concept of microbe/infection to be accepted. One interesting potential reason as to why TCM does not have a significant input in terms of microbial disease treatment (*i.e.*, modern antibiotics), is that even today, there are no antibiotics in use that come from plant sources (Chao et al., 2017). Once some of the causative microbes could be purified, a simple assay enabled potential treatments to be tested directly as demonstrated by the discovery of penicillin. One might be tempted to ascribe the concept of drug/target in the West to these initial discoveries.

This does not mean that TCM did not recognize diseases caused by external forces. Influenza, malaria and other epidemic diseases were recognized over 2000 years ago with potential treatments reported in TCM, though the causes were not identified for millennia.

In this review, major examples will be given as to how data from TCM have led to novel treatments for malaria and other viral diseases, and leukemias. These examples will also show how using modern concepts of medicinal chemistry and pharmacology, the "base chemical structure(s)" from TCM (investigations under the rubric of SCM) have been or are being used to extend the initial biological activities into other diseases. Finally, there will be a discussion of the application of modern concepts of systems pharmacology (also biology and chemistry); *i.e.*, approaches with the aims of elucidating the component or components that are the "active principles" of TCM formulae in particular diseases. The ultimate aim of such systems approaches is to be able to identify the multiple cellular targets of the active principle(s) and thus be able to tune the medication to the disease. This latter approach will hopefully demonstrate how the Western concept of one drug/one target has now become closer to the Chinese approach of potentially multiple targets for a given medication.

The emphasis in the rest of this short review on antitumor and infectious diseases is primarily due to the scientific background of the author being in natural product-derived antibiotics and antitumor agents, but choices have been made as to the agents discussed due to their importance in World-wide diseases today. The prime example being the utility of the artemisinin base chemical skeleton as a treatment for malaria but also for its potential in the derivation of compounds for treatment for other diseases, as can be seen in Sections 2.2.2.1 and 2.2.2.5 for potential use in antitumor studies. The discussions around Danggui Longhui Wan and its subsequent leads to treatment of leukemia are also designed to show that such agents, though not used in the West for disease treatments, were known over 2000 years ago but their medicinal applications were not known. The discussion on the use of arsenic-based antitumor treatments that effectively came directly from recent TCM studies and were approved for use in the USA as arsenious trioxide, is also used to demonstrate that arsenicals had been used in Western medicine for over 2000 years, and at the turn of the 20th Century, led to the development of the first effective treatment for syphilis.

These aptly demonstrate that classical TCM is a treasure-trove of medicinal agents that will add very significantly to the armamentarium of "drug hunters" and lead to the ultimate development of these traditional remedies in disease areas that were not medically identifiable (in Western terms) when they were first introduced to Chinese patients.

2. Artemisinin, initial discovery

The history of the discovery of a 2000 plus years old potential treatment for malaria, has been told a fair number of times by many authors, but the definitive discussions are You-You Tu's Nobel Lecture in 2016 (Tu, 2016) and her very recent paper in 2019 (Wang et al., 2019). Records of fevers in TCM that nowadays were probably malaria, dated back some thousands of years. Similar timings were also true for the use of extracts from plants of the genus *Artemisia* (Chinese Qinghao) as medicinal agents. Such extracts were initially mentioned as a specific remedy for what are now recognized as malarial symptoms in Ge Hong's Zhouhou Beiji Fang (or Handbook of Prescriptions for Emergency) that dates back to the Eastern Jin Dynasty (317–420 CE), and later works such as the Bencao Gangmu (Compendium of Materia Medica) by Li Shizhen (Ming Dynasty, 1368–1644 CE) recommended application of "Qinghao and other techniques" for relief of what were almost certainly malarial symptoms. It was not until the discovery of the malarial parasites by Laveran in 1880 and mosquitoes as the vectors for avian malaria by Ross in 1897, and then for human malaria by Battista et al. by 1900 (Cox, 2010) that the true causes of malaria were identified.

In You-You Tu's Nobel lecture, she emphasized that use of the conventional TCM methodology of using hot to boiling water extractions gave variable results, and that on searching the ancient TCM literature, she realized that warm water extracts were the recommended method. Following that system finally yielded ART (Fig. 1, **1**) though her preferred method to avoid heat-induced loss was to use ether as the extractant. Later work determined that of the six *Artemisia* species, only one, *Artemisia annua* actually contained ART. Inspection of the definitive structure of artemisinin showed why the group had very variable results, as the internal peroxide is a heat-labile group, and at above roughly 45 °C would decompose. Her 2016 Nobel lecture paper contained only 25 references, but the 2019 paper is much more inclusive with 145 up to date citations. Further information as to her role and others was published in 2017 by Liu (2017). This paper contains references to earlier work by Chinese investigators working with Professor Tu, that are not easily available to Western scientists, thus this paper is an excellent historical resource.

2.1 Artemisinin: Production via biochemical engineering

Once the compound established its superiority over the then conventional antimalarials, which were loosely based upon part of the structure of quinine, the requirement for large amounts became a major problem to overcome. Since the plant is slow growing and is destroyed by the then current extraction method, either very large plantations were required, which is what was done in the US under the auspices of the US Army, or methods to produce either the final compound or an intermediate were

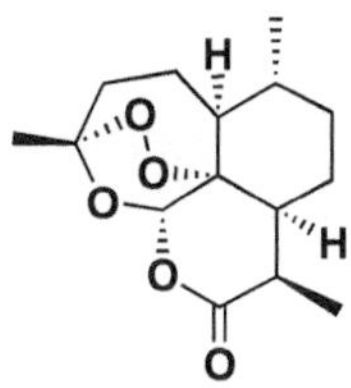

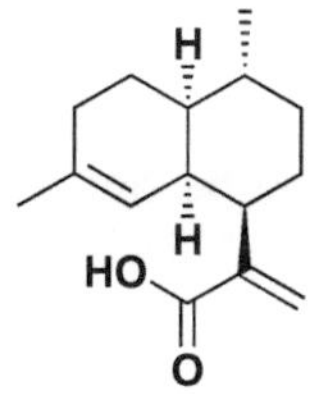

1. (+)-Artemisinin **2. Artemisinic Acid**

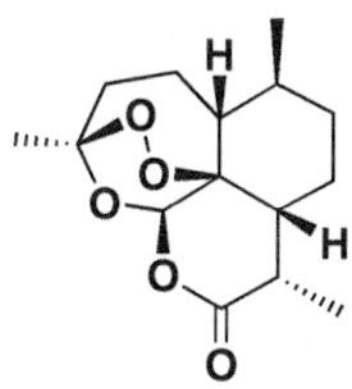

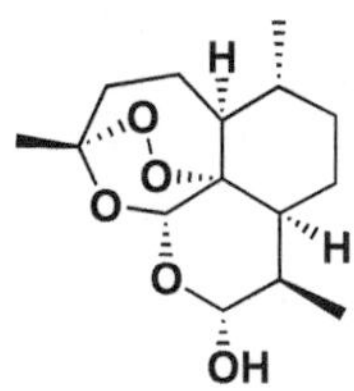

3. (-)-Artemisinin **4. Dhydroartemisinin**

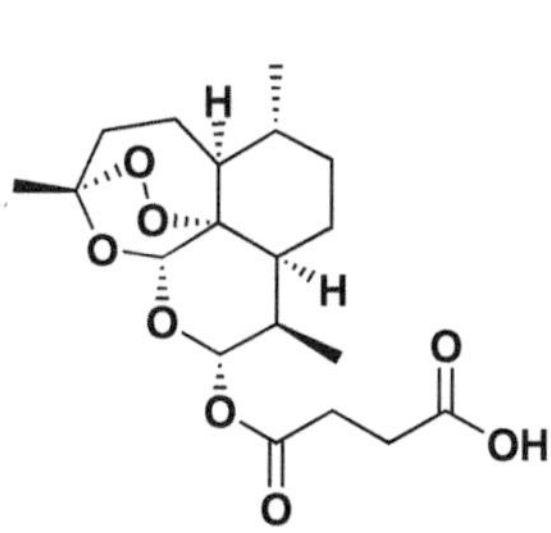

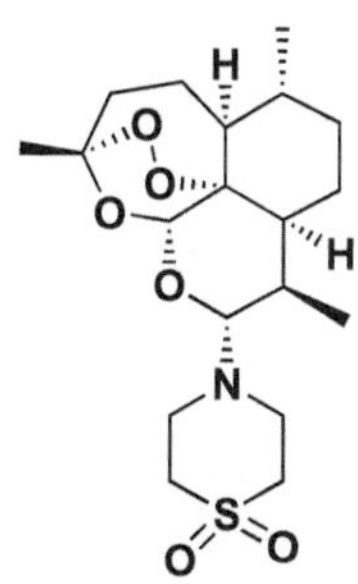

5. Artesunate **6. Artemisone**

Fig. 1 Artemisinin and derivatives.

necessary. To shorten a long story, in 2004 the Gates Foundation initially funded work by the Keasling group at Berkeley, and then its later spin-off, Amyris, continued the work, ending up with a process based on bio-engineered *Saccharomyces cerevisiae* to produce the essential intermediate artemisinic acid (Fig. 1, **2**) in large quantities and established a subsequent semi-synthetic process to produce ART. The method involved moving the necessary genes from *A. annua*, expressing them in a suitably prepared host and then developing the subsequent chemical conversion of artemisinic acid to ART (Paddon & Keasling, 2014; Paddon et al., 2013). The process was then licensed to Sanofi for large-scale production with the ultimate aim of reducing the cost to $1 US per dose for use mainly by WHO.

2.2 Properties of chemically modified artemisinin derivatives

2.2.1 Stereochemistry of artemisinin

Though this may appear to be out of sequence, modification of ART by groups in the West occurred almost from the beginning, as ART though active, had significant pharmacological flaws, particularly solubility. Since ART has stereochemistry, there was always the question at the back of a chemist's mind as to whether or not there was a stereospecific aspect to artemisinin's antiparasitic activity. The native molecule is the (+) antipode, so in order to determine if there is a stereospecificity in its antimalarial activity, the (−) antipode had to be synthesized *de novo* and then tested alongside its natural partner. Although there had been a number of synthetic routes to the (+) isomer, none had been reported on the (−) isomer (Fig. 1, **3**) prior to the 2018 paper by Krieger et al. (2018).

In this paper, the authors demonstrated that the antimalarial activity is independent of the stereochemistry, which is not the norm, as most interactions with protein targets are stereospecific and at times, the presence of the wrong antipode acts as an inhibitor of the desired interaction. They also make the point that artemisinin is reported by a number of authors to bind to a significant number of different plasmodial proteins, thus casting doubt upon the hypothesis that artemisinin bound only to a specific plasmodial protein. They also checked the activity of both antipodes against the *P. falciparum* parasite and within error the activities were identical.

When tested for cytotoxic activity against CCRF-CEM leukemia cells and adriamycin resistant CEM cells, in both cases the (+) antipode was approximately twice as active as the unnatural (−) antipode, though the SEM values did not overlap so these may be genuine but subtle differences, at least in the reported experiments. What is of import however, is that the synthetic steps yielding both the unnatural antipode and the natural antipode can be easily modified to produce previously unreported compounds which may well lead to molecules active against resistant parasites.

2.2.2 Artemisinin and derivatives activities in multiple diseases

2.2.2.1 Antitumor activities of first-generation derivatives

Before 2004, there was evidence that the metabolite dihydroartemisinin (DHA: Fig. 1, **4**) which had been synthesized by Tu, might be beneficial for the treatment of Lupus erythematosus-related nephritis, by inhibiting of the production of anti-ds-DNA antibodies, and concomitantly inhibiting the secretion of TNF-α and the NF-κB pathway (Li, Dong, Tu, & Lin, 2006). Though dated 2006, this work was almost certainly performed earlier, as mentioned by Efferth in a 2017 review (Efferth, 2017).

In his 2017 review, Efferth provided an excellent series of tables that show the published data up to the end of 2016 covering the effects of ART (Fig. 1, **1**), DHA (Fig. 1, **4**) and artesunate (Fig. 1, **5**) which was synthesized relatively early on to overcome some of the pharmaceutical problems with the pure natural product. These compounds cover a wide range of potential interactions with mammalian cancer cells including, but not limited to; oxidative stress, induction of DNA lesions, arrest of the cell cycle, inducing various modes of programmed cell death, antiangiogenesis and some interactions with signal-transduction processes.

As of the middle of July 2019, the NIH Clinical Trials database though having over 170 citations for "artemisinins" only 5 have any link to neoplasms, and four of these are at Phase I/II in the USA, China, Vietnam and the EU, but recruiting. Only one Phase I trial against metastatic breast cancer using artesunate (**5**) under NCT00764036 has completed and no results have been published, even though the trial started in 2008.

2.2.2.2 Activities of amino-artemisinin-derivatives

All of the first-generation artemisinins produced DHA (Fig. 1, **4**) as their first metabolite on treatment. However, if a molecule did not have an oxygen group at position C^{10} then this metabolite could be avoided. In 2006 Haynes et al. demonstrated that a very active antimalarial with an amino-substituted group at C^{10} was active *in vivo* and was given the name artemisone (Fig. 1, **6**) (Haynes et al., 2006). This compound was modified by use of a piperazine substituent (Fig. 2, **7**) and then used as the basis to produce the ferrocene-linked molecules (Fig. 2, **8–10**) which differ by the linkages to the ferrocene ring. These molecules showed excellent selectivity against the asexual blood stages of three *Pf* strains, one sensitive and two resistant, and demonstrated some selectivity when assayed against normal and tumor cells. The compounds still need refinement but aptly demonstrate that such molecules have potential (de Lange et al., 2018a, 2018b).

2.2.2.3 Artemisinin-based compounds with antiviral and antiparasitic activities

Although ART-based compounds demonstrated a variety of activities as mentioned above, the base molecule has a multiplicity of biological activities when chemically modified. These include activity against a variety of viruses, other parasitic diseases such as toxoplasmosis (Radke, Burrows, Goldberg, & Sibley, 2018) and their extension to mainly leukemias. There have been many variations on the base molecule and only a few will be alluded to in this review. Data up through early 2014 including an excellent chart of the levels of reports from 1980 through early 2013, was published by

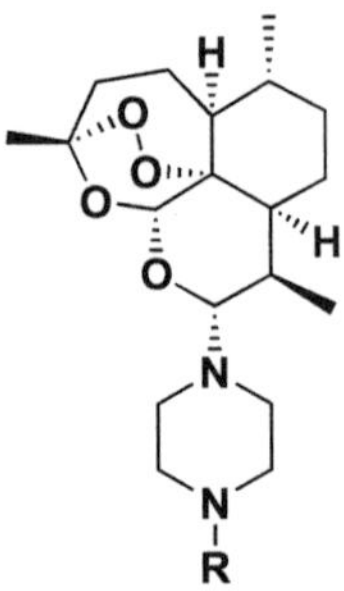

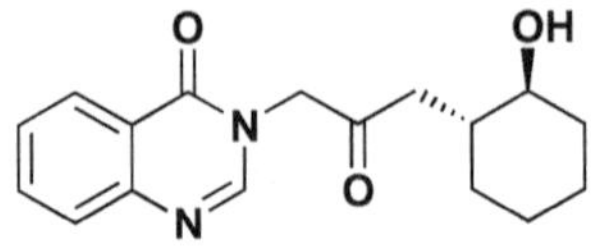

11. Febrifugine

7. Piperazine Base Compound, R = H

8. R = -CH_2-CH_2-CO-Fc
9. R = -CH_2-Fc
10. R = -CH_2-CH_2-CH2-Fc

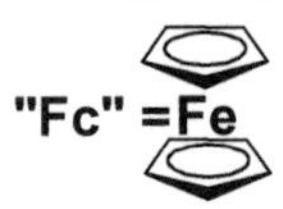

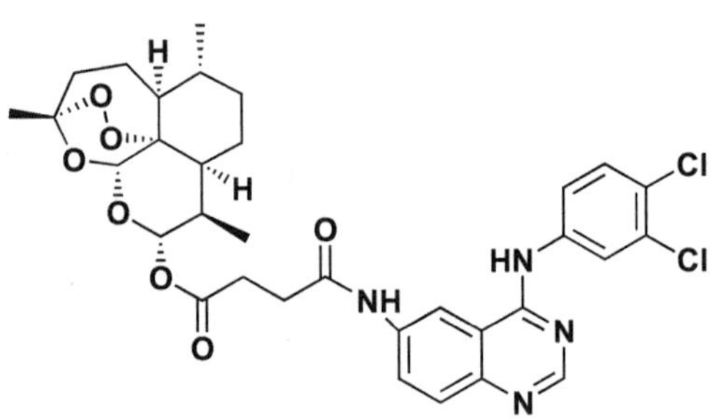

12

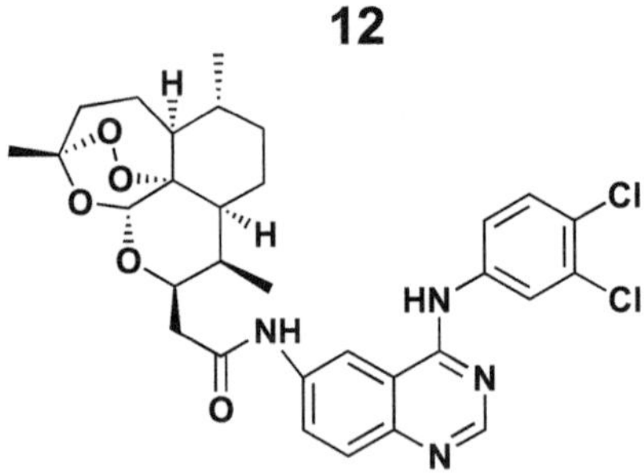

13

Fig. 2 Artemisinin derivatives with unusual substitutions and biological activities.

Ho et al. from the National University of Singapore in 2014 (Ho, Peh, Chan, & Wong, 2014). A chart close to the beginning of their paper, shows that approximately 30–40% of published reports from as early as 1982, extended into pharmacological areas other than antimalarials.

There is reasonable evidence from *in vitro* studies for the activity of ART and some of its derivatives against DNA viruses of the Herpesviridae and Hepadnaviridae families such as the cytomegaloviruses, including human herpesvirus 6, herpes simplex viruses 1 and 2, Epstein-Barr virus and Hepatitis B virus. However, with polyomaviruses and papilloma viruses the evidence for activity is somewhat weaker. Little to no *in vitro* inhibitory activity has been reported for RNA viruses such as HIV 1 and 2, hepatitis C virus, influenza virus. The 2018 review by Efferth (Efferth, 2018) contains tables showing the effects of the various "first-generation" ART derivatives, that should be consulted to see the results from these agents.

Recent papers that demonstrate how relatively simple modifications (dimers and trimers of artemisinin), or modifications to the first-generation agents by coupling to other potential pharmacophores, can extend their activities to antiviral targets are discussed in the following sections.

2.2.2.4 Artemisinin coupled to quinazoline

Quinazolines are fused six membered rings composed of benzene and pyrimidine can trace their origin as a bioactive agent to febrifugine (Fig. 2, **11**) a naturally occurring alkaloid which was reported close to 70 years ago from the Chinese plant "aseru" (*Dichroa febrifuga* Lour), which had been used as an antimalarial in TCM for over 2000 years under the name Ch'ang Shan (Koepfli, Mead, & Brockman, 1947; Kuehl, Spencer, & Folkers, 1948).

In a 2017 paper in the journal ACS Omega, Frolich et al. reported the syntheses and biological activities of a series of artemisinin-quinazoline hybrids based upon the core structure of febrifugine with different linkers to the same quinazoline derivative, giving constructs (Fig. 2, **12**, **13**) (Frohlich et al., 2017). These two constructs demonstrated excellent *in vitro* activities against the *P. falciparum* 3D7 parasite with compound **13** being superior, but against HCMV, their activities overlapped when the SEM values were taken into account. The differences in activity may relate to the different linkages used with the C^{10} acetal in (Fig. 2, **12**) being 30 times more active as an antimalarial than the C^{10} nonacetal-link in (Fig. 2, **13**). When tested against both wild type and doxorubicin resistant CRRF-CEM leukemia cells, (Fig. 2, **13**) demonstrated no significant activity, but in contrast, (Fig. 2, **12**) was comparable to artesunic acid (Fig. 1, **5**) which is the same molecule as artesunate.

2.2.2.5 Artemisinin dimers, trimers and dendrimers

An excellent recent paper by Frohlich et al. (2018) demonstrated the power of linking such molecules to rigid beads, then using these to "catch" the biological target(s), and subsequently identify the "captured protein(s)" by mass spectroscopic techniques. This is not a new technique as can be seen by reviewing the recent article by Laraia, Robke, and Waldmann (2018), but it is a very useful method to identify potential pharmacological targets of the chemical construct. In addition, the use of ART-based dimers and trimers with varying linkers between the molecules and their observed biological activities, which included significant activity against tumor cell lines, though often with very significant toxicity against normal cells, has been well described since the late 1990s.

Using excellent synthetic chemistry, the group produced a number of molecules, based on linkages to artenusic acid (Fig. 1, **5**). Of the 13 linked compounds, the dimer (Fig. 3, **14**) and the trimer (Fig. 3, **15**) and investigated their binding to proteins from total lysates of human fibroblasts infected with HCMV. Table 3 in their paper shows the multiplicity of both cellular proteins and HCMV related proteins that bound. Are these all primary targets? The initial experiments cannot tell at this point, but the process can be repeated with timed infection experiments to further identify the pathway(s).

2.2.2.6 Artemisinin derivatives coupled to thymoquinone, egonal and homoegonol

In a 2018 paper, Karagöz et al. (2018) from the same group as Frolich, linked the three natural products, thymoquinone (Fig. 3, **16**), egonal (Fig. 3, **17**), and homoegonal (Fig. 3, **18**), to ART derivatives, yielding a variety of compounds that were assayed against their usual targets, CCRF-CEM, its doxorubicin resistant companion (CEM/ADR), *P. falciparum* 3D7 in human erythrocytes and HCMV. When compared on a molar basis the hybrid of artesunic acid and egonal (Fig. 3, **19**) was four times more active against HCMV than either of its parts, even taking into account the doubling of molecular weight. However, against the other targets, none of the hybrids showed significant differences when compared to their individual components.

2.2.2.7 A relevant comment on interpretation of biological data in papers quoted

The data above brings up an important point when comparing results within biological assays. Using molar quantification rather than grams per

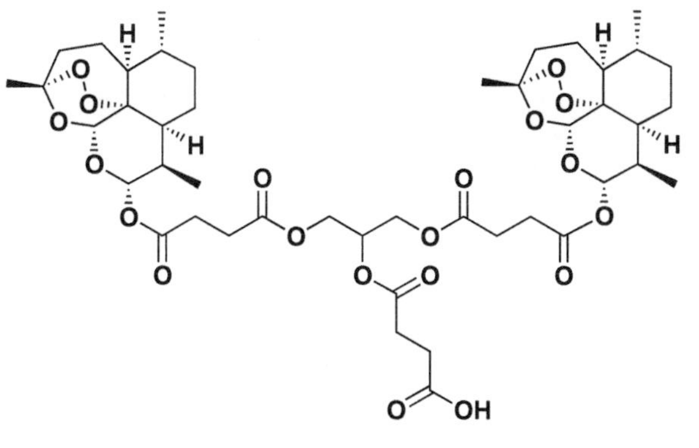

14

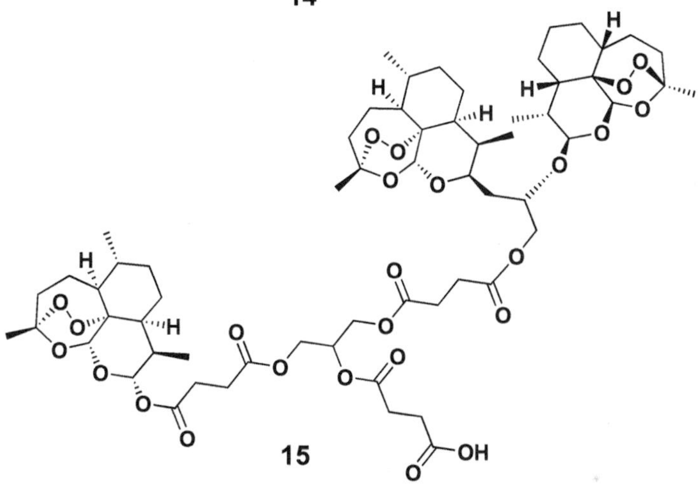

15

Fig. 3 Artemisinin dimers, trimers, and hybrid molecules with other natural products.

unit volume is ideal, as long as the individual molecular weights are also given in the table. In the paper by Karagöz et al. (2018) the hybrids were roughly twice the molecular weights of the individual components, thus comparable activities in molar units need to be taken into account. For example, if the hybrid's activity measured as the EC_{50}, is 10% that of the parental molecules, *i.e.*, parental 10 nM; hybrid 1 nM, then it is significantly more potent, but a control experiment where comparable quantities of both agents, but not linked are used in the same well, is needed for proper comparison. This may seem a minor point, but it is essential in being able to make a true comparison.

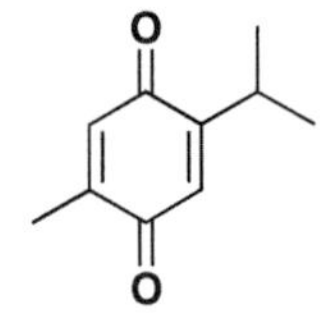

16. Thymoquinone

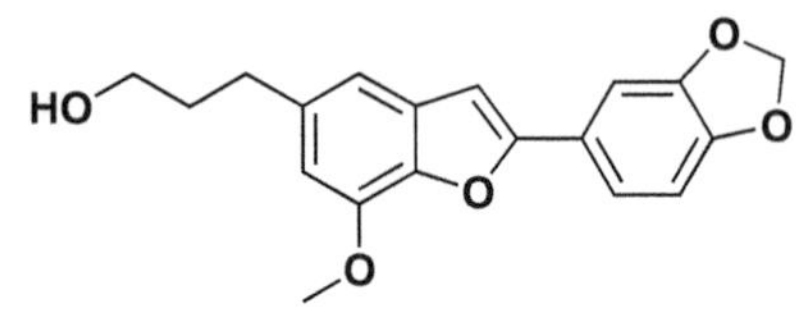

17. Egonal

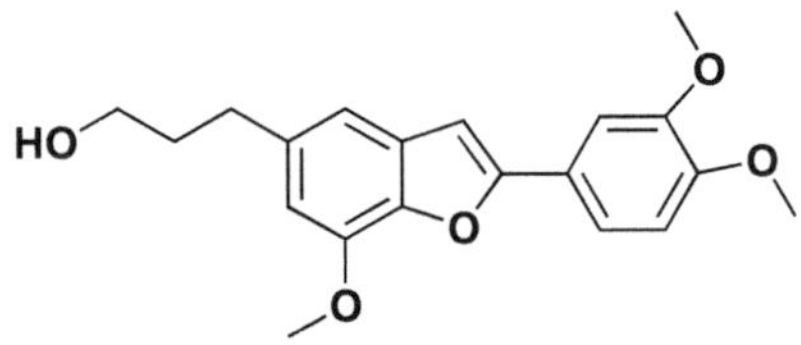

18. Homoegonal

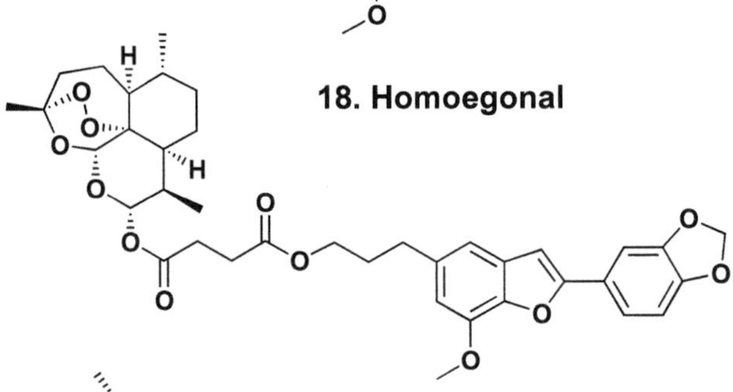

19. Artesunic acid-egonal hybrid

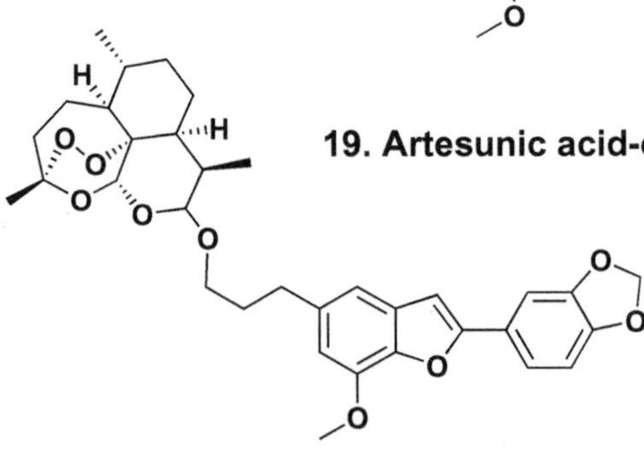

20. DHA-egonal hybrid

Fig. 3—cont'd

One good example of this is shown by the data for hybrid **20** (Fig. 3), which has DHA (Fig. 1, **4**) coupled to egonal (Fig. 3, **17**) *via* an ether-linkage. In this case, DHA is inactive and egonal's EC_{50} is 2380 nM against HCMV. In contrast, the standard for treatment, ganciclovir has an EC_{50} comparable to egonal whereas the hybrid **20** (Fig. 3) has an EC_{50} value of 170 nM or approximately 15 times more potent in the same assay.

2.2.2.8 HCMV-active artesunate-based drug candidates

Two papers from the same scientific group as those discussed above were recently published in the journal Antiviral Research. The first was one by Hahn et al. (2018) demonstrating syntheses of molecules related to the trimeric TF 27 (Fig. 4, **21**) that demonstrated excellent *in vitro* activity comparable to that of TF 27 (Fig. 4, **21**) with an EC_{50} value of 40 nM ±10 nM with low cytotoxicity when measured by an LDH release assay. However,

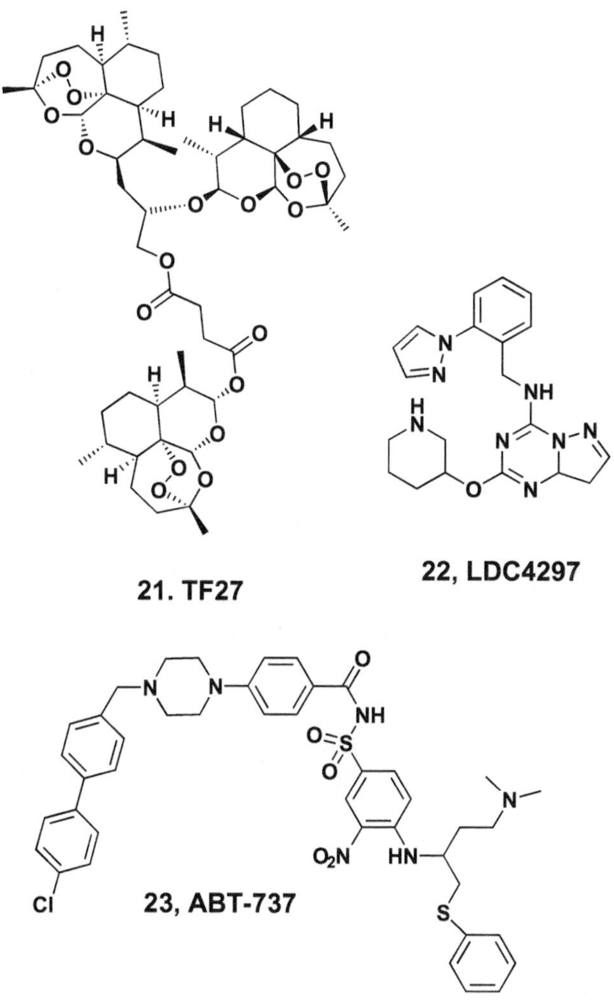

Fig. 4 Artemisinin derivatives and synthetic compounds based upon the trioxane pharmacophore.

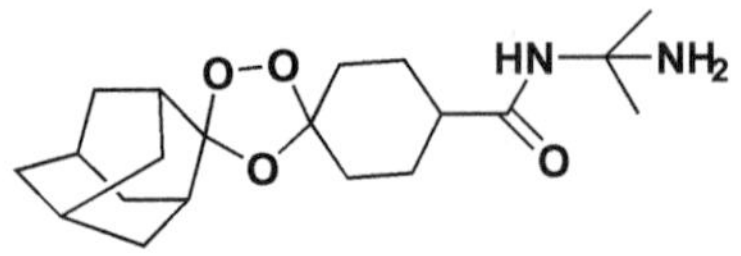

24. OZ277

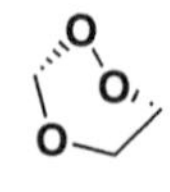

25. 1,4,4-Trioxane Pharmacophore

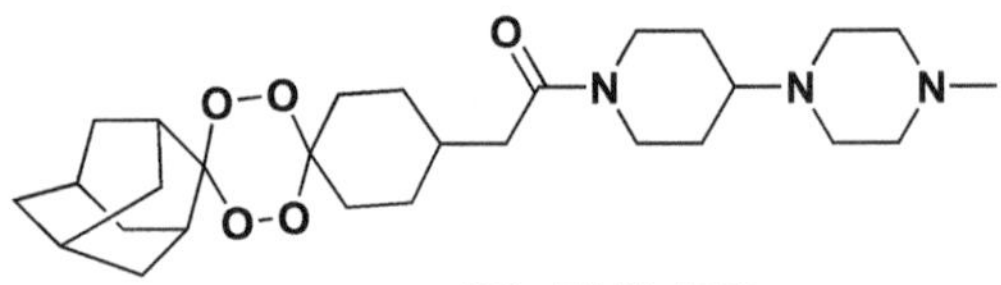

26. RKA182

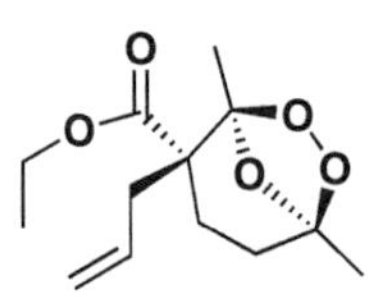

27

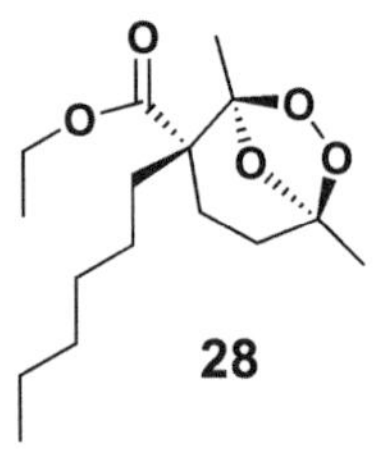

28

Fig. 4—cont'd

the later paper from the same group (Sonntag et al., 2019) demonstrated *in vivo* activity utilizing bioluminescence to quantify effects. What is of interest is that at the end of the experiment 7 days post-injection of the drug, no compound could be found in the plasma. This could well imply that the trimeric structure in TF 27 (Fig. 4, **21**) is broken down into active metabolites, in contrast to another drug, LDC4297 (Fig. 4, **22**) with a non-ART but pyrazolotriazine structure, did show the drug in the plasma compartment at the end of the experiment. The anti-cytomegaloviral activity *in vivo*, appeared to result from a restriction of the viral replication to the site of infection, thus preventing subsequent organ dissemination. In addition, the absence of any major compound-associated adverse effects is encouraging, though it should be emphasized that the experiment was only 7 days in length and was not designed to investigate delayed toxicity. However, as a start this is a very encouraging result. Another paper from the same group plus other collaborators was published in 2018 reporting the antileukemia activity of artesunate-based hybrids, that aptly demonstrated the potential for these hybrid molecules and is well worth consulting (Gruber et al., 2018).

2.2.2.9 BAD, a human target of artesunate

In a very recent paper, a group from Macquarie University in Australia, reported the identification by use of reverse chemical proteomics, of an unanticipated human target for artesunate (Gotsbacher et al., 2019). By using a phage expression system that permitted unbiased interrogation of several human cDNA libraries, displayed on a bacteriophage T7 vector, they demonstrated that probably the human target of artesunate was the cell death promoter BAD. Under the experimental conditions artesunate inhibited the phosphorylation of BAD, which then causes the formation of the proapoptotic BAD/Bcl-xL complex. The subsequent intrinsic apoptotic cascade involves cytochrome *c* release, PARP cleavage, subsequent caspase activation, and ultimately leads to cell death.

The unexpected role of BAD as a possible drug target of artesunate can be utilized for clinical exploitation of ART derivatives in the Bcl-xL life/death switch. The cytotoxicity of artesunate can be abrogated in HeLa cells if BAD is knocked down by siBAD (see Watts and Corey for a discussion of ways to prove specific interactions), which is suggestive that binding of artesunate is required for its apoptotic effect, and also suggests that its anticancer activity might well be independent of reactive oxygen species (Watts & Corey, 2012). If treated with ABT-737 (Fig. 4, **23**), a known BH3 mimic that binds to various components of the Bcl-cascade, demonstrated a synergistic activity in HeLa cells when artesunate was present. HeLa cells are constitutively resistant to ABT-737 due to high intrinsic levels of Mcl-1. Thus, previous experiments that invoked ferreptosis when cell lysates contained large amounts of free hemin, are not biochemically relevant as artesunate reacts with free hemin. This work now opens up a whole new area for studying the interactions of artemisinin-derived compounds with human cell lines.

2.3 Synthetic peroxy compounds that reverse treatment expectations

After the initial discovery of the peroxy bridge structure of artemisinin, in addition to exploring the features of this natural product, synthetic chemists also began to design and make potential compounds that had that particular motif or extended variations of it, as potential antimalarial agents. These led to a series of compounds, some like the trioxolane OZ277 (Fig. 4, **24**) were based upon the 1,2,4-trioxane pharmacophore (Fig. 4, **25**) in artemisinin, and others like RKA182 (Fig. 4, **26**) were based on a tetraoxane ring system.

In a 2018 paper Coghi et al. (2018) reported on their current work with such systems. They evaluated the *in vitro* antimalarial and antitumor activities on the human liver HepG2 and lung cancer A549 cell lines, of a set of peroxides that included bridged 1,2,4,5-tetraoxanes, bridged 1,2,4-trioxolanes, and tricyclic monoperoxides. The effects of all compounds were tested against *P. falciparum* 3D7 and effects against the non-tumor cell lines Hepatic LO2 and bronchial BEAS-2B lines were used as controls, together with the normal human fibroblast line CCD19Lu.

From studies involving 26 compounds split into 11 tetraoxanes, 6 trioxolanes (3 sets of stereoisomers) and 9 monoperoxides, with ART, artesunic acid, chloroquine and taxol as controls, the following compounds were emphasized. In the present work, synthetic ozonides were shown to have high cytotoxicity *in vitro* and selectivity, in particular ethyl (1*R*,2*R*,5*S*)-2-allyl-1,5-dimethyl-6,7,8-trioxabicyclo[3.2.1]octane-2carboxylate (Fig. 4, **27**) with a selectivity index of ~20, and ethyl (1*R*,2*S*,5*S*)-2-hexyl-1,5-dimethyl6,7,8-trioxabicyclo[3.2.1]octane-2-carboxylate (Fig. 4, **28**) with a selectivity index of 28 against the HepG2 cancer cell line compared to the LO2 cell line. In contrast, artesunic acid had a selectivity index of 0.3 against the same cell lines. From an antimalarial aspect all of the compounds tested were several orders of magnitude less active than the controls.

Although designed around what were thought to be active antimalarial pharmacophores from previously published data from a number of laboratories, these compounds turned out to be potential anticancer leads with IC_{50} values between 360 and 590 nM against HepG2.

3. Treatment of chronic myelogenous leukemia with Danggui Longhui Wan

This TCM treatment was originally composed of a mixture of plant components from 11 sources. Although the original references are not available to the author, the story is given in the introduction to the 1999 paper by Hoessel et al. (1999) noting that the original mixture contained a high level of the blue dye indigo (Fig. 5, **29**). The indigo was almost certainly from three of the components of the original 11, *Isatis indigotica* (Brassicaceae), *Indigofera suffrutticosa* (Fabaceae) and *Indigofera tinctoria* (Fabaceae. However, later work implicated that the active principle was the red colored isomer of indigo, indirubin (Fig. 5, **30**). Confusion can exist in the literature as the two compounds indirubin (isoindigotin or indigo red) and indigo (indigotin) are themselves produced from colorless intermediates. As shown in the Hoessel paper, there have been clinical trials of indirubin in China against leukemias with reportedly good results. A current search of the NIH NCT database lists only two trials of indirubin, under the name Couroupitine B. One in

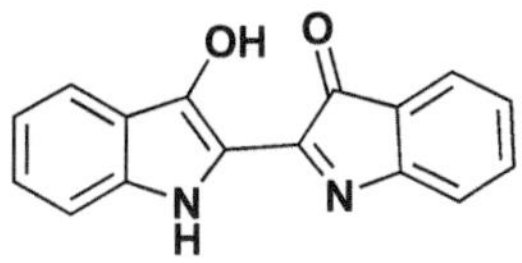

29. Indigo or Indigotin

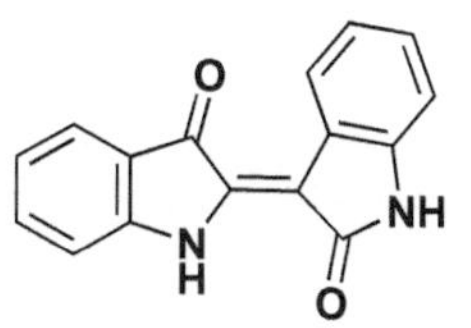

30. Indirubin

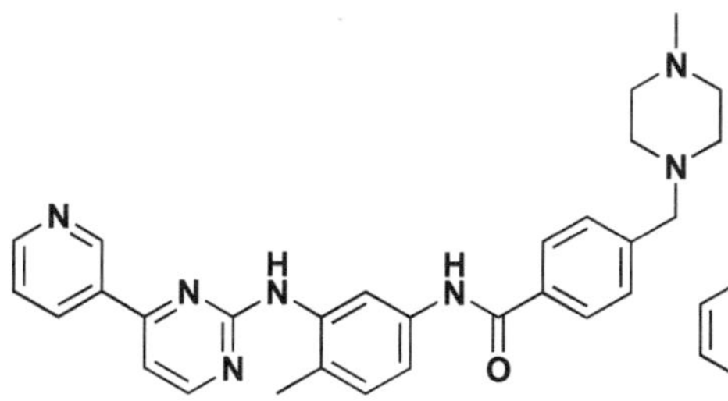

31. Gleevec or Imatinib

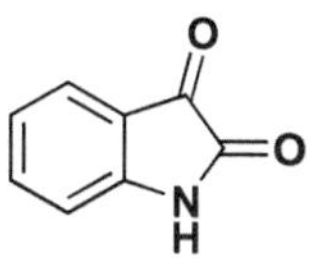

34 Isatin

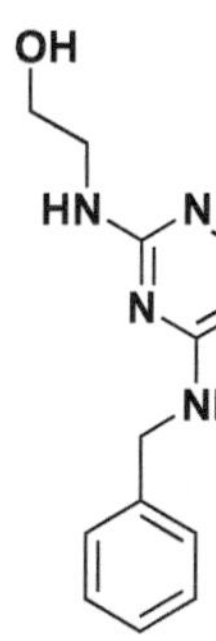

32. Olomoucine

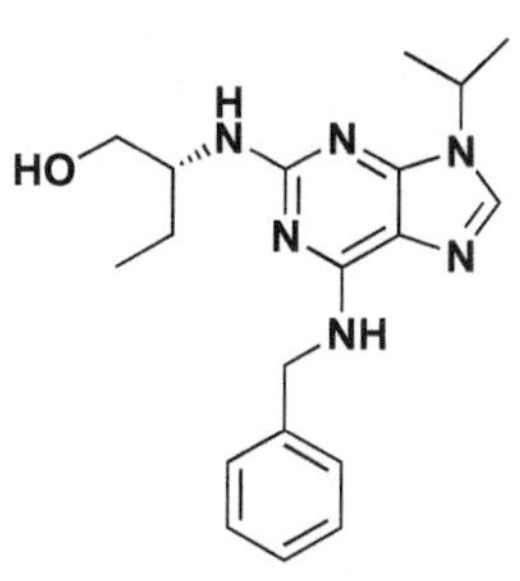

33. Roscovitine or Selicilib

Fig. 5 Indirubin and derivatives.

2012 and one currently recruiting, but these appear to be under the auspices of a group in Taiwan, investigating the compound as an oil extract of the plant for use in psoriasis. Some coverage before 2012 of the potential for indirubin treatment in this disease, is given in following sections.

3.1 Cellular targets of the indirubin(s)

While searching for antineoplastic compounds derived from TCM-related plants, Hoessel et al. (1999) discovered that simple indirubin derivatives and close analogs, selectively inhibited cyclin-dependent kinases in particular

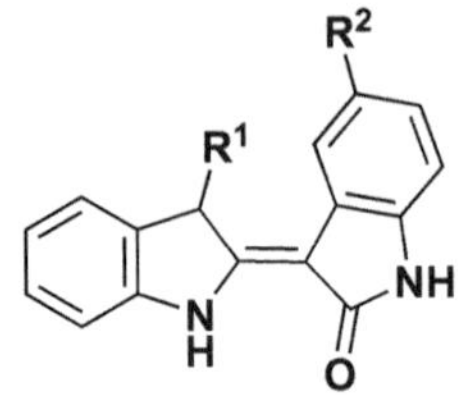

35. Indirubin-3'-monoxime. R^1 = NOH, R^2 = H aka "IO"
36. 5-Chloro-Indirubin. R^1 = O, R^2 = Cl
37. Indirubin-3'-monoxime. R^1 = O, R^2 = SO_3H

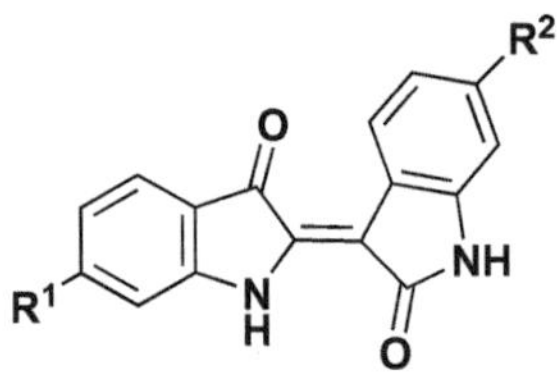

38. 6'-Bromo-indirubin, R^1 = Br, R^2 = H
39. 6-Bromo-indirubin, R^1 = H, R^2 = Br
40. 6,6'-Dibromo-Indirubin, R^1 = R^2 = Br

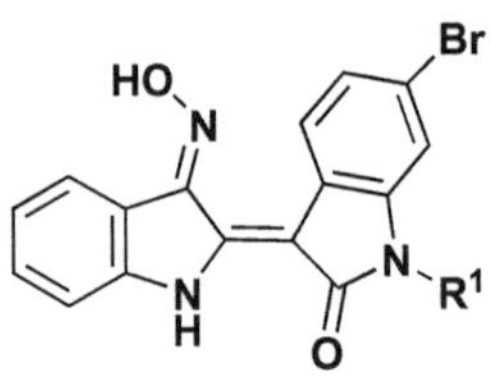

41. BIO, R^1 = H
42. MeBIO, R^1 = CH_3

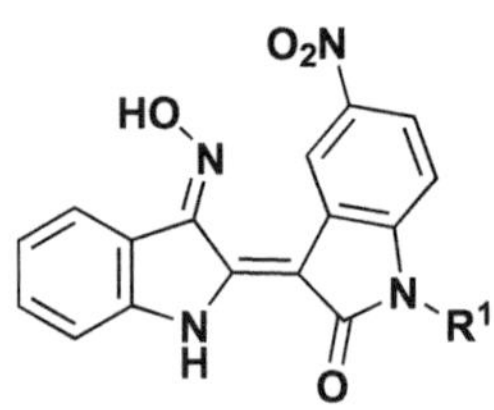

43.

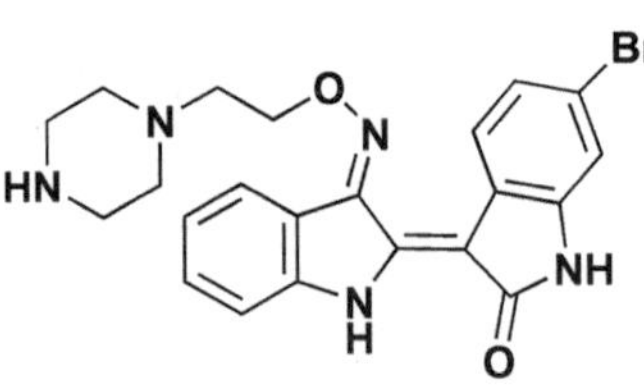

44. MLS-2384
Neutral form

Fig. 5—cont'd

CDK2. Such inhibitors were not only relevant for cancer, but also may well have activity in human diseases such as psoriasis, cardiovascular problems, glomerulonephritis, parasitism, viral infections and also neurodegenerative disorders. It should be emphasized that this work was being performed in the early days of investigations of kinase inhibitors as drug entities, with the first clinical PTK inhibitor, Gleevec (Fig. 5, **31**) being approved in 2001 by the US FDA. It should also be emphasized that the Meijer laboratory (Meijer being the lead author in the Hoessel paper), had been working on the CDKs using starfish as the source of these proteins for a number of years, and had identified active kinase inhibitors such as olomoucine (Fig. 5, **32**) (Vesely et al., 1994) and roscovitine (Fig. 5, **33**) (De Azevedo et al., 1997; Meijer et al., 1997) 2–5 years earlier.

Although the base indigo-related structures, indigo (Fig. 5, **29**), isatin (Fig. 5, **34**) and indirubin (Fig. 5, **30**) were effectively inactive against CDK1-cyclin B, three quite simple modifications of indirubin, the 3′-oxime (Fig. 5, **35**), 5-chloro (Fig. 5, **36**), and 5-sulfonic acid (Fig. 5, **37**), had IC_{50} values between 0.4 and 0.055 μM, which are comparable to roscovitine's value of 0.45 μM. Although the 5-sulfonate was slightly more active in terms of IC_{50} values, the antiproliferation activities showed that the 3′-oxime derivative "IO" (Fig. 5, **35**) was more active, possibly due to transport/solubility differences. What was also of significance, was that the 5′-sulfonate and 3′-oxime bound at the ATP site in CDK-2 when co-crystallized.

3.2 Further biochemical developments based on indirubin derivatives

3.2.1 Brominated derivatives from Tyrian purple

The work described above demonstrated that the basic chemical skeleton from these plant-sourced materials could be described as a potential "privileged structure" using the nomenclature pioneered by Evans et al. (1988). Four years after the Hoessel paper, the Meijer group demonstrated this. They reported the discovery of GSK-3 selective inhibitors derived from the indigo-indirubin-based dyes used over 2500 years ago as the Phoenician dyestuff, "Tyrian Purple." These inhibitors were isolated from this mixture, which was originally obtained from the Mediterranean gastropod mollusk, *Hexaplex trunculus,* but the compounds were later known from bacterial sources (Meijer et al., 2003).

These molecules were chemically similar to the indirubins reported above from plant sources. But in addition, had bromine substitution on the benzene ring portion of the molecule as shown (Fig. 5, **38–40**). The Meijer group then synthesized a variety of simple modifications, including two oxime derivatives, 6-bromoindirubin-3′-oxime (BIO, Fig. 5, **41**) a direct analog of the compound published in 1999 from TCM plants, (Hoessel et al., 1999) and its *N*-methylated counterpart 1-methyl-6-bromoindirubin-3′-oxime (MeBIO, Fig. 5, **42**) in addition to others.

When screened against CDK1/Cyclin B, CDK5/p25 and GSK-3 Kinase, both of the 3′-oxime derivatives (**IO**, Fig. 5, **35**; **BIO**, Fig. 5, **41**) demonstrated excellent activities with IC_{50} values against GSK-3 α/β being 5 nM for BIO and 22 nM for IO, with the corresponding 1-*N*-methylated derivatives being >40 μM. Similar nanomolar activities were seen for CDK1/Cyclin B and CDK5/p25 but in those assays the figures for IO and BIO were comparable but in the 83 to 320 nM range. By linking indirubin to a suitable linker in a pull-down experiment using a porcine brain lysate as a protein source, the bound protein was identified as GSK-3 by Western blotting and the bound protein was competed off by BIO. Following on from these *in vitro* studies, the effect(s) of BIO on *Xenopus laevis* embryos was investigated, and here it was shown that there was *in vivo* inhibition of GSK-3.

In 2017, Sklirou et al. published an interesting paper in Scientific Reports that demonstrated that BIO (Fig. 5, **41**) can activate cytoprotective cellular models. When human diploid fibroblasts from skin were exposed for significant lengths of time to this agent, there was a reduced oxidative load which could confer protection against oxidative stress-mediated DNA damage. There was also promotion of activation of the antioxidant and proteostatic modules. These effects were almost certainly due to inhibition of GSK-3, since the effects could be mimicked by genetic inhibition of GSK-3. BIO can thus be considered a novel activator of antioxidant responses in cells (Sklirou, Gaboriaud-Kolar, Papassideri, Skaltsounis, & Trougakos, 2017).

3.2.2 Inhibitors of DYRK1A based on BIO

This kinase, known as dual specificity, tyrosine phosphorylation regulated kinase 1A, is thought to play a key role in Alzheimer's disease and Down's syndrome. CDKs, GSK-3, CK1s, and DYRK1A are involved in the two key molecular features of Alzheimer's disease, production of amyloid-β peptides (extracellular plaques) and hyperphosphorylation of the microtubule-binding protein *Tau* (intracellular neurofibrillary tangles). Though from current knowledge, as early 2019, the direct involvement of plaque formation in Alzheimer's disease may not be as originally thought, due to the multiple failures of drugs designed to interdict such formation in man. However, this current opinion does not detract from the experimental data that will be shown.

Using data from earlier work, Meijer's group synthesized variations on the BIO structure (Fig. 5, **41**) including nitro-substituted variants and screened them *in vitro* against a series of kinases. From these studies, one compound (Fig. 5, **43**), with a 5-nitrogroup and a 3′oxime, which was effectively a modification of **IO** (Fig. 5, **36**) did show modest activity against DYRK1A but the activity against GSK-3 and other kinases were up to 2 orders of magnitude more sensitive. None demonstrated higher activity in antiproliferation assays against a variety of cells than that shown by roscovitine (Fig. 5, **33**) (Beauchard et al., 2009).

3.2.3 Antileukemia BIO-based agents

Although the use of Gleevec (imatinib) as the first line treatment of CML patients eclipsed the use of indirubin-based drugs at least in the West, there are still CML variants that are resistant to this agent due to specific mutations in the *Bcr-Abl* kinase domain, leading to the expression of the mutant protein T315I *Abl*. In this, the threonine is substituted by isoleucine at position 315. In a 2016 paper Gaboriaud-Kolar et al. (2016) reported the results from screening 95 analogs of BIO against two cell lines, KCL-22 and its corresponding T315I mutant line. In order to determine the most sensitive analogs, the initial concentration started at 1 μM. From both *in vitro* cell studies and also inhibition of individual kinases, the ethylpiperazine moiety in (Fig. 5, **44**) appeared to be a key substitution, giving comparable results against the two cell lines with IC_{50} values of 330 nM for WT and 430 nM for T315I. When tested against a battery of relevant isolated kinases, this compound was the only one of nine related compounds to inhibit all 6 kinases (*Abl*1, *Abl* T315I, *Aur* A, *c-Src*, *JAK*2 *GSK*-3) with IC_{50} values ranging from 0.5 to 9 nM for 5 of the kinases, and 234 nM for *JAK*2. The other compounds tested were between 10 and 1000 times less active depending upon the particular kinase, but in every case, this construct was the compound with the lowest IC_{50}. Only in the case of *Aur*A was there a compound with a similar potency.

Docking studies were performed using available geometries for three binding modes with the T315I mutant structure. The closest fit was one similar to the *Src*-like inactive *Abl* structure. This gave a computerized fit that corresponded with the observed activities, in contrast to the other two models considered. This compound together with others that may be developed from its basic structure, when explored on an experimental basis, may lead to the development of inhibitors rationally targeting specific resistant mutants of this kinase that will be based on the bis-indole scaffold of this compound (Fig. 5, **44**). This may lead to a new molecular class of agents targeting the T315I mutant *Bcr-Abl* in imatinib-resistant CML.

3.3 Structures beyond the basic indirubins

3.3.1 Search for DYRK-specific inhibitors

From earlier work on DYRK kinases, in particular DYRK2, it was known that the ATP-binding pockets of CLK1 and DYRK1A are similar in terms of both amino acid sequence and their nominal surface shape. In both, the gatekeeper residue leading to the binding site is a phenylalanine, plus the three following amino acids are either identical in terms of the next after phenylalanine, or similar, with the third being leucine in CLK1 and methionine in DYRK1A (Walter et al., 2018).

Given the structural similarity of the two kinase families, the *de novo* design of specific inhibitors of the ATP-binding pocket would be difficult, but using accumulated information from earlier work with indirubins and topographically similar heterocyclic compounds, the dihydropyrrolo[3,4-*g*]indol-8(1*H*)-ones such as (Fig. 6, **45**), which contain a pyrrole connected to a γ-butyrolactam ring *via* a double bond, is related chemically to the GSK/CDK inhibitor indirubin (Fig. 5, **30**).

Using multiple *in vitro* assays in both isolated kinase preparations and in the NCI 60 cell line, a series of compounds that demonstrated very good activity against the CLK series in the submicromolar range (Fig. 6, **46**) without any activity at the highest level tested (10 μm) against the DYRK series. A close relative, with a hydroxy substituent in place of the chlorine (Fig. 6, **47**) demonstrated activity at submicromolar levels against most of the kinases tested, though none were found to be only DYRK active.

3.3.2 Combination of indirubin and podophyllotoxin

A recent paper from Wang, Long, Chen, Xu, and Zhang (2018) reported on an interesting series of compounds where podophyllotoxin (Fig. 6, **48**) was linked to one of the nitrogen atoms in indirubin, *via* a series of methylene spacers as shown in structures (Fig. 6, **49–52**). These compounds were then tested *in vitro* against two chronic CML cell lines K562 and its vincristine-resistant line, K562/VCR. When tested, the compound with the shortest linker (Fig. 6, **49**) was the most active against both lines with IC_{50} values of 34 nM against the WT *versus* 76 nM against the resistant strain with the ratio being 2.23. This construct was significantly more active than etoposide

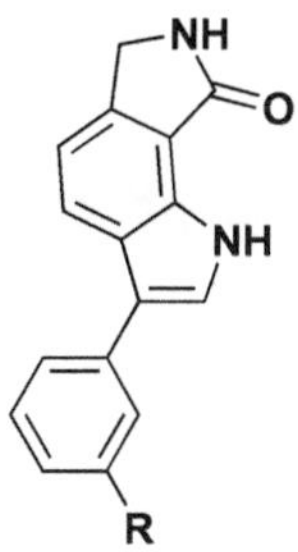

45. R = H
46. R = Cl
47. R = OH

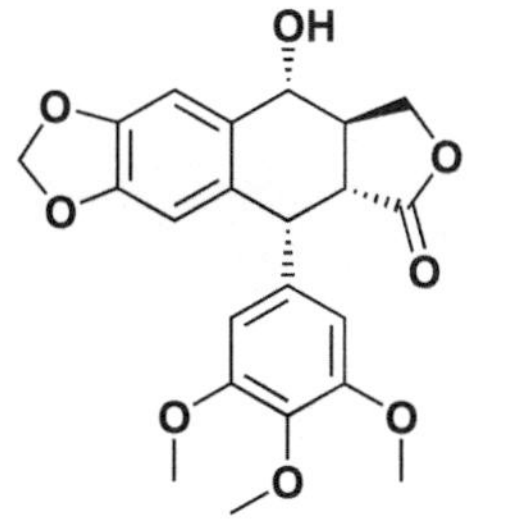

48. Podophyllotoxin

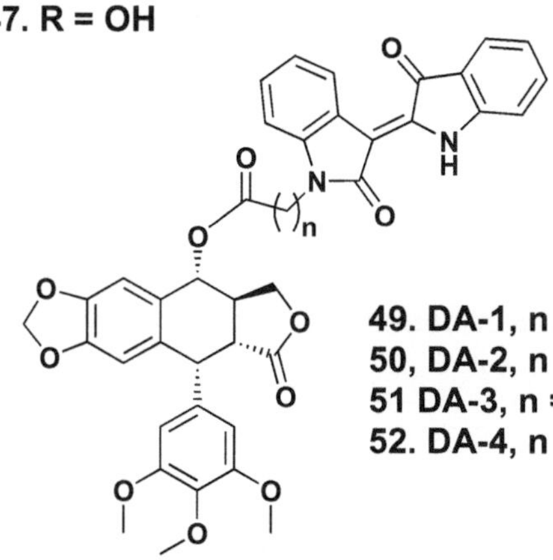

49. DA-1, n = 1
50, DA-2, n = 2
51 DA-3, n = 3
52. DA-4, n = 4

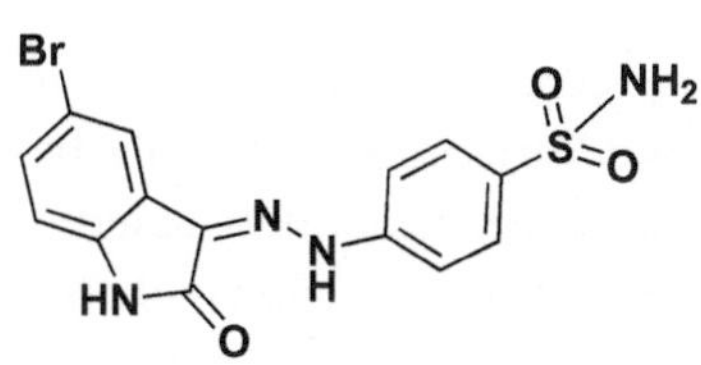

53

Fig. 6 Indirubin-related and other natural product-related kinase inhibitors.

or vincristine but was less active than the parent podophyllotoxin, and indirubin had no activity at the concentrations used. Though it appeared to have the same nominal activity, when cell cycle studies were performed, there were significant differences in the profiles. There were also indications that apoptosis was increased on treatment in the vincristine-resistant cells and that the construct interacted with tubulin in a somewhat different manner to podophyllotoxin itself.

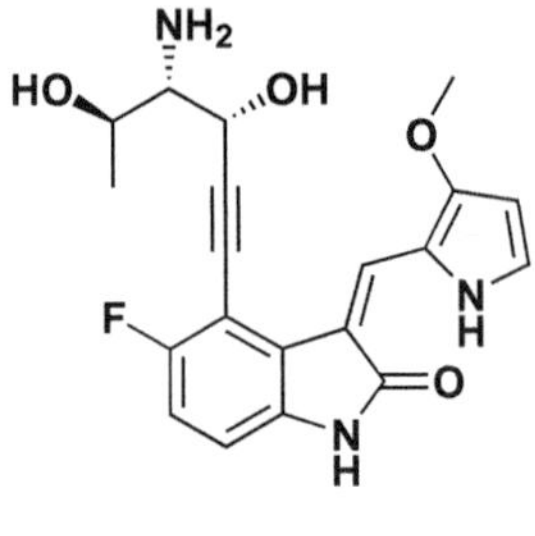

54

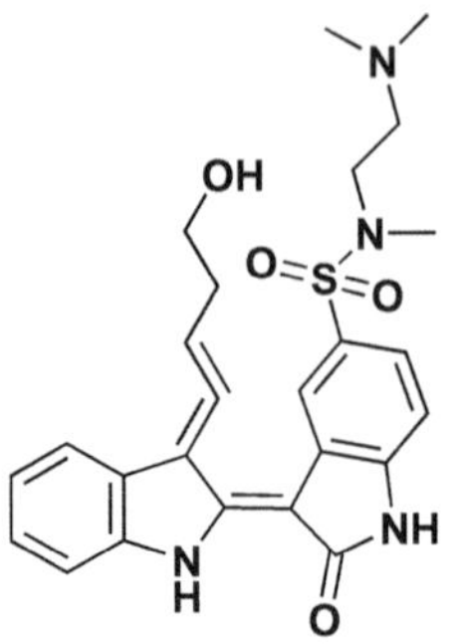

55

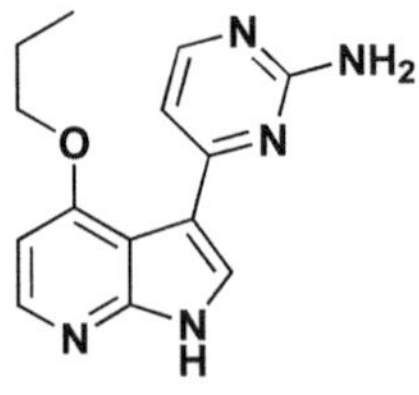

57, Meridianin-based

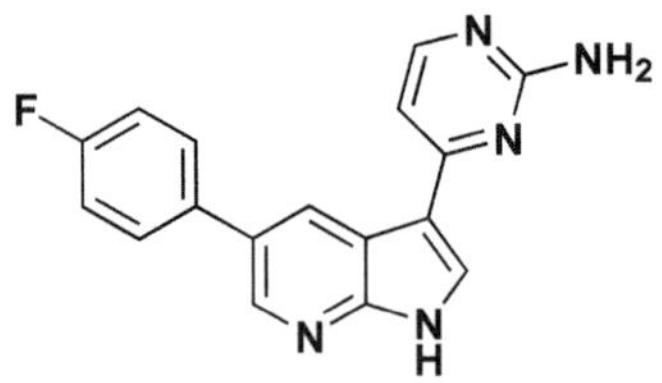

58. Variolin-based

Fig. 6—cont'd

3.3.3 A 2019 update on CDK 2 inhibitors

A very recent paper by Tadesse, Caldon, Tilley, and Wang (2019) brings up to date data on the various structures that can inhibit CDK2 and other CDKs. Among the core pharmacophores discussed is a short but excellent discussion of two variations on indole-based CDK2 inhibitors. The first series, showing three structures based on indirubin (Fig. 6, **53–55**), have IC_{50} values of 60, 3, and 40 nM, respectively, against CDK2, and the second set, based on other marine natural products, the meridianins and variolins, led to (Fig. 6, **57** and **58**) with IC_{50} values of 3 and 5.5 nM, respectively.

3.4 Final comments on the indirubins

The initial data from TCM and the Phoenicians has led to novel series of molecules that though currently not in clinical trials as pure compounds, have led to a much deeper understanding of how such molecules interact with cellular targets. It should be noted that effectively all of results of these early studies were first seen in phenotypic screens, be they in man from TCM, or in cell lines or by following cell cycling in starfish.

In addition to the results discussed above, very recently a review was published by Varun et al. covering syntheses around the simpler molecule, isatin (Fig. 5, **34**), that demonstrated multiple activities, both pharmacological and industrial linked to derivatives of this simple molecule, that were not covered above as they did not come from either TCM or other medicinal systems (Varun, Sonam, & Kakkar, 2019).

Though the paper by Zhou et al. (2018) may seem to be out of contextual order, it was inserted here rather than in the later section on systems biology and metabolomics, as it appears to be unusual in that the targets of the indirubins and their role in potential treatment of specific leukemias were initially described as shown in the above sections in the late 1990s. This paper effectively gave the same results as described earlier in this section, and therefore it is listed for completeness.

It must be pointed out that it cannot be determined from the paper if the results were simply force-fitting from already known and well described data, or was it intended to be thought of as an exemplar of a nominally new technique? Due to lack of evidence either way, no further discussion of the results from this paper will be made.

4. Use of arsenic compounds in TCM and old and current western medicine

Perhaps the first notification of the use of arsenicals in TCM dates from roughly 200 BCE, with the publication of *Shennong Bencaojing* which extensively covered the usages of arsenic compounds at that time (from reference 12 in Hoonjan, Jadhav, and Bhatt, 2018). However, Hippocrates over 200 years earlier had published the use of sulfides of arsenic, realgar or As_4S_4, to treat abscesses and topical ulcers, with contemporary usage under the Indian Ayurvedic medical system. There is an excellent table in Hoonjan et al.'s, 2018 paper (Hoonjan et al., 2018) that shows the usage of arsenicals as medicine (not poisons), from ~200 BCE to date, and what is very interesting, is that similar treatments for similar diseases appeared to be "in fashion" in both the East and the West at similar times. Since the Ayurvedic system was well known in the Middle East, there is a possibility that there was unrecognized, or perhaps it might be better to say, "undocumented" interactions among the various plant/mineral based treatment systems in the middle ages (~900–1500 CE).

The first real notice of arsenic by the public as what might be considered a true compound as a drug entity, though not from a plant source, would be the discovery of compound 606 or salvarsan (Fig. 7, **59**) for the treatment of syphilis. The structure of this compound was published as a bis-arsenic compound with a double bond between the two "As" atoms. It was often postulated that the actual active species was not the compound as written. In 2005, a New Zealand group synthesized salvarsan and investigated its structure by electrospray ionization mass spectroscopy, proving that the compound was actually a mixture of cyclic species with one ring being a triplet of As atoms and the other a quintet of As atoms (Fig. 7, **60**)

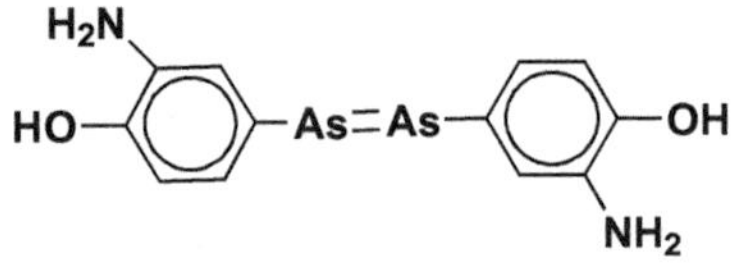

59. Salvarsan

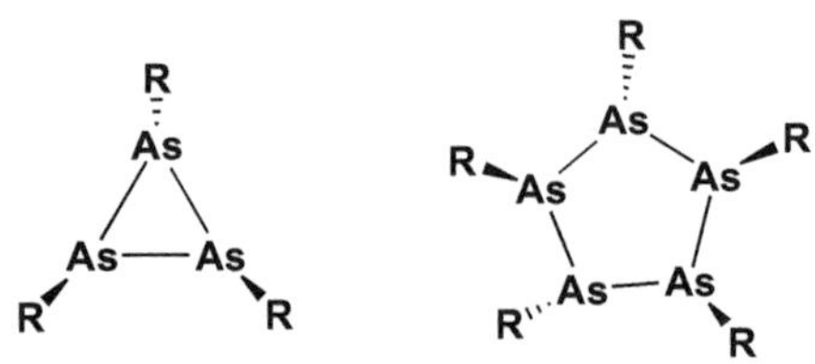

60. Salvarsan Revised 2005,

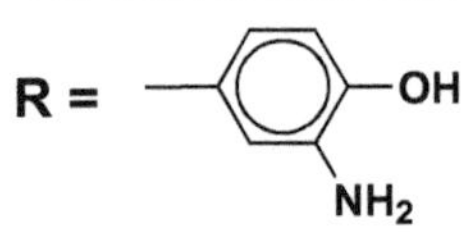

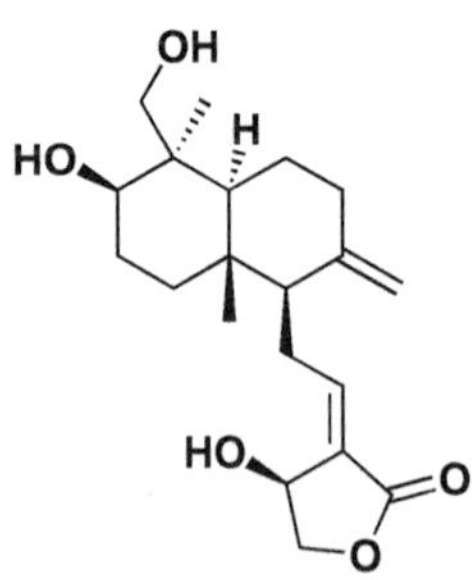

61. Andrographolide

Fig. 7 Arsenicals and natural product "modulators" of their activities.

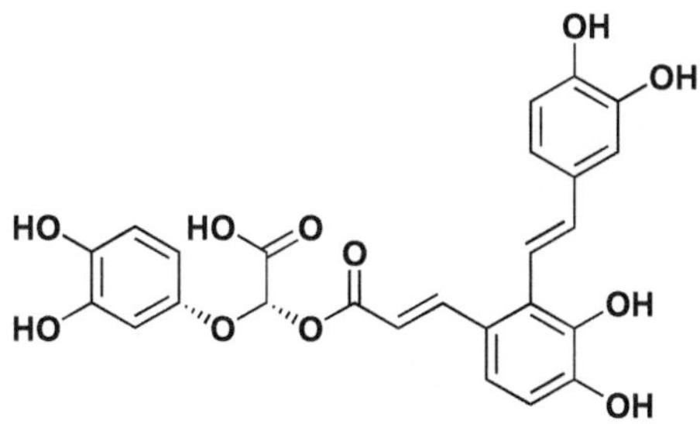

62. Salvianolic Acid A

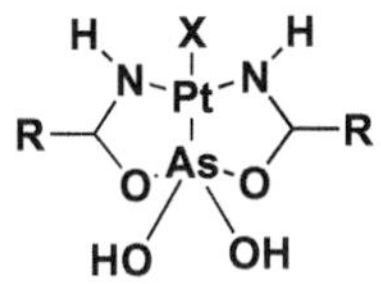

63. AP-1, R = CH_3, X = $Cl^{\ominus}$
64. AP-2, R = CH_2CH_3, X = $Cl^{\ominus}$

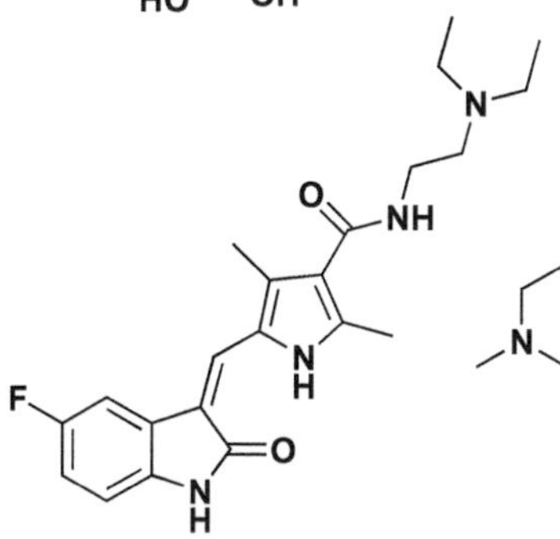

65. Sunitinib

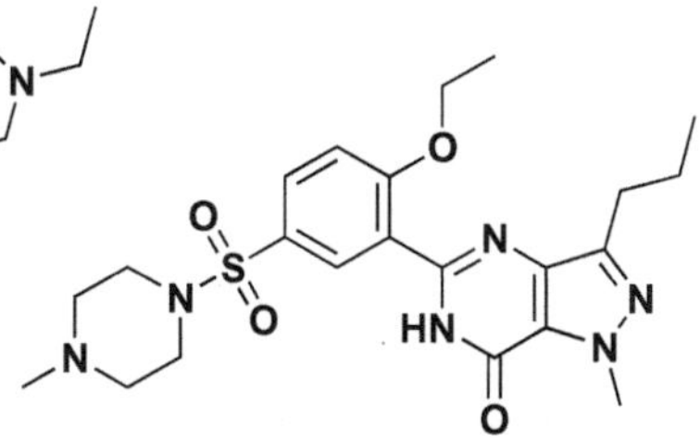

66. Sildenafil

Fig. 7—cont'd

(Lloyd, Morgan, Nicholson, & Ronimus, 2005). A less chemical description was given by Yarnell in the American Chemical Society's Chemical and Engineering News in 2005 (volume 83, issue 25) as part of a special issue on "Pharmaceuticals that Changed the World."

4.1 Arsenic trioxide (trisenox)

In 1878 there was a report that Fowler's solution (potassium arsenite) reduced white cells in normal blood and significantly reduced the white cell level in a leukemia patient (Cutler & Bradford, 1878). In the 1930s there were sporadic reports of the use of arsenic trioxide in the treatment of leukemias in the USA, (Forkner & Scott, 1931) together with a later report of arsenical poisoning in some patients (Kandel & LeRoy, 1937). Thus this treatment modality was shelved in the USA.

However, in contrast, a long tradition of the use of arsenicals in TCM led to the introduction of "Ailing-1," a solution of crude As_2O_3 and herbal extracts for the treatment of patients with APL, which is the M3 subtype of AML. Today a major difference in treatment modalities is that AML treatments usually include chemotherapeutic drugs such as cytarabine, plus an anthracycline such as idarubicin. In contrast, modern treatment of APL includes all trans retinoic acid and arsenic trioxide.

Following an initial clinical trial with As_2O_3 at the Harbin Medical College in the PRC, a larger controlled trial at the Shanghai Second Medical University documented very good clinical efficacy in patients with both freshly diagnosed APL and also relapsed APL (Niu et al., 1999; Shen et al., 1997). The effects of this agent were not lost on the rest of the world, with the compound being approved for APL treatment by the US FDA in 2000. A short history up through 2000 was published by Waxman and Anderson in 2001 that makes interesting reading (Waxman & Anderson, 2001).

A recent paper from Hong Kong gave data on long-term remission of APL patients after trisenox therapy, with an almost 60% 10-year survival rate. Checking the NIH clinical trials database at the end of May 2019, there are 24 active trials at the recruiting or active stage, including 10 that are in the PRC with two of these being Phase 3 trials, plus a significant number at Phase 2. One covers modifications of the treatment for APL and myelodysplastic syndrome (Phase 3 trial NCT03377725 at Ruijin Hospital in Shanghai), and another is the trial using Realgar-*Indigo naturalis* for APL treatment that has a trisenox arm, under the Phase 3 trial NCT 02899169 at the First Affiliated Hospital of Xi'an Jiaotong University.

4.1.1 Combination of natural products with trisenox treatment

Two recent papers have demonstrated enhancement of the antitumor effects of trisenox in leukemias and on hepatocellular carcinoma, a major disease in China. In a 2017 report in Oncotarget, Duan et al. (2017) demonstrated that andrographolide (Fig. 7, **61**), a plant-derived natural product from the traditional medicinal herb *Andrographis paniculata* Nees (transliterated name being Chuan Xin Lian from data in Yan, Zhou, & Xie, 1999) which was reported to exhibit several pharmacological effects, demonstrated synergistic effects in both *in vitro* and *in vivo* studies in murine models utilizing HepG2 cells. Initial *in vitro* studies in HepG2 sells demonstrated that andrographolide synergistically increased As_2O_3-induced apoptosis in HepG2 cells in a caspase-dependent manner.

These studies were followed up by determining the expression levels of 37 genes under various related conditions and demonstrated that the level of EphB4 decreased under treatment with the combination, indicating that the EphB4 level was influenced by the synergy between andrographolide and As_2O_3. EphB4 is a member of the receptor tyrosine kinase family, but other studies in HCC have shown variable relationships between expression level and apoptosis. On performing similar experiments *in vivo* in suitable murine hosts with the same cell line, definitive reductions in tumor weight were demonstrated together with reduction in expression of EphB4 in the treated groups, and using the TUNEL assay technique, greater apoptosis was shown with the combination in the *in vivo* studies. Even bearing in mind the caveat on the relationship of expression of EphB4 mentioned above, this is an excellent example of well-controlled studies opening up novel areas for future work.

A report in 2018 by Zhang et al. (2018) extended the use of another TCM component salvianolic acid A (Fig. 7, **62**) to address the cardiac side effects of As_2O_3. *Salviae miltiorrhizae* (Danshen) is a frequently used TCM remedy and is believed to have effects on cardiovascular diseases (Yan, Jiang, Bi, Yang, & Chen, 2015). Salvianolic acids were reported to exhibit potent antioxidative capabilities due to their polyphenolic structure (Wang, Liu, Meng, & Lin, 2012), with Sal A (Fig. 7, **62**) reported to be the most potent antioxidant of the series (Zhang et al., 2011).

Zhang et al. determined the effects of As_2O_3 and/or Sal A in H9c2 cardiomyocytes *in vitro*, demonstrating the cascade of deleterious effects that occurred following treatment with As_2O_3. These included induced structural damage to mitochondria, abnormal permeability transition pore (mPTP) opening in the mitochondria, overproduction of ROS, and concomitantly decrease in the ATP content. Pretreatment with Sal A alleviated the As_2O_3 induced mitochondrial damage. Extending the combination treatment to other cell lines *in vitro* including SGC7901, HepRG, K562 and HL60 cells, increased (*i.e.*, decreased the IC_{50} values) the cytotoxicity of As_2O_3. The results imply that Sal A may protect the heart from the side effects of As_2O_3 treatment, though as yet no *in vivo* studies have been reported using this combination.

4.1.2 Network pharmacology with trisenox

The paper by Dawood, Hamdoun, and Efferth (2018) extended the investigation into the pharmacology of As_2O_3 by utilizing a combination of classical pharmacology and coupled studies to utilize "Network Pharmacology." An excellent presentation of the basis behind network pharmacology was given by Rask-Andersen et al. in 2011 using examples from known drugs (Rask-Andersen, Almen, & Schioth, 2011), with a short discussion of the earlier days by Ainsworth the same year (Ainsworth, 2011). Although there will be a later section covering such usages with TCM "mixtures" toward the end of this review, the Dawood et al. paper gives a relevant demonstration of what can be done just looking at one compound.

This paper is a complex one and various aspects deserve to be discussed but readers should peruse the paper themselves, to better understand how data from the NCI 60 cell line screen, the cancer genome project and many of the tools derived by NCI from both of these major projects, have enabled researchers to both pose questions at a molecular level, and then gain further insight from the results of statistical and network techniques. One of the major messages from this paper is best expressed by quoting directly from some of the authors' conclusions.

> *In the case of As_2O_3, we found several major functional groups using manual curated network analysis to be involved in cellular responsiveness to the drug, i.e., oxidative stress response, DNA repair, regulation of cell cycle/proliferation, signal transduction, drug transporter, cytoskeletal elements, tumor suppressors/oncogenes, metabolic pathways, and apoptosis. On the other hand, we found many other important pathways using IPA network analysis, e.g., molecular mechanisms of cancer, axonal guidance signaling, signaling by Rho family GTPases, protein kinase A signaling, phospholipase signaling, actin cytoskeleton signaling etc. The manually curated and the IPA approaches revealed comparable findings.*

Then from the neurotoxic aspect the authors stated. "Moreover, axonal guidance signaling, neuroregulin signaling and agrin interaction at neuromuscular junction pathways may demonstrate the neurotoxicity of As_2O_3." This last point is an interesting finding, since neurotoxicity is a known problem from arsenic treatment.

4.1.3 Clinical trials with trisenox

An interesting aspect of the work with trisenox is whether or not its antitumor activity can be extended to solid tumors. As mentioned by Hoonjan et al. in their 2018 review (Hoonjan et al., 2018), there have been a significant number of reports of *in vitro* studies where it induces apoptosis in both small cell and non-small cell lung cancer lines, in particular showing a relationship with levels of anoxia. With breast cancer lines such as MDA-MB-231, MCF-7, T47D and BT-20 earlier reports referenced by Hoonjan et al. (2018) demonstrated apoptosis.

Consulting the NIH's database of reported clinical trials using trisenox as the drug, and looking for all reported trials irrespective of status, currently there are 128 records. Among these are some relatively recent trials at the Phase 2 level including one, NCT02956772, that is investigating its effect in primary hepatocellular carcinoma with 190 patients. It is currently listed as not yet recruiting and is being performed in Guizhou Cancer Hospital in the PRC, with no information after early February 2017. In 2015, a report was published by Wang et al. on the use of trisenox plus TACE surgical treatment for hepatocellular carcinoma (Wang et al., 2015), which was the report of the ChiCTR-TRC-13004547 trial, and demonstrated a significant increase in a therapeutic response in the cohort that had trisenox plus TACE.

A number of trials listed had only abstracts published, and in general, one needs to wait anywhere up to five to 6 years for more detailed discussions of results from trials. Until recently, negative trial results were usually not published, but then the NIH changed their rules on clinical trial data, in that now they require data on both successful and unsuccessful human trials to be published. To date only relatively few pharmaceutical companies (who sponsor the majority of such trials) have begun to comply. Thus, it appears that careful use of this agent may well extend its utility well beyond APL and related hematological cancers.

4.2 Realgar or As_4S_4

This compound has almost as long a history as trisenox in TCM and similarly has efficacy in the treatment of APL (Liu, Lu, Wu, Goyer, & Waalkes, 2008; Lu et al., 2002). Three arsenicals, two of which contain sulfides of arsenic and one that contains the trioxide are known in TCM; orpiment (As_2S_3), realgar (As_4S_4), and arsenolite (contains arsenic trioxide, As_2O_3, discussed earlier). Realgar was frequently included as an ingredient in oral TCM mixtures for its antipyretic, anti-inflammatory, antiulcer, anti-convulsive, and anti-schistosomiasis actions, but the pharmacological basis for such an inclusion has not been be fully justified.

In 2018, Wang et al. published an interesting article (Wang et al., 2018) demonstrating that by treating realgar with acidophilic bacteria, they obtained what they have named "realgar transforming solution or RTS," where the active ingredient is inorganic trivalent arsenic, though they reported a significant number of other inorganic entities related to arsenic in the mixture. By using the K562 WT cell line and its Adriamycin-resistant mutant line, K562/ADR, they demonstrated that RTS strongly induced apoptosis in both cell lines, plus there was induction of autophagy at much lower doses of RTS (measured as As III) than from using realgar or trisenox. Thus, they consider that their RTS is a viable option for treatment. It certainly produces a more soluble form than the regular involved treatment methodologies, but no data is currently available comparing the actual inorganic components in these cases.

4.3 An inorganic dual pharmacophore anticancer agent

Unlike the serendipitous discovery of the antitumor activities of the platinates, recently a group composed of both American and Italian inorganic chemists, published a very interesting paper in the Journal of the American Chemical Society, reporting the synthesis of two closely related compounds that they have named arsenoplatins (Fig. 7, **63**, **64**) (Miodragovic et al., 2019). The two compounds differ simply by the use of methyl substituents in AP-1 *versus* ethyl substituents in AP-2. Extensive analyses using the NCI 60 cell line data, demonstrated activity of AP1 across the nine major classes of cell lines in that panel, including examples within the eight solid tumor panels. It should be emphasized that the data is expressed as percentage of growth with respect to control as this data was from the NCI's one-dose assay conventionally run at 10 μM, not the five-dose system.

Synergy was shown with the individual components at a 1:1 ratio in the triple-negative breast cancer line MDA-MB-231 that is resistant to cisplatin. The levels of Pt and As bound to DNA on treatment are similar at 4 h but at 8 h, the As level decreases relative to Pt and may well be the reason for the higher cytotoxicity of AP1 due to the release of $As(OH)_2$ moieties within the cell. Further investigation of this and similar molecules is definitely warranted, particularly against solid tumors.

5. Modern analytical and computerized techniques applied to TCM medicines

As has been mentioned earlier, the particular combinations of plants and/or mineral-derived substances that compose the basis of "TCM," contain many different chemical substances, and these can differ in specific TCM medications depending upon the techniques used to prepare them. An excellent example was in the story of artemisinin, where what turned out to be six plants of the genus *Artemisia* were possibilities as "producing the active principle(s)." When one adds to this the requirements for growth and harvesting, then in the late 20th Century, it became apparent that if the "active principle(s)" of a given TCM preparation could be identified by combining current metabolomic and annotating techniques, a rational basis for the use of the cornucopia of potential treatments could progress not only within TCM, but also spread into medicinal systems based more on the modern concepts of Western treatments, which were initially built on the principle of "one target: one drug."

5.1 Demise of the one target one drug concept in the west and the evolution of polypharmacology

An example of the conversion in the West to what has been termed polypharmacology, or expressed in more simpler words; "a drug may have many targets, some related to what it was approved for, and others that bear no nominal relationship to the initial approved one," with a current drug would be imatinib (Gleevec®; Fig. 5, **31**), which was originally approved as a treatment for CML in 2001 and was designed to inhibit the Abelson kinase in the *BCR-ABL* translocation in this disease.

A paper in the IUPHAR Review Series by Fabbro, Cowan-Jacob, and Moebitz (2015) demonstrated the multitarget effects of this drug just among the PTKs, with excellent diagrams showing the number of targets known as of 2015 in the human kinome for this one compound. This added PDGFR, PDGF, SCF and c-Kit to the approved kinase, thus adding gastrointestinal stromal tumors to the list. In the same paper, the polypharmacology of sunitinib (Fig. 7, **65**) is also shown diagrammatically; effectively every kinase family in the human kinome has at least one representative that binds this promiscuous compound. It is of interest that in this molecule the influence of the indigo/indirubin pharmacophore can be seen. For further information on kinase polypharmacology, one may consult the eurofins/discoverX web site at https://www.discoverx.com/tools-resources/interaction-maps.

Another example, but not from kinase inhibition is the PDE5 inhibitor sildenafil (Fig. 7, **66**) which is used to treat erectile dysfunction, but also can restore genitive defects in animal models (Ganesan, 2016). That paper is part of a special 2016 issue of ChemMedChem that dealt with polypharmacology and the whole issue is freely available, as mentioned in the editorial by Bolognesi and Cavalli (2016) A more recent (2019) editorial by Bolognesi is also worth reading as there she covers, albeit in a short format, the requirements for multitarget drug entities (Bolognesi, 2019). Another very interesting and recent paper on the topic of multiple unrecognized activities, is the one by Gilberg and Bajorath (2019) in which they demonstrate the capability of using X-ray structural data to determine if a particular interaction with a compound is due to an artifact, promiscuous binding or is genuinely another target of the drug entity. The X-ray structures of the potential targets have to be available but many can be approximated by utilizing data from similar targets.

Following on from these papers, in 2019, Proschak, Stark, and Merk (2019) published an excellent perspective in the Journal of Medicinal Chemistry that gave some of the history of promiscuous drug compounds, including what is probably the best example from the end of the 19th Century, aspirin, whose full gamut of targets is still not known, even though it is almost certainly the most used drug in the world.

They claim that the following diseases are the current focus of multitarget drugs, and state: "Currently, neurodegenerative and psychiatric disorders, infectious diseases, cancer and metabolic/cardiovascular diseases are in the focus of multitarget drug discovery due to their multifactorial nature or because of therapeutic resistance development."

This quote could almost be a description of the concepts behind TCM as they emphasize phenotypic screening of drug combinations, and cover the various computational and chemical techniques that can be used to determine the targets of such compounds, then from a synthetic chemistry viewpoint, how modifications of pharmacophores can lead to multitargeted drug candidates, and point out the various biological systems that can be useful, which includes high content screening (HCS) which will be covered later.

5.2 The chemical content of TCM preparations

Possibly the major non-scientific "problem" that TCM has in its relationship to Western concepts, is that the identity of the chemical components of particular preparations were not usually available in a non-Chinese format until relatively recently. An initial attempt to produce a usable compendium that linked the PinYin transliteration, the Linnean binomial identification and the chemical structure/ "usual" name was the publication in 1999 of the book by Yan et al., entitled "Traditional Chinese Medicines" (Yan et al., 1999). Although there were reference lists in this 1000 plus page volume, covering names in English and Chinese, taxonomy and compound structures, the lack of a true-cross referencing system meant that one had to manually investigate compounds or activities using multiple printed lists.

Although an excellent "reference source" for individual questions, it was not searchable in this age of digitized databases. However, in the last 2 or

3 years, a number of web-based databases, covering the "content" of TCM from various aspects, have been listed in the literature and the references are given at the end of this paragraph. There is one point, however, and that is that some of the databases, though they have what appear to be legitimate web addresses, do not open on a search from an US based IP address. This does not seem to be linked to the year published, and it is quite possible that they will open easily from Europe or from Eastern countries.

These databases include: TCM analyzer by Liu et al. (2018); YaTCM by Li et al. (2018) and SymMap by Wu et al. (2019). Thus consulting these databases will materially aid in determining what is known from a natural product chemistry aspect in a given TCM preparation.

In addition to these databases directly linked to TCM, there are also two interesting reviews that can add to the information available, once a given chemical identity is known. These are the review by Chen et al. published in the Journal of Chemical Information and Modeling in 2017 which covers the varied databases, both commercial and free use, that can be consulted, including three more TCM-oriented databases (Chen, de Bruyn Kops, & Kirchmair, 2017). In 2018 Chen et al. extended their review to include the chemical space covered by the available natural products, so this paper is an excellent extension of the earlier one (Chen, de Lomana, Friedrich, & Kirchmair, 2018). There is also a Korean-sourced database, NPCARE by Choi et al., specifically designed to look for cancer-related information, that crosses over to some extent with the earlier ones listed, but does have information about the gene targets *etc.* (Choi et al., 2017).

5.3 The potential of metabolomics and molecular network systems in TCM

Approximately ten to twelve years ago, natural product chemists began to utilize collaborative computerized networks to identify relationships among metabolite data. The data used was obtained from large-scale HPLC-MS^n analyses of samples from microbes and marine invertebrates (Quinn et al., 2017). It is probable that the first report of such a system, minus the analytical systems which had not yet been invented, was a paper by Horning and Horning in 1970, reporting on linkages from using analytical methods available in the late 1960s for determining a variety of metabolites in man (Horning & Horning, 1970).

Using the techniques described by Quinn et al., investigators have established the world's largest repository of data from natural products, and concomitant data analysis tools utilizing tandem mass spectroscopy

(MS^2 or MS/MS). This repository is the "Global Natural Products Social Molecular Networking" or GNPS and can be freely accessed at https://gnps.ucsd.edu. The system is continuously updated by users, and the necessary analytical tools are also available together with explanations of the methodologies for searching *etc.*

In addition to the previous paper, a preprint in "bioRxiv" was first published on 31st May 2019 under the title "MolNetEnhancer," that provides an enhanced set of tools for further integration of metabolome mining and subsequent annotation of the results. This is designed for the interrogation of HPLC-MS^n data sets from metabolic experiments and promises to be a very useful set of tools in unraveling the effects of TCM preparations on cell line and animal metabolic data. Since this is a freely available preprint, the examples in Fig. 1 in the preprint gives an excellent overview of the process (Ernst et al., 2019).

A recent paper in 2019 from the PRC by Zhang, Lin, Zou, Zhang, and Xiao (2019) demonstrated how natural products that were not always from TCM, can be utilized to determine optimal lead structures for compounds with anti-inflammatory activities by investigating "chemical space" and the corresponding biological targets.

By coupling these tools to metabolomic studies, the current analytical techniques and computational power can be utilized to identify TCM-sourced compounds from both pharmacology and chemistry properties. An excellent example of the coupling of TCM preparations, in this case from ginseng, to the identification of active components using data from pharmacodynamic studies, was recently published in Talanta by Feng et al. (2019) and the following quote from their paper's abstract makes very interesting reading.

> *Based on the* in vivo *metabolites, network pharmacology analysis was applied to screen the PCs (pharmacodynamic constituents) of ginseng and clarified the action mechanism of ginseng for the treatment of Alzheimer's disease (AD). A total of 27 herbal constituents and 64 related targets shared commonly by compounds and AD were integrated via target network pharmacology analysis. These results demonstrated that this original approach will greatly improve high–throughput screening of metabolites and PCs on AD. It also can explicate the mechanism of action of TCM. Furthermore, this strategy is practicable to identify metabolites and screen PCs in other herbal medicines.*

In 2019 another group from the PRC published an excellent paper in the journal Mass Spectroscopy Reviews, on the use of mass spectroscopy coupled to metabolomics (Wang et al., 2019). This paper demonstrates the power of these coupled techniques to identify the targets and active principles in TCM, thus allowing physicians and scientists to utilize the information to ameliorate disease. The paper also contains very well documented tables linking TCM preparations to MS^n analyses of their components to the initial reports, which are of definite value in determining what is or is not known in a particular TCM preparation.

Other recent relevant papers that cover the topic of metabolomics linked to chemical identification of active principles that also will not be formally discussed, but provide relevant data are: Liu et al., Network Pharmacology (Liu et al., 2015); Gao et al., Compound Kushen (Gao et al., 2018); Niu et al., *Angelica sinensis* and infarction (Niu et al., 2018); Zhu et al., TCM and Colorectal Cancer (Zhu et al., 2018); Zuo et al., Yu Ping Feng decoction (Zuo et al., 2018); Lin et al., TCM and lung cancer cells (Lin et al., 2019) and Ren et al., Caowu/Yunnan Baiyao (Ren et al., 2019).

5.4 High content screening

The recent review by Wang et al., published in Chinese Medicine (Wang, Wu, Tan, Li, & Lu, 2019) demonstrates that the technique of HCS can be applied to TCM, and as shown in the following quote from their paper, they appreciate both the potential usefulness, but most importantly, also what else has to be known in order to fulfill the promise of this technique and its linkage to the other modern analytical techniques.

> *The advent of high content screening technology has absolutely contributed to a breakthrough in compound discovery and influenced the evolution of technology in the screening field. The review introduces the concept and principle of high content screening, lists and compares the currently used HCS instruments, and summarizes the examples from ours and others research work which applied HCS in TCM-derived compound screening. Meanwhile, this article also discusses the advantages and limitations of HSC technology in drug discovery from TCM libraries.*

6. Conclusion

This review has hopefully demonstrated that TCM-derived medications derived from nominally ancient knowledge, still has relevance in the 21st Century. Though the examples discussed are few in number, compared to the numbers of natural product preparations/compounds in TCM, they have been chosen to demonstrate that TCM has had a significant influence in world-wide treatments for malaria and some specific leukemias to date. What has also been aptly demonstrated, is that once a particular compound has been identified that has a good pharmacological activity in one disease area, the compound itself, and/or its pharmacophore can be further developed by chemistry and lead to potential drug leads in other diseases.

Thus, artemisinin and simple derivatives have been developed into potential treatments for viral diseases and some cancers. The trioxy pharmacophore from artemisinin has also led to the production of totally synthetic drug candidates in malaria, and others with potential in cancer treatment.

The application of modern analytical techniques coupled to metabolomics and network pharmacology which though often assumed to be separate "disciplines and/or techniques," are basically the application of analytical data to computerized analysis, utilizing knowledge from a variety of "semi-disciplines" including molecular pharmacology. Molecular pharmacology, which came into being in the 1978–82 time frame, was really the application of applied biochemical techniques, at that time mainly based on analyses of proteins, to interactions between chemical entities and their potential receptors, which led to the identification of the kinase/phosphatase cascades that underpin cellular signaling mechanisms.

What is of significant import is that TCM was always involved in interactions between multiple pharmacologic targets, in contrast to the Western "one drug/one target mantra," which now has definitively moved to the concept of pluripotent drug entities, as demonstrated in this review.

In the future, with the increased knowledge from modern analytical techniques, in particular the use of HPLC-MS^n systems, and linkage with the tools already in use to help dereplicate natural products discovered from many sources, the impact of TCM-related information on modern drug discovery and development can only increase, world-wide. As mentioned earlier, the "treasure-trove" of bioactive materials that is encompassed by TCM when coupled to modern techniques of identification of both the bioactive compound(s) in classical TCM medicaments, and their potential targets in cells, means that the "melding" of this information with current Western drug concepts bodes well for the future.

Conflict of interest

This entire article was self-funded and there are no conflicts of interest involved.

References

Ainsworth, C. (2011). Networking for new drugs. *Nature Medicine*, *17*, 1166–1168.

Beauchard, A., Laborie, H., Rouillard, H., Lozach, O., Ferandin, Y., Le Guével, R., et al. (2009). Synthesis and kinase inhibitory activity of novel substituted indigoids. *Bioorganic & Medicinal Chemistry*, *17*, 6257–6263. https://doi.org/10.1016/j.bmc.2009.07.051.

Bolognesi, M. L. (2019). Harnessing polypharmacology with medicinal chemistry. *ACS Medicinal Chemistry Letters*, *10*, 273–275. https://doi.org/10.1021/acsmedchemlett.9b00039.

Bolognesi, M. L., & Cavalli, A. (2016). Multitarget drug discovery and polypharmacology. *ChemMedChem*, *11*, 1190–1192. https://doi.org/10.1002/cmdc.201600161.

Chao, J., Dai, Y., Verpoorte, R., Lam, W., Cheng, Y.-C., Pao, L.-H., et al. (2017). Major achievements of evidence-based traditional Chinese medicine in treating major diseases. *Biochemical Pharmacology*, *139*, 94–104. https://doi.org/10.1016/j.bcp.2017.06.123.

Chen, Y., de Bruyn Kops, C., & Kirchmair, J. (2017). Data resources for the computer-guided discovery of bioactive natural products. *Journal of Chemical Information and Modeling*, *57*, 2099–2111. https://doi.org/10.1021/acs.jcim.7b00341.

Chen, Y., de Lomana, M. G., Friedrich, N.-O., & Kirchmair, J. (2018). Characterization of the chemical space of known and readily obtainable natural products. *Journal of Chemical Information and Modeling*, *58*, 1518–1532. https://doi.org/10.1021/acs.jcim.8b00302.

Choi, H., Cho, S. Y., Pak, H. J., Kim, Y., Choi, J.-Y., Lee, Y. J., et al. (2017). NPCARE: Database of natural products and fractional extracts for cancer regulation. *Journal of Cheminformatics*, *9*, 2. https://doi.org/10.1186/s13321-016-0188-5.

Coghi, P., Yaremenko, I. A., Prommana, P., Radulov, P. S., Syroeshkin, M. A., Wu, Y. J., et al. (2018). Novel peroxides as promising anticancer agents with unexpected depressed antimalarial activity. *ChemMedChem*, *13*, 902–908. https://doi.org/10.1002/cmdc.201700804.

Cox, F. E. G. (2010). History of the discovery of the malaria parasites and their vectors. *Parasites & Vectors*, *3*, 5. https://doi.org/10.1186/1756-3305-3-5.

Curran, J. (2008). The yellow Emporer's classic of medicine. *British Medical Journal*, *336*, 777.

Cutler, E. G., & Bradford, E. H. (1878). Action of iron, cod-liver oil, and arsenic on the globular richness of the blood. *The American Journal of the Medical Sciences*, *75*, 74–84.

Dawood, M., Hamdoun, S., & Efferth, T. (2018). Multifactorial modes of action of arsenic trioxide in cancer cells as analyzed by classical and network pharmacology. *Frontiers in Pharmacology*, *9*, 143. https://doi.org/10.3389/fphar.2018.00143.

De Azevedo, W. F., Leclerc, S., Meijer, L., Havlicek, L., Strnad, M., & Kim, S. H. (1997). Inhibition of cyclin-dependent kinases by purine analogues: Crystal structure of human cdk2 complexed with roscovitine. *European Journal of Biochemistry*, *243*(1–2), 518–526.

de Lange, C., Coertzen, D., Smit, F. J., Wentzel, J. F., Wong, H. N., Birkholtz, L.-M., et al. (2018a). Synthesis, antimalarial activities and cytotoxicities of amino-artemisinin-1,2-disubstituted ferrocene hybrids. *Bioorganic & Medicinal Chemistry Letters*, *28*, 3161–3163. https://doi.org/10.1016/j.bmcl.2018.08.037.

de Lange, C., Coertzen, D., Smit, F. J., Wentzel, J. F., Wong, H. N., Birkholtz, L.-M., et al. (2018b). Synthesis, *in vitro* antimalarial activities and cytotoxicities of amino-artemisinin-ferrocene derivatives. *Bioorganic & Medicinal Chemistry Letters*, *28*, 289–292. https://doi.org/10.1016/j.bmcl.2017.12.057.

Dobell, C. (1932). *Antony van Leeuwenhoek and his "Little animals"* New York: Harcourt, Brace & Co.

Duan, X., Li, T., Han, X., Ren, J., Chen, P., Li, H., et al. (2017). The antitumor effect of arsenic trioxide on hepatocellular carcinoma is enhanced by andrographolide. *Oncotarget*, *8*, 90905–90915.

Efferth, T. (2017). From ancient herb to modern drug: *Artemisia annua* and artemisinin for cancer therapy. *Seminars In Cancer Biology*, *46*, 65–83. https://doi.org/10.1016/j.semcancer.2017.02.009.

Efferth, T. (2018). Beyond malaria: The inhibition of viruses by artemisinin-type compounds. *Biotechnology Advances*, *36*, 1730–1737. https://doi.org/10.1016/j.biotechadv.2018.01.001.

Ernst, M., Kang, K. B., Caraballo-Rodríguez, A. M., Nothias, L.-F., Wandy, J., Wang, M., et al. (2019). MolNetEnhancer: Enhanced molecular networks by integrating metabolome mining and annotation tools. *Metabolites*, *9*, 144. https://doi.org/10.1101/654459.

Evans, B. E., Rittle, K. E., Bock, M. G., DiPardo, R. M., Freidinger, R. M., Whitter, W. L., et al. (1988). Methods for drug discovery: Development of potent, selective, orally effective cholecystokinin antagonists. *Journal of Medicinal Chemistry*, *31*, 2235–2246.

Fabbro, D., Cowan-Jacob, S. W., & Moebitz, H. (2015). Ten things you should know about protein kinases: IUPHAR review 14. *British Journal Of Pharmacology*, *172*, 2675–2700. https://doi.org/10.1111/bph.13096.

Feng, G., Sun, Y., Liu, S., Song, F., Pi, Z., & Liu, Z. (2019). Stepwise targeted matching strategy from *in vitro* to *in vivo* based on ultra–high performance liquid chromatography tandem mass spectrometry technology to quickly identify and screen pharmacodynamic constituents. *Talanta*, *194*, 619–626. https://doi.org/10.1016/j.talanta.2018.10.074.

Forkner, C. E., & Scott, T. F. M. (1931). Arsenic as a therapeutic agent in chronic myelogenous leukemia. *JAMA*, *97*(1), 3–5. https://doi.org/10.1001/jama.1931.02730010007002.

Frohlich, T., Hahn, F., Belmudes, L., Leidenberger, M., Friedrich, O., Kappes, B., et al. (2018). Synthesis of artemisinin-derived dimers, trimers and dendrimers: Investigation of their antimalarial and antiviral activities including putative mechanisms of action. *Chemistry—A European Journal*, *24*, 8103–8113. https://doi.org/10.1002/chem.201800729.

Frohlich, T., Reiter, C., Ibrahim, M. M., Beutel, J., Hutterer, C., Zeittrager, I., et al. (2017). Synthesis of novel hybrids of quinazoline and artemisinin with high activities against *Plasmodium falciparum*, human cytomegalovirus, and leukemia cells. *ACS Omega*, *2*, 2422–2431. https://doi.org/10.1021/acsomega.7b00310.

Gaboriaud-Kolar, N., Myrianthopoulos, V., Vougogiannopoulou, K., Gerolymatos, P., Horne, D. A., Jove, R., et al. (2016). Natural-based indirubins display potent cytotoxicity toward wild-type and T315I-resistant leukemia cell lines. *Journal of Natural Products*, *79*, 2464–2471. https://doi.org/10.1021/acs.jnatprod.6b00285.

Ganesan, A. (2016). Multitarget drugs: An epigenetic epiphany. *ChemMedChem*, *11*, 1227–1241. https://doi.org/10.1002/cmdc.201500394.

Gao, L., Wang, K.-X., Zhou, Y.-Z., Fang, J.-S., Qin, X.-M., & Du, G.-H. (2018). Uncovering the anticancer mechanism of compound Kushen injection against HCC by integrating quantitative analysis, network analysis and experimental validation. *Scientific Reports*, *8*, 624. https://doi.org/10.1038/s41598-017-18325-7.

Gilberg, E., & Bajorath, J. (2019). Recent progress in structure-based evaluation of compound promiscuity. *ACS Omega*, *4*, 2758–2765. https://doi.org/10.1021/acsomega.8b03639.

Goodman, L. S., & Gilman, A. (1941). *The pharmacological basis of therapeutics: A textbook of pharmacology, toxicology, and therapeutics for physicians and medical students.* New York: Macmillan.

Gotsbacher, M. P., Cho, S. M., Kim, N. H., Liu, F., Kwon, H. J., & Karuso, P. (2019). Reverse chemical proteomics identifies an unanticipated human target of the antimalarial Artesunate. *ACS Chemical Biology*, *14*, 636–643. https://doi.org/10.1021/acschembio.8b01004.

Gruber, L., Abdelfatah, S., Fröhlich, T., Reiter, C., Klein, V., Tsogoeva, S. B., et al. (2018). Treatment of multidrug-resistant leukemia cells by novel artemisinin-, egonol-, and thymoquinone-derived hybrid compounds. *Molecules*, *23*, 841. https://doi.org/10.3390/molecules23040841.

Hahn, F., Fröhlich, T., Frank, T., Bertzbach, L. D., Kohrt, S., Kaufer, B. B., et al. (2018). Artesunate-derived monomeric, dimeric and trimeric experimental drugs-their unique mechanistic basis and pronounced antiherpesviral activity. *Antiviral Research*, *152*, 104–110. https://doi.org/10.1016/j.antiviral.2018.02.013.

Haynes, R. K., Fugmann, B., Stetter, J., Rieckmann, K., Heilmann, H.-D., Chan, H.-W., et al. (2006). Artemisone-a highly active antimalarial drug of the artemisinin class. *Angewandte Chemie, International Edition*, *45*, 2082–2088. https://doi.org/10.1002/anie.200503071.

Ho, W. E., Peh, H. Y., Chan, T. K., & Wong, W. S. F. (2014). Artemisinins: Pharmacological actions beyond antimalarial. *Pharmacology & Therapeutics*, *142*, 126–139. https://doi.org/10.1016/j.pharmthera.2013.12.001.

Hoessel, R., Leclerc, S., Endicott, J. A., Nobel, M. E. M., Lawrie, A., Tunnah, P., et al. (1999). Indirubin, the active constituent of a Chinese antileukaemia medicine, inhibits cyclin-dependent kinases. *Nature Cell Biology*, *1*, 60–67.

Hoonjan, M., Jadhav, V., & Bhatt, P. (2018). Arsenic trioxide: Insights into its evolution to an anticancer agent. *Journal of Biological Inorganic Chemistry*, *23*, 313–329. https://doi.org/10.1007/s00775-018-1537-9.

Horning, E. C., & Horning, M. G. (1970). Metabolic profiles: Chromatographic methods for isolation and characterization of a variety of metabolites in man. *Methods in Medical Research*, *12*, 369–371.

Kandel, E. V., & LeRoy, G. V. (1937). Chronic arsenical poisoning during the treatment of chronic myeloid leukemia. *Archives of Internal Medicine*, *60*, 846–866.

Karagöz, A. C., Reiter, C., Seo, E.-J., Gruber, L., Hahn, F., Leidenberger, M., et al. (2018). Access to new highly potent antileukemia, antiviral and antimalarial agents via hybridization of natural products (homo)egonol, thymoquinone and artemisinin. *Bioorganic & Medicinal Chemistry*, *26*, 3610–3618. https://doi.org/10.1016/j.bmc.2018.05.041.

Kirsch, D. R., & Ogas, O. (2017). *The drug hunters*. New York: Arcade Publishing.

Koepfli, J. B., Mead, J. F., & Brockman, J. A., Jr. (1947). An alkaloid with high antimalarial activity from *Dichroa febrifuga*. *Journal of the American Chemical Society*, *69*, 1837. https://doi.org/10.1021/ja01199a513.

Krieger, J., Smeilus, T., Kaiser, M., Seo, E.-J., Efferth, T., & Giannis, A. (2018). Total synthesis and biological investigation of (−)-artemisinin: The antimalarial activity of artemisinin is not stereospecific. *Angewandte Chemie, International Edition*, *57*, 8293–8296. https://doi.org/10.1002/anie.201802015.

Kuehl, F. A., Jr., Spencer, C. F., & Folkers, K. (1948). Alakaloids of *Dichroa febrifuga* Lour. *Journal of the American Chemical Society*, *70*, 2091–2093. https://doi.org/10.1021/ja01186a031.

Laraia, L., Robke, L., & Waldmann, H. (2018). Bioactive compound collections: From design to target identification. *Chem*, *4*, 705–730.

Li, W. D., Dong, Y. J., Tu, Y. Y., & Lin, Z. B. (2006). Dihydroarteannuin ameliorates lupus symptom of BXSB mice by inhibiting production of TNF-alpha and blocking the signaling pathway NF-kappa B translocation. *International Immunopharmacology*, *6*, 1243–1250. https://doi.org/10.1016/j.intimp.2006.03.004.

Li, B., Ma, C., Zhao, X., Hu, Z., Du, T., Xu, X., et al. (2018). YaTCM: Yet another traditional Chinese medicine database for drug discovery. *Computational And Structural Biotechnology Journal*, *16*, 600–610.

Lin, Y.-J., Liang, W.-M., Chen, C.-J., Tsang, H., Chiou, J.-S., Liu, X., et al. (2019). Network analysis and mechanisms of action of Chinese herb-related natural compounds in lung cancer cells. *Phytomedicine: International Journal Of Phytotherapy And Phytopharmacology*, *58*, 152893. https://doi.org/10.1016/j.phymed.2019.152893.

Liu, C.-x. (2017). Discovery and development of artemisinin and related compounds. *Chinese Herbal Medicines*, *9*(2), 101–114. https://doi.org/10.1016/S1674-6384(17)60084-4.

Liu, Z., Du, J., Yan, X., Zhong, J., Cui, L., Lin, J., et al. (2018). TCMAnalyzer: A chemo- and bioinformatics web service for analyzing traditional Chinese medicine. *Journal of Chemical Information and Modeling*, *58*, 550–555. https://doi.org/10.1021/acs.jcim.7b00549.

Liu, C.-X., Liu, R., Fan, H.-R., Xiao, X.-F., Chen, X.-P., Xu, H.-Y., et al. (2015). Network pharmacology bridges traditional application and modern development of traditional Chinese medicine. *Chinese Herbal Medicines*, 7(1), 3–17. https://doi.org/10.1016/S1674-6384(15)60014-4.

Liu, J., Lu, Y., Wu, Q., Goyer, R. A., & Waalkes, M. P. (2008). Mineral arsenicals in traditional medicines: Orpiment, realgar, and arsenolite. *The Journal Of Pharmacology And Experimental Therapeutics*, *326*(2), 363–368. https://doi.org/10.1124/jpet.108.139543.

Lloyd, N. C., Morgan, H. W., Nicholson, B. K., & Ronimus, R. S. (2005). The composition of Ehrlich's Salvarsan: Resolution of a century-old debate. *Angewandte Chemie, International Edition*, *44*, 941–944. https://doi.org/10.1002/anie.200461471.

Lu, D.-P., Qiu, J.-Y., Jiang, B., Wang, Q., Liu, K.-Y., Liu, Y.-R., et al. (2002). Tetra-arsenic tetra-sulfide for the treatment of acute promyelocytic leukemia: A pilot report. *Blood*, *99*, 3136–3143. https://doi.org/10.1182/blood.V99.9.3136.

Meijer, L., Borgne, A., Mulner, O., Chong, J. P., Blow, J. J., Inagaki, N., et al. (1997). Biochemical and cellular effects of roscovitine, a potent and selective inhibitor of the cyclin-dependent kinases cdc2, cdk2 and cdk5. *European Journal of Biochemistry*, *243*(1–2), 527–536.

Meijer, L., Skaltsounis, A.-L., Magiatis, P., Polychronopoulos, P., Knockaert, M., Leost, M., et al. (2003). GSK-3-selective inhibitors derived from Tyrian purple indirubins. *Chemistry & Biology*, *10*, 1255–1266. https://doi.org/10.1016/j.chembiol.2003.11.010.

Miodragovic, D., Merlino, A., Swindell, E. P., Bogachkov, A., Ahn, R. W., Abuhadba, S., et al. (2019). Arsenoplatin-1 is a dual pharmacophore anticancer agent. *Journal of the American Chemical Society*, *141*, 6453–6457. https://doi.org/10.1021/jacs.8b13681.

Moosavi, J. (2009). The place of Avicenna in the history of medicine. *Avicenna Journal Of Medical Biotechnology*, *1*(1), 3–8.

Niu, C., Yan, H., Yu, T., Sun, H.-P., Liu, J.-X., Li, X.-S., et al. (1999). Studies on treatment of acute promyelocytic leukemia with arsenic trioxide: Remission induction, follow-up, and molecular monitoring in 11 newly diagnosed and 47 relapsed acute promyelocytic leukemia patients. *Blood*, *94*(10), 3315–3324.

Niu, X., Zhang, J., Ni, J., Wang, R., Zhang, Z., Sun, S., et al. (2018). Network pharmacology-based identification of major component of *Angelica sinensis* and its action mechanism for the treatment of acute myocardial infarction. *Bioscience Reports*, *38*, 0519. https://doi.org/10.1042/BSR20180519.

Paddon, C. J., & Keasling, J. D. (2014). Semi-synthetic artemisinin: A model for the use of synthetic biology in pharmaceutical development. *Nature Reviews. Microbiology*, *12*, 355–367. https://doi.org/10.1038/nrmicro3240.

Paddon, C. J., Westfall, P. J., Pitera, D. J., Benjamin, K., Fisher, K., McPhee, D., et al. (2013). High-level semi-synthetic production of the potent antimalarial artemisinin. *Nature*, *496*, 528–532.

Proschak, E., Stark, H., & Merk, D. (2019). Polypharmacology by design: A medicinal chemist's perspective on multitargeting compounds. *Journal of Medicinal Chemistry*, *62*, 420–444. https://doi.org/10.1021/acs.jmedchem.8b00760.

Quinn, R. A., Nothias, L.-F., Vining, O., Meehan, M., Esquenazi, E., & Dorrestein, P. C. (2017). Molecular networking as a drug discovery, drug metabolism, and precision medicine strategy. *Trends In Pharmacological Sciences*, *38*(2), 143. https://doi.org/10.1016/j.tips.2016.10.011.

Radke, J. B., Burrows, J. N., Goldberg, D. E., & Sibley, L. D. (2018). Evaluation of current and emerging antimalarial medicines for inhibition of *Toxoplasma gondii* growth *in vitro*. *ACS Infectious Diseases*, *4*(8), 1264–1274. https://doi.org/10.1021/acsinfecdis.8b00113.

Rask-Andersen, M., Almen, M. S., & Schioth, H. B. (2011). Trends in the exploitation of novel drug targets. *Nature Reviews. Drug Discovery*, *10*, 579–590.

Ren, J.-I., Sun, H., Dong, H., Yang, L., Zhang, A.-H., Han, Y., et al. (2019). A UPLC-MS-based metabolomics approach to reveal the attenuation mechanism of Caowu compatibility with Yunnan Baiyao. *RSC Advances*, *9*, 8926–8933. https://doi.org/10.1039/c8ra09894h.

Shen, Z.-X., Chen, G.-Q., Ni, J.-H., Li, X.-S., Xiong, S.-M., Qiu, Q.-Y., et al. (1997). Use of arsenic trioxide (As_2O_3) in the treatment of acute promyelocytic leukemia (APL): II. Clinical efficacy and pharmacokinetics in relapsed patients. *Blood*, *89*(9), 3354–3360.

Sklirou, A. D., Gaboriaud-Kolar, N., Papassideri, I., Skaltsounis, A.-L., & Trougakos, I. P. (2017). 6-bromo-indirubin-3′-oxime (6BIO), a glycogen synthase kinase-3β inhibitor, activates cytoprotective cellular modules and suppresses cellular senescence-mediated biomolecular damage in human fibroblasts. *Scientific Reports*, *7*, 11713. https://doi.org/10.1038/s41598-017-11662-7.

Sonntag, E., Hahn, F., Bertzbach, L. D., Seyler, L., Wangen, C., Müller, R., et al. (2019). *In vivo* proof-of-concept for two experimental antiviral drugs, both directed to cellular targets, using a murine cytomegalovirus model. *Antiviral Research*, *161*, 63–69. https://doi.org/10.1016/j.antiviral.2018.11.008.

Tadesse, S., Caldon, E. C., Tilley, W., & Wang, S. (2019). Cyclin-dependent kinase 2 inhibitors in cancer therapy: An update. *Journal of Medicinal Chemistry*, *62*(9), 4233–4251. https://doi.org/10.1021/acs.jmedchem.8b01469.

Tu, Y. Y. (2016). Artemisinin-a gift from traditional Chinese medicine to the world (Nobel lecture). *Angewandte Chemie, International Edition*, *55*(35), 10210–10226.

Varun, Sonam, & Kakkar, R. (2019). Isatin and its derivatives: a survey of recent syntheses, reactions, and applications. *Medicinal Chemistry Communications*, *10*, 351–368. https://doi.org/10.1039/c8md00585k.

Vesely, J., Havlicek, L., Strnad, M., Blow, J. J., Donella-Deana, A., Pinna, L., et al. (1994). Inhibition of cyclin-dependent kinases by purine analogues. *European Journal of Biochemistry*, *224*(2), 771–786. https://doi.org/10.1111/j.1432-1033.1994.00771.x.

Walter, A., Chaikuad, A., Helmer, R., Loaec, N., Preu, L., Ott, I., et al. (2018). Molecular structures of cdc2-like kinases in complex with a new inhibitor chemotype. *PLoS One*, *13*(5). e0196761https://doi.org/10.1371/journal.pone.0196761.

Wang, X., Chen, B., Zhao, L., Zhi, D., Hai, Y., Song, P., et al. (2018). Autophagy enhanced antitumor effect in K562 and K562/ADM cells using realgar transforming solution. *Biomedicine & Pharmacotherapy*, *98*, 252–264. https://doi.org/10.1016/j.biopha.2017.12.038.

Wang, B., Liu, J. X., Meng, H. X., & Lin, C. R. (2012). Blocking effect of salvianolic acid A on calcium channels in isolated rat ventricular myocytes. *Chinese Journal of Integrative Medicine*, *18*, 366–370. https://doi.org/10.1007/s11655-011-0707-1.

Wang, H., Liu, Y., Wang, X., Liu, D., Sun, Z., Wang, C., et al. (2015). Randomized clinical control study of locoregional therapy combined with arsenic trioxide for the treatment of hepatocellular carcinoma. *Cancer*, *121*(17), 2917–2925. https://doi.org/10.1002/cncr.29456.

Wang, J., Long, L., Chen, Y., Xu, Y., & Zhang, L. (2018). Design, synthesis and antineoplastic activity of novel hybrids of podophyllotoxin and indirubin against human leukaemia cancer cells as multifunctional anti-MDR agents. *Bioorganic & Medicinal Chemistry Letters*, *28*, 1817–1824. https://doi.org/10.1016/j.bmcl.2018.04.019.

Wang, X.-J., Ren, J.-L., Zhang, A.-H., Sun, H., Yan, G.-L., Han, Y., et al. (2019). Novel applications of mass spectrometry-based metabolomics in herbal medicines and its active ingredients: Current evidence. *Mass Spectrometry Reviews*, *9999*, 1–23. https://doi.org/10.1002/mas.21589.

Wang, J., Wu, M.-Y., Tan, J.-Q., Li, M., & Lu, J.-H. (2019). High content screening for drug discovery from traditional Chinese medicine. *Chinese Medicine, 14*, 5. https://doi.org/10.1186/s13020-019-0228-y.

Wang, J., Xu, C., Wong, Y. K., Liao, F., Jiang, T., & Tu, Y. Y. (2019). Artemisinin, the magic drug discovered from traditional Chinese medicine. *Engineering, 5*, 32–39. https://doi.org/10.1016/j.eng.2018.11.011.

Watts, J. K., & Corey, D. R. (2012). Gene silencing by siRNAs and antisense oligonucleotides in the laboratory and the clinic. *The Journal of Pathology, 226*(2), 365–379. https://doi.org/10.1002/path.2993.

Waxman, S., & Anderson, K. C. (2001). History of the development of arsenic derivatives in cancer therapy. *The Oncologist, 6*(suppl 2), 3–10.

Wu, Y., Zhang, F., Yang, K., Fang, S., Bu, D., Li, H., et al. (2019). SymMap: An integrative database of traditional Chinese medicine enhanced by symptom mapping. *Nucleic Acids Research, 47*, D1110–D1117. https://doi.org/10.1093/nar/gky1021.

Yan, X., Jiang, Z., Bi, L., Yang, Y., & Chen, W. (2015). Salvianolic acid A attenuates TNF-alpha- and D-GalN-induced ER stress-mediated and mitochondrial dependent apoptosis by modulating Bax/Bcl-2 ratio and calcium release in hepatocyte LO2 cells. *Naunyn-Schmiedeberg's Archives of Pharmacology, 388*, 817–830. https://doi.org/10.1007/s00210-015-1116-3.

Yan, X., Zhou, J., & Xie, G. (1999). Traditional Chinese medicines; molecular structures, natural sources and applications. In G. W. A. Milne (Ed.), *Traditional Chinese medicines; molecular structures, natural sources and applications*. Aldershot, UK: Ashgate.

Zhang, R., Lin, J., Zou, Y., Zhang, X.-J., & Xiao, W.-L. (2019). Chemical space and biological target network of anti-inflammatory natural products. *Journal of Chemical Information and Modeling, 59*, 66–73. https://doi.org/10.1021/acs.jcim.8b00560.

Zhang, J.-Y., Wang, M., Wang, R.-Y., Sun, X., Du, Y.-Y., Ye, J.-X., et al. (2018). Salvianolic acid A ameliorates arsenic trioxide-induced cardiotoxicity through decreasing cardiac mitochondrial injury and promotes its anticancer activity. *Frontiers in Pharmacology, 9*, 487. https://doi.org/10.3389/fphar.2018.00487.

Zhang, L., Zhang, W., Zhao, Y., Yang, X., Fang, L., Wang, S., et al. (2011). Research progress of salvianolic acid A. *Zhongguo Zhong Yao Za Zhi, 36*(19), 2603–2609.

Zhou, C., Liu, L.-J., Zhuang, J., Wei, J.-Y., Zhang, T.-T., Gao, C.-D., et al. (2018). A systems biology-based approach to uncovering molecular mechanisms underlying effects of Traditional Chinese Medicine Qingdai in chronic myelogenous leukemia, involving integration of network pharmacology and molecular docking technology. *Medical Science Monitor, 24*, 4305–4316. https://doi.org/10.12659/MSM.908104.

Zhu, H., Hao, J., Niu, Y., Liu, D., Chen, D., & Wu, X. (2018). Molecular targets of Chinese herbs: A clinical study of metastatic colorectal cancer based on network pharmacology. *Scientific Reports, 8*, 7238. https://doi.org/10.1038/s41598-018-25500-x.

Zuo, H., Zhang, Q., Su, S., Chen, Q., Yang, F., & Hu, Y. (2018). A network pharmacology-based approach to analyse potential targets of traditional herbal formulas: An example of Yu Ping Feng decoction. *Scientific Reports, 8*, 11418. https://doi.org/10.1038/s41598-018-29764-1.

CHAPTER SIX

LW-AFC, a new formula from the traditional Chinese medicine Liuwei Dihuang decoction, as a promising therapy for Alzheimer's disease: Pharmacological effects and mechanisms

Xiaorui Cheng[a,b], Yan Huang[a,b], Yongxiang Zhang[a,b], Wenxia Zhou[a,b,*]

[a]Beijing Institute of Pharmacology and Toxicology, Beijing, China
[b]State Key Laboratory of Toxicology and Medical Countermeasures, Beijing, China
*Corresponding author: e-mail address: zhouwx@bmi.ac.cn

Contents

Abstract

LW-AFC is a new formula derived from the Liuwei Dihuang decoction, a classical traditional Chinese medicine prescription. Based on our research, LW-AFC is a promising drug for Alzheimer's disease (AD). The studies were conducted primarily in two typical AD mouse models: SAMP8 and APP/PS1 mice. The results showed that LW-AFC could improve many cognitive behaviors, such as spatial learning and memory ability, passive and active avoidance response, and object recognition memory capability. In addition, LW-AFC could also alleviate the AD-like pathology in animal models, such as neuron loss

Advances in Pharmacology, Volume 87
ISSN 1054-3589
https://doi.org/10.1016/bs.apha.2019.10.005

and Aβ deposition. Subsequent studies found that LW-AFC could rebalance hypothalamic-pituitary-adrenal (HPA) axis and hypothalamic-pituitary-gonadal (HPG) axis, and modulate the disturbance of immune system and gut flora. These data suggested that the anti-AD effects of LW-AFC might be mainly *via* modulating the neuroendocrine immunomodulation (NIM) network. As inhibiting the immune function by immunosuppressant could abolish the protective effects of LW-AFC against long-term potentiation (LTP) impairment model, it is likely that LW-AFC balancing the NIM network is initiated by modulating the immune system.

Abbreviations

Aβ	amyloid-beta peptide
ACTH	adrenocorticotropic hormone
AD	Alzheimer's disease
APP/PS1 mouse	double-transgenic *PrP-h*A*β*PPswe/PS1$^{\Delta E9}$ mouse
CRH	corticotropin releasing hormone
FAD	familial AD
FSH	follicle-stimulating hormone
G-CSF	granulocyte colony stimulating factor
GM-CSF	granulocyte-macrophage colony stimulating factor
GnRH	gonadotropin-releasing hormone
HPA	hypothalamic-pituitary-adrenal
HPG	hypothalamic-pituitary-gonadal
IFN	interferon
IL	interleukin
LH	luteinizing hormone
LTP	long-term potentiation
LW	Liuwei Dihuang decoction
MCP	monocyte chemotactic protein
MIP	macrophage inflammatory protein
NFTs	neurofibrillary tangles
NIM	neuroendocrine immunomodulation
RANTES	regulated upon activation normal T cell expressed and secreted factor
SAD	sporadic AD
SAMP8	senescence-accelerated mouse prone 8 strain
SAMR1	senescence-accelerated mice resistant-1 strain
T	testosterone
TNF	tumor necrosis factor

1. Introduction

Alzheimer's disease (AD) is a widespread and devastating neurodegenerative disease, characterized by a progressive loss of episodic memory and other cognitive functions. Although there is now a significant debate as to the relationship between amyloid-beta peptide (Aβ) and AD, the specific and typical neuropathological hallmarks of AD are brain atrophy due to neuronal and synapse loss, extracellular senile plaques (SP) composed largely of Aβ and intraneuronal neurofibrillary tangles (NFTs) caused by intracellular aggregates of hyperphosphorylated tau protein in the brain. The gold standard for diagnosis of AD still is brain atrophy, SP and NFT in the brain of autopsy. The etiology of the disease is elusive, and disease-modifying treatment remains beyond reach.

The senescence-accelerated mouse prone 8 (SAMP8) strain is a spontaneous animal model of accelerated aging. Conversely, the senescence-accelerated mouse resistant 1 (SAMR1) strain presents a normal aging pattern. SAMP8 strain is considered a robust model for exploring the etiopathogenesis of sporadic AD (SAD) and a plausible experimental model for developing preventative and therapeutic treatments for late-onset/age-related AD, which accounts for the vast majority of cases (Cheng, Zhou, & Zhang, 2014). The transgenic mouse models, such as over-producing human APP and associated secretases, tau and Apo E, are more suitable for familial AD (FAD). Among the gene-modified models, the double-transgenic *PrP-hAβ*PPswe/PS1$^{\Delta E9}$ (APP/PS1) mouse is the most popular one.

Liuwei Dihuang decoction (LW), a classical prescription in traditional Chinese medicine (TCM), has been used for nearly 1000 years for various diseases with characteristic features of *kidney Yin* deficiency (Zhou, Cheng, & Zhang, 2016). LW consists of six herbs, including Dihuang (prepared root of *Rehmannia glutinosa*), Shanyao (rhizome of *Dioscorea opposita*), Shanzhuyu (fruit of *Cornus officinalis*), Mudanpi (root bark of *Paeonia suffruticosa*), Zexie (rhizome of *Alisma plantago-aquatica*), and Fuling (sclerotia of *Poria cocos*). Our previous studies have revealed that modulating the NIM network plays an important role on the pharmacological effects of LW, such as improving the cognitive ability and neuronal synaptic function in aging or AD animal models (Huang, Hu, Liu, Zhou, & Zhang, 2012; Huang, Zhang, et al., 2012; Yang, Zhou, Zhang, Yan, & Zhao, 2006; Zhou et al., 2016; Zhou, Zhang, Liu, & Zhou, 1999; Zhou, Zhang, & Zhou, 1999). LW-AFC (LW-active fraction combination) is prepared from LW, composing of a polysaccharide fraction (LWB-B), a glycoside fraction (LWD-b), and an oligosaccharide fraction (CA-30) (Wang, Lei, et al., 2016). LW-AFC has been approved by the Chinese Food and Drug Administration for clinical trial on menopausal syndrome with *kidney Yin* deficiency

(Huang et al., 2019). Our previous results indicated that the pharmacological effects of LW-AFC are similar to LW (Cheng et al., 2015; Cheng, Qi, Wang, Zhou, & Zhang, 2019; Zhou et al., 2016). Hypothalamic-pituitary-adrenal (HPA) axis dysfunction play an important role in AD patients (Swanwick et al., 1998), and our previous studies also showed that the HPA axis is abnormal in AD animal models (Li, Chen, Zhang, Fu, & Wang, 2017; Wang, Zhang, et al., 2017), indicating that AD is related to a disturbance of the NIM network. So LW-AFC might have beneficial effects on AD. To evaluate the effects of LW-AFC on AD, SAMP8 and APP/PS1 mouse model were utilized in our studies. This chapter summarizes the progress of LW-AFC in treating AD.

2. The anti-AD effects of LW-AFC

2.1 Preparation and quality control of LW-AFC

LW-AFC was prepared from Liuwei Dihuang decoction and includes polysaccharide fraction (LWB-B), glycosides fraction (LWD-b) and oligosaccharide fraction (CA-30). LW-AFC was prepared as follows (Fig. 1).

(1) The six individual medicinal materials of Liuwei Dihuang decoction, including *Rehmannia glutinosa* Libosch., *Cornus officinalis* Sieb., *Dioscorea opposita* Thunb., *Alisma orientale* (G. Samuelsson) Juz, *Poria cocos* (Schw.) Wolf and *Paeonia suffruticosa* Andrews (Tongrentang drug store, Beijing, China) were mixed according to the dry weight ratio of 8:4:4:3:3:3. Then the mixture of material was decocted within 10 volume of deionized water with boiling refluxing thrice, 2h per time. After finishing the extraction, the materials were 6-layer gauze filtered to yield three extraction solutions at 50 °C, allowed them to room temperature, centrifuged (2500 rpm/min, 25 min). The supernatants were combined and then concentrated under reduced pressure (relative density was 1.09 at 20 °C) into quintessence (Fig. 1).

(2) The quintessence was left in 30% ethanol overnight at room temperature. After centrifugation (2500 rpm/min, 25 min) and washing sedimentation with 30% ethanol three times, the sedimentation was decanted. All the supernatant was collected and combined, then concentrated under reduced pressure (relative density was 1.17 at 20 °C) (Fig. 1).

(3) The concentrated extract was left in 60% ethanol overnight at room temperature, then centrifuged (2500 rpm/min, 25 min), the supernatant (LWD) was collected, the sedimentation left in deionized water and

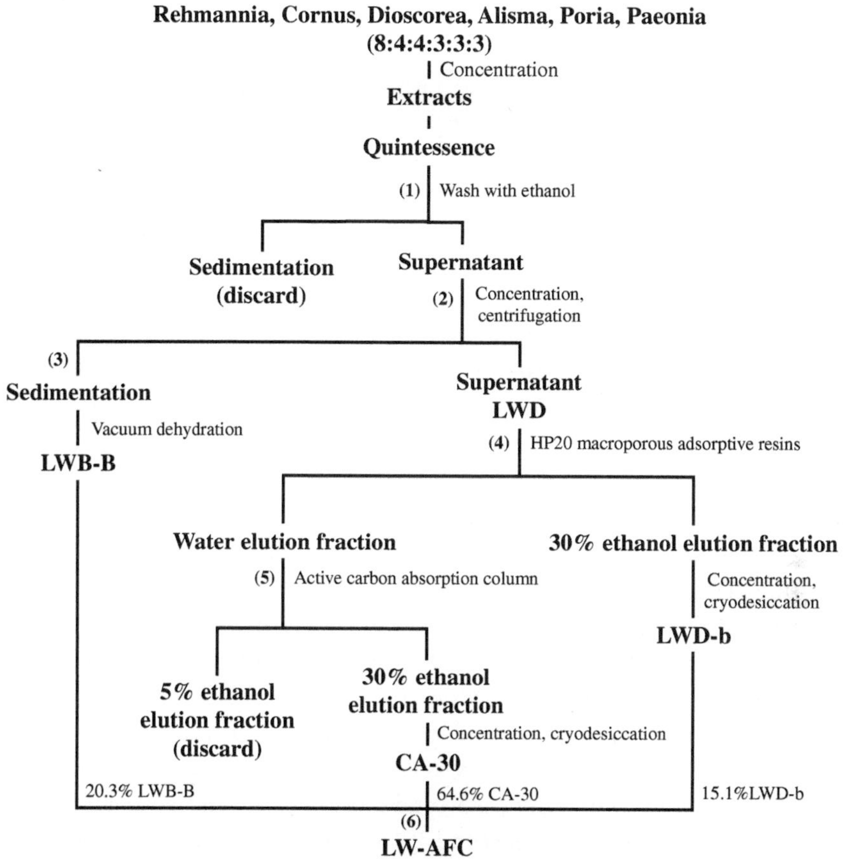

Fig. 1 The schematic diagram of LW-AFC preparation. *Reproduced with permission from Wang, J., Zhang, X., Cheng, X., Cheng, J., Liu, F., Xu, Y., et al. (2017). LW-AFC, a new formula derived from Liuwei Dihuang decoction, ameliorates cognitive deterioration and modulates neuroendocrine-immune system in SAMP8 mouse.* Current Alzheimer Research, 14*(2), 221–238. https://doi.org/10.2174/1567205013666160603001637.*

concentrated under reduced pressure (relative density was 1.09 at 20 °C) three times, then dried at 70 °C to obtain polysaccharide fraction (LWB-B) (Fig. 1).

(4) The supernatant (LWD) was left in 60% ethanol and concentrated to 1/10 original volume under reduced pressure, then added 20% of its original volume of deionized water, concentrated three times (relative density was 1.285 at 20 °C), then dissolved in a sufficient quantity of deionized water and eluted in turn by deionized water (6 column volume) and 30% ethanol (4 column volume) on macroporous adsorptive resins (DIAION HP20, Φ150 × 1500 mm, diameter height ratio was 1/9) (Mitsubishi Chemical Corporation, Minato-ku, Tokyo, Japan) with 19.1 cm/h sample flow rate and 19.1 cm/h eluent flow rate. 30% ethanol elution of LWD was concentrated (relative density was 1.05 at 20 °C), cryodesiccated to obtain glycosides fraction (LWD-b) (Fig. 1).

(5) Water elution of LWD was concentrated (relative density was 1.192 at 20 °C), eluted in turn by 5% ethanol (6 column volume) and 30% ethanol (2 column volume) on active carbon absorption column (GH-15, Φ150 × 1500 mm, diameter height ratio was 1/9) (Guanghuajingke Activate Carbon Ltd., Beijing, China) with 19.1 cm/h sample flow rate and 25.0 cm/h eluent flow rate. 5% ethanol elution was decanted. 30% ethanol elution was concentrated to 1/20 of its original volume under reduced pressure, then added 20% of its original volume of deionized water, concentrated three times (relative density was 1.10–1.15 at 20 °C), cryodesiccated to obtain oligosaccharide fraction (CA-30) (Fig. 1).

(6) LW-AFC was composed of 20.3% polysaccharide fraction (LWB-B), 15.1% glycosides fraction (LWD-b) and 64.6% oligosaccharide fraction (CA-30) in the dry weight ratio (Fig. 1).

For pharmacognosy identification of LW-AFC, high-performance liquid chromatography (HPLC) method was used to analysis and control the quality of LW-AFC. For mixture of CA-30 and LWD-b, the chromatographic separation was obtained on a Diamond C18 (250 × 4.6 mm, 5 μm) column in Agilent 1100 (Agilent Technologies). Mobile phase consisted of CH_3CN-H_2O and purified water. A gradient program was performed as follows: 0–25 min, 0–15% A; 25–50 min, 15–35% A; 50–60 min, 35–56% A. Fig. 2A showed the typical HPLC fingerprint of CA-30 and LWD-b mixture. There are 17 chromatogram peaks and the No. S peak represents loganin in fingerprint of CA-30 and LWD-b mixture (Fig. 2A). For LWB-B, the chromatographic separation was obtained on a NucleosilNH_2 100 Å (250 × 4.6 mm, 5 μm) column in Agilent 1100.The effluent was monitored on the differential refractive index detector. The mobile phase consisted of 70% CH_3CN-H_2O and 30% purified water. Column temperature was 35 °C and flow rate was 1.0 mL/min. Fig. 2B showed the typical HPLC fingerprint of LWB-B. There are five chromatogram peaks and these five peaks represent fructose, glucose, sucrose, mannotriose and stachyose, the retention times of them were 6.260, 6.829, 8.186, 18.305 and 21.506 min, respectively (Fig. 2B).

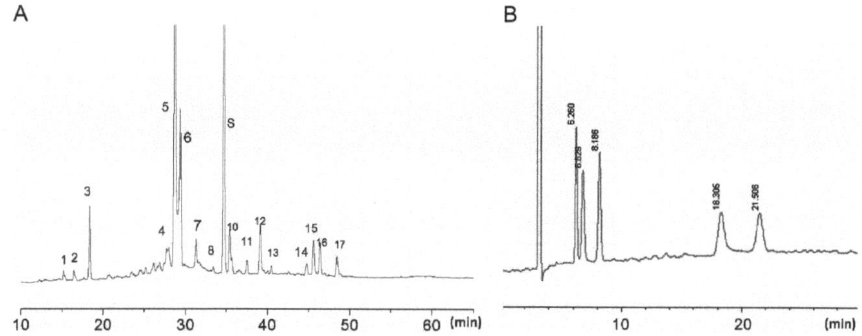

Fig. 2 The HPLC fingerprint of LW-AFC. (A) The HPLC fingerprint of LWD-B. The peak S is loganin. (B) The HPLC fingerprint of LWB-B and CA30 mixture. The peak at 6.26, 6.83, 8.19, 18.30 and 21.50 min is, respectively, fructose, glucose, sucrose, mannotriose and stachyose. *Reproduced with permission from Wang, J., Zhang, X., Cheng, X., Cheng, J., Liu, F., Xu, Y., et al. (2017). LW-AFC, a new formula derived from Liuwei Dihuang decoction, ameliorates cognitive deterioration and modulates neuroendocrine-immune system in SAMP8 mouse.* Current Alzheimer Research, *14(2), 221–238. https://doi.org/10.2174/1567205013666160603001637.*

2.2 Effects on learning and memory behaviors

Our studies showed that LW-AFC diminished the impairment of learning and memory and anti-aging. In the step-down test, LW-AFC administration significantly decreased the number of errors in the SAMP8 and APP/PS1 mouse models, and shortened the training time in the APP/PS1 mouse model (Wang, Lei, et al., 2016; Wang, Zhang, et al., 2017). The SAMP8 or APP/PS1 mice treated with LW-AFC showed significant increase on the successful avoidance times in the training and testing phases of the shuttle-box test (Wang, Lei, et al., 2016; Wang, Zhang, et al., 2017). In the Morris water maze test, LW-AFC treatment remarkably shortened the latency in the learning task and probe trial, increased the number of times that the mice crossed the removed platform in the probe trial of SAMP8 and APP/PS1 mice, and extended the swimming time within the target quadrant in the probe trial in APP/PS1 mice (Wang, Lei, Cheng, Zhang, et al., 2016; Wang, Zhang, et al., 2017). The administration of LW-AFC helped SAMP8 and APP/PS1 mice obtain a better discrimination index score in the novel object recognition memory test (Wang, Lei, et al., 2016; Wang, Zhang, et al., 2017). After receiving an intragastric administration of LW-AFC (1.6 g/kg) once a day for over 3 months, AD mice exhibited an amelioration of impairment in object recognition memory, spatial learning and memory, active and passive avoidance (Table 1). In addition,

Table 1 Effects of LW-AFC on cognitive behaviors.

The ability of learning and memory	Behavioral detection	Index	6-month-old SAMP8 mouse		9-month-old APP/PS1 mouse	
			SAMP8 *vs* SAMR1	SAMP8+ LW-AFC *vs* SAMP8	APP/PS1 mice *vs* wild type	APP/PS1 + LW-AFC *vs* APP/PS1 mice
Passive avoidance	Step-down test	Number of errors	↑↑	↓	↑↑↑	↓↓
		Training time	↑↑	–	↑↑↑	↓↓
Active avoidance	Shuttle-box test	The successful avoidance times in training phase	↓↓↓	↑↑↑	↓↓↓	↑↑↑
		The successful avoidance times in testing phase	↓↓↓	↑↑↑	↓↓↓	↑↑↑
The ability of spatial learning and memory	Morris water maze test	Latency in the learning task	↑↑↑	↓↓↓	↑↑↑	↓↓
		Latency in the probe trial	↑↑	↓↓	↑↑↑	↓↓
		Numbers of crossing the plate in the probe trial	↓↓↓	↑↑	↓↓↓	↑↑↑
		The swimming time within the target quadrant in the probe trial	↓	–	↓↓↓	↑↑↑
The object recognition memory	The novel object recognition memory test	The discrimination index	↓↓↓	↑↑	↑↑↑	↑↑↑

"↓" and "↑" means decrease and increase respectively; "↓", $P < 0.05$; "↑↑" or "↓↓", $P < 0.01$; "↑↑↑" or "↓↓↓", $P < 0.001$; "--", means no difference.

LW-AFC treatment decreased the grading score of senescence, increased the body weight, prolonged average life span and ameliorated spatial memory impairment in 12- and 24-month-old SAMR1 mice (Wang, Cheng, Zhang, Cheng, et al., 2016).

2.3 Effects on the typical pathological signs of AD

LW-AFC treatment alleviates Aβ deposition in the brain of APP/PS1 mice. LW-AFC-treated APP/PS1 mice had a significantly smaller area of Aβ deposits in the whole brain and hippocampus, and lower $A\beta_{1-42}$ levels in the hippocampus and plasma of APP/PS1 mice than in untreated APP/PS1 mice (Wang, Lei, et al., 2016). The administration of LW-AFC significantly increased the density of healthy neurons in the hippocampus and CA3 region of APP/PS1 mice (Wang, Lei, et al., 2016). These results indicated that LW-AFC had the effects of lessening AD-like pathological damage (Table 2).

3. The anti-AD mechanisms of LW-AFC

3.1 Modulating immune function play an important role

The immune system plays an important role in modulating cognition. Many causes of induced immune deficits can lead to cognitive impairment. Anti-thymocyte serum (Barnard, Collins, Daisley, & Behnke, 2009) and thymectomy can impair not only the immune response but also the learning ability (Zhang, Saito, & Nishiyama, 1994); nude mice have impaired cognitive ability (Kipnis, Cohen, Cardon, Ziv, & Schwartz, 2004; Ziv et al., 2006) and restoring the immune function can improve their cognitive ability (Kipnis et al., 2004; Ziv et al., 2006). Recent research has suggested that the disruption of immune function might be an important factor in AD (Cashman, Ghirmai, Abel, & Fiala, 2008; Liu et al., 2013; Song et al., 1999). Three fractions of LW-AFC were screened by immune activity to determine whether LW-AFC achieves its anti-AD effects *via* immune modulation.

To investigate this issue, we used corticosterone (Cort) treated animals as a synaptic plasticity impaired model. Administration, e.g., for 7 days of LW-AFC and its three active fractions could ameliorate Cort-induced LTP impairment. Single administration of any one of the active fractions, even directly injected into the lateral ventricles, had no effect on Cort-induced LTP impairment. Cyclophosphamide, an immune immunosuppressant, was able to abolish the protective effect of LW-AFC against Cort-induced LTP impairment

Table 2 The effects of LW-AFC on typical pathological signs of AD in APP/PS1 mouse.

Pathological sign	Method	Index	APP/PS1 mice *vs* wild type	APP/PS1 + LW-AFC *vs* APP/PS1 mouse
Aβ deposits	Immunofluorescence staining	Aβ deposits in the brain	↑↑↑	↓
		Aβ deposits in the hippocampus	↑↑↑	↓↓
	AlphaLISA	The concentration of Aβ1-42 in hippocampus	↑↑↑	↓↓
		The concentration of Aβ1-40 in hippocampus	↑↑	–
		The concentration of Aβ1-42 in plasma	↑↑↑	↓↓
		The concentration of Aβ1-40 in plasma	↓↓↓	–
Neuron loss	Nissl staining	IOD of Nissl bodies in the hippocampus	↓↓↓	↑↑
		IOD of Nissl bodies in the CA3 regions	↓↓↓	↑

"↓" and "↑" means decrease and increase respectively; "↓", $P<0.05$; "↑↑" or "↓↓", $P<0.01$; "↑↑↑" or "↓↓↓", $P<0.001$; "--", means no difference.

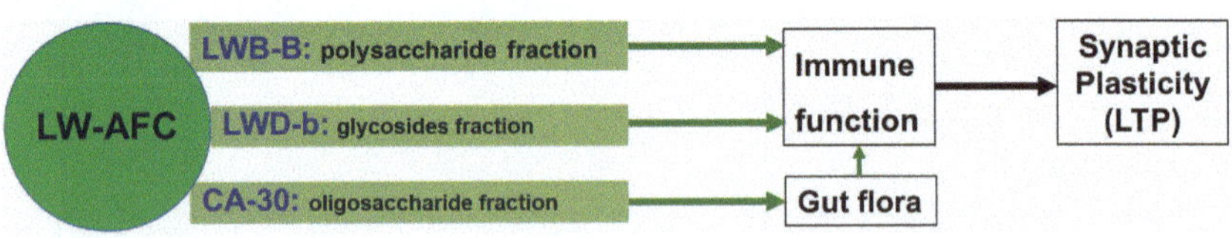

Fig. 3 The schematic diagram for the pathway of LW-AFC's neural protective effects.

(Huang et al., 2019). These results suggest that the neural protective effects of LW-AFC are unlikely activated through a direct route, and that immune modulation might be the common pathway (Fig. 3) (Huang et al., 2019).

3.2 Modulating the balance of NIM network

The neuroendocrine immunomodulation (NIM) network maintains the processes of adaptation, homeostasis, and defense against hostile environmental factors (Bellavance & Rivest, 2012; Masek, Slansky, Petrovicky, & Hadden, 2003; Wang et al., 2018). Anomalous secretions of neurotransmitters, hormones, or cytokines in a dysregulated NIM network stimulate or aggravate Aβ deposits (Sanchez-Ramos et al., 2009; Verdile et al., 2014), tau hyperphosphorylation (Brureau et al., 2013; Green, Billings, Roozendaal, McGaugh, & LaFerla, 2006), neuronal cell loss (Tan et al., 2014; Tripathy, Thirumangalakudi, & Grammas, 2010), neuroinflammation (Jiang et al., 2010), and cognitive deterioration (Bowen, Perry, Xiong, Smith, & Atwood, 2015; Green et al., 2009; Wang, Cheng, Zhang, Wang, et al., 2016) in AD animal models and patients. Because AD is related to a disturbance of the NIM network, and due to regulating the rebalance of the NIM work network might play an important role in the anti-AD effects of LW-AFC. Modulating the NIM network should be the advantage of LW-AFC over other single-target drugs.

The LW-AFC treatment decreased the concentrations of corticotropin releasing hormone (CRH) in hypothalamus and adrenocorticotropic hormone (ACTH) in pituitary of hypothalamic-pituitary-adrenal (HPA) axis, gonadotropin-releasing hormone (GnRH) in hypothalamus, follicle-stimulating hormone (FSH) and luteinizing hormone (LH) in pituitary and increased the level of testosterone (T) in plasma of hypothalamic-pituitary-gonadal (HPG) axis in SMP8 mice. The administration of LW-AFC increased the numbers of CD^{3+} CD^{4+} T helper cells, $CD^{8+}CD^{28+}$ T cells, CD^{19+} and CD^{19+} CD^{80+} B cells, reduced CD^{4+} $CD^{25+}Foxp^{3+}$ regulatory T cells of spleen lymphocytes in SAMP8 mice. Moreover, the LW-AFC treatment reduced the levels of interleukin (IL-1β; IL-2; IL-6; IL-23), Colony stimulating factor (GM-CSF), Interferon (IFN-γ), Tumor necrosis factor (TNF-α; TNF-β), Chemotactic factor (RANTES; Eotaxin), but increased the levels of Chemotactic factor MCP-1 and anti-inflammatory factor IL-5 in the blood plasma of SAMP8 mice (Wang, Zhang, et al., 2017).

In APP/PS1 mice, LW-AFC treatment decreased the concentrations of CRH in hypothalamus and ACTH in pituitary of HPA axis, GnRH in hypothalamus, LH and FSH in pituitary of HPG axis. LW-AFC administration increased $CD8^+$ $CD28^+$ T cells and decreased $CD4^+$ $CD25^+Foxp3^+$ regulatory T cells in the spleen lymphocytes. In addition, the LW-AFC reduced the concentrations of pro-inflammatory factor IL-1β, IL-2, IL-6,

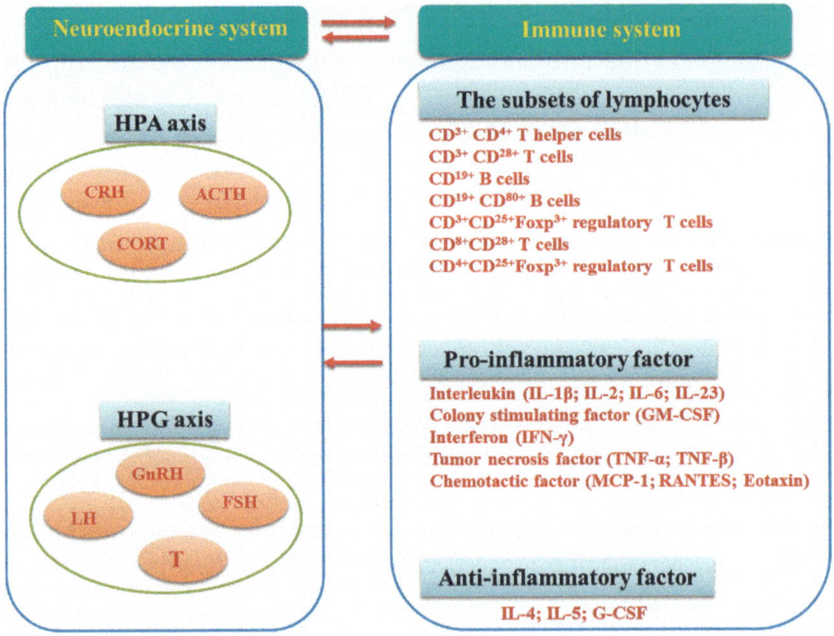

Fig. 4 The modulation of LW-AFC on neuroendocrine system and immune system.

IL-23, GM-CSF, TNF-α, TNF-β and eotaxin, increased anti-inflammatory factor IL-4 and G-CSF in the blood plasma (Wang, Lei, et al., 2016).

These results indicated that LW-AFC treatment suppressed the hyperactivity of HPA and HPG axis, increased the secretion of anti-inflammatory factor and decreased the secretion of pro-inflammatory factor. LW-AFC regulated abnormal subsets of spleen lymphocytes in an AD mouse model. Modulating and restoring the balance of the NIM network might be one of the mechanisms LW-AFC utilizes to offset AD symptoms (Fig. 4).

3.3 Effects on the intestinal flora and protein glycosylation in the brain

The results from 16S rRNA amplicon sequencing of gut microbiota showed that the LW-AFC treatment altered 22 (16 increased and 6 decreased) OTUs in SAMP8 mice. Among them, 15 OTUs could be reversed by LW-AFC resulting in a microbial composition similar to that of SAMR1 mice. There were seven (three negative and four positive correlation) OTUs significantly correlated with spatial learning and memory ability, active avoidance response, and object recognition memory capability, at the order level, including *Bacteroidales*, *Clostridiales*, *Desulfovibrionales*, *CW040*, and two unclassified orders (Wang, Ye, et al., 2016). This indicated that LW-AFC influenced bacterial taxa in correlation with the abilities of learning and memory in SAMP8 mice and restored them to SAMR1 mice.

The oligosaccharide fraction CA-30 is one of components of LW-AFC. The results from metagenomic sequencing showed that CA-30 mainly altered the abundance of 4 genera and 10 newborn genera. Seven genera were significantly correlated with the NIM network and cognitive performance (Moalem et al., 2000). CA-30 only showed protective effects against corticosterone induced LTP impairment *via* intragastric administration and the protective effects could be blocked by an unsortable antibiotic cocktail (pimaricin 2.5 mg/kg, bacitracin 50 mg/kg, and neomycin 50 mg/kg) according to as Verdu's study (Verdu et al., 2006), and the cocktail itself had little effects on LTP (Huang et al., 2019). These data suggest that CA-30 provides its protective effects *via* modulation of the intestinal flora. LW-AFC contains many ingredients that could not be absorbed into blood nor penetrate the blood-brain barrier, so must be taken for a long time to be effective. Recently, a lot of researches focus on the relation between AD and gut flora. It has believed that disturbance of gut flora may significantly contribute to the pathogenesis of AD (Bostanciklioglu, 2019; Kowalski & Mulak, 2019; Szablewski, 2018). Serotonin (5-HT) play an important role in cognition and mood (Jenkins, Nguyen, Polglaze, & Bertrand, 2016). Gut flora is the main resource of 5-HT, about 95% 5-HT is derived from the gut. In the germ-free (GF) mice, the 5-HT decreased about 60% in the blood, and reconstruction of gut flora can restore the 5-HT level (Yano et al., 2015). Similarly, tryptophan (Trp), precursors of 5-HT, decreased in the cerebrum of GF mice (Matsumoto et al., 2013). Therefore, we speculate regulating intestinal microbiome is one of the central mechanisms for the anti-AD effects of LW-AFC.

The transcriptome in the hippocampus and cerebral cortex of SAMP8 mice is different from one of SAMR1 mice, and there was a specific genetic sub-network in the brains of SAMP8 mice (Cheng et al., 2013). The results from RNA-seq analysis by an Illumina HiSeq 2500 sequencer showed that LW-AFC reversed the transcriptome in the hippocampus of SAMP8 mice. The specific investigation of altered gene expression in subtypes defined by cognitive profiles indicated that the systemic lupus erythematosus pathway, spliceosomes, amyotrophic lateral sclerosis, and insulin signaling were involved in the improvement of cognitive ability by LW-AFC. The expression of genes Enpp2, Etnk1, Epdr1, and Gm5900 in the hippocampus were correlated with that of LW-AFC's ameliorating cognitive impairment, including spatial learning and memory abilities, active avoidance response capability, and object recognition memory in SAMP8 mice (Wang, Liu, et al., 2017). We infer that LW-AFC has direct or indirect effects on altering gene expressions and regulating pathways in the hippocampus of SAMP8 mice.

Glycosylation is one of the most common eukaryotic post-translational modifications. The protein glycosylation is defective in AD. LW-AFC treatment modulated the abundance of 21 and 6 *N*-glycan in the cerebral cortex and serum of SAMP8 mice, respectively. The abundance of (Hex)3 (HexNAc)5(Fuc)1(Neu5Ac)1 and (Hex)2(HexNAc)4 decreased in the cerebral cortex and serum of SAMP8 mice compared with SAMR1 mice, decreases that were significantly correlated with learning and memory measures. The administration of LW-AFC could reverse or increase these levels in SAMP8 mice (Wang, Cheng, et al., 2017).

4. Conclusion

LW is composed of 6 herbs, and there are at least 224 identified compounds produced in it (Wang, Bai, et al., 2017; Zhang, Yu, Bai, & Ning, 2017). LW-AFC is extracted from LW and composed of three fractions: a polysaccharide fraction (LWB-B), a glycoside fraction (LWD-b) and an oligosaccharide fraction (CA-30). Our phytochemical study showed that the glycosides fraction contained more than 30 compounds, which could be separated into (at least) 5 categories: iridoid glycosides, paeoniflorin, phenylpropionic acid and phenethanol-glycosides, 5-hydroxymethyl-furaldehyde and derivant, and others. There were levidulinose, TMAN, and stachyose in the oligosaccharide fraction. The polysaccharide fraction contained more than 16 compounds, which could be subdivided into 4 categories: polygalacturonic acid, rhamnogalacturonic acid polysaccharide, arabinogalactan, and dextran. To our knowledge, the total number of compounds and the identities of the bioactive or therapeutic constituents in LW-AFC are still unknown.

Our studies indicated LW-AFC had anti-AD effects. We speculate the pharmacologic mechanisms might be due to a synergistic effect by multilayered, multi-dimensional networks of the potential combination of components in LW-AFC. Then we analyzed the relationship between intestinal flora and the NIM network. Our analysis showed an abundance of 68 genera in intestinal flora, 24 molecular in the NIM network, 21 *N*-glycan in the cerebral cortex and expressions of 170 genes in hippocampus respectively correlation with object recognition memory, spatial learning and memory, active or passive avoidance. The edge was defined as the significant correlation between the different types among flora, molecular, gene and glycan. The multi-layered network regulated by LW-AFC had 370 edges. Therefore, we infer the mechanism of LW-AFC anti-AD might be that LW-AFC target on intestinal flora, then restore the balance of NIM network, next regulate gene expression and protein glycosylation in brain, ultimately improve cognitive function (Fig. 5).

To our knowledge, oligosaccharides and polysaccharides are hardly be absorbed and across the blood-brain barrier (BBB) to affect the brain function directly. It is likely that LW-AFC play its anti-AD effects *via* an indirect way. Our study showed that suppressing immune function could abolish the neural protective effects of LW-AFC, and disturb the intestinal flora could

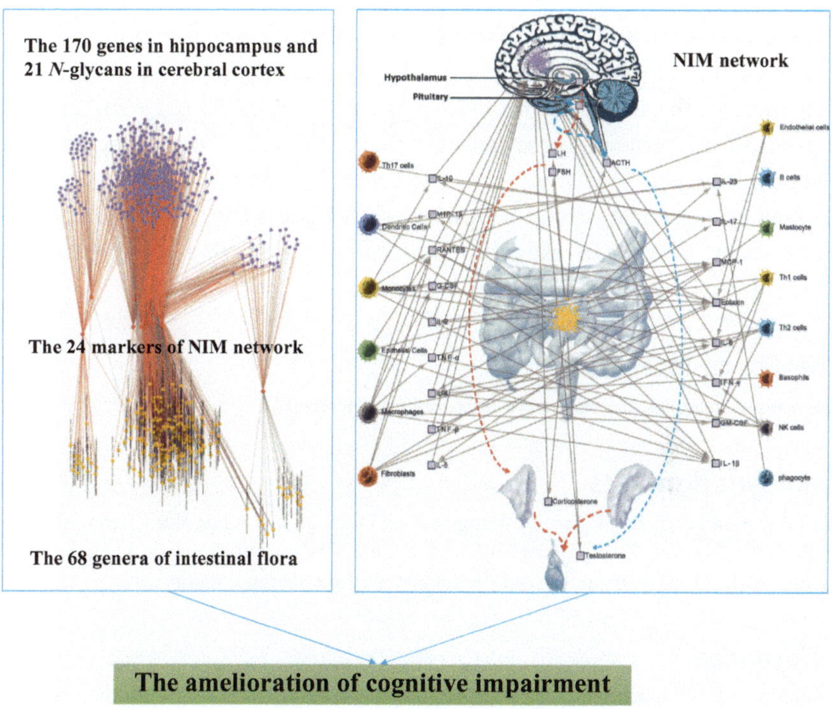

Fig. 5 The relationship of intestinal flora and the NIM network and the possible mechanism of LW-AFC: The nodes represent genes, markers of NIM network, genera of intestinal flora, immune cells or endocrine organs. Among nodes, the yellow circle node indicates genera of intestinal flora, the red circle node indicates markers of NIM network, the blue circle node indicates genes. The edges represent affiliation or interaction relationship. In the figure, there are 68 genera in intestinal flora, 24 molecular in the NIM network, and 170 genes in hippocampus.

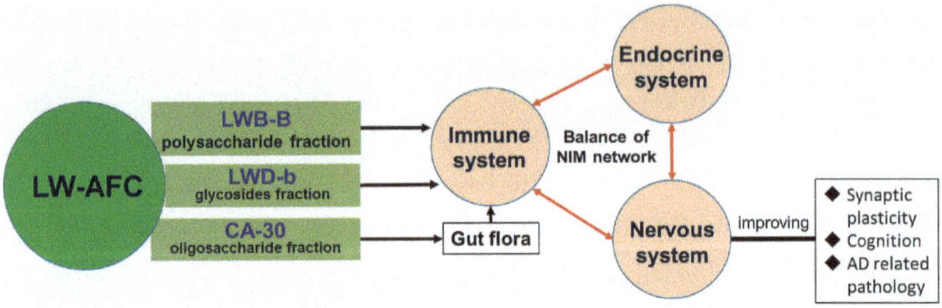

Fig. 6 The schematic diagram of the anti-AD effects of LW-AFC.

block the neural protective effects of CA-30 with little influence on the protective effects of LWB-B and LWD-b (Huang et al., 2019). Previous study showed that LWB-B and LWD-b could act on immune system directly and CA-30 could only affect the immune system *via* gut flora (Zhou et al., 2016). Therefore, we propose that modulation of the immune function and intestinal flora might be the *Start Button* for the anti-AD effect of LW-AFC, which then initiates the modulation of the balance of the NIM network and gene expression and protein glycosylation in brain, ultimately improving cognitive function (Fig. 6).

Due to its intricate composition, we can imagine the LW-AFC as a complex system. Further investigation is needed to achieve a complete understanding of the pharmacology of LW-AFC.

Conflict of interest

The authors confirm that they have no conflicts of interest.

Acknowledgments

We want to sincerely thank Jianhui Wang, Xi Lei, Dong Li, Gang Liu, Bin Cheng, Yang Liu, Fuqiang Ye, Xiaorui Zhang, Jiangbei Yuan, Zhongfu Wang, Ju Zeng, Lu Han, Fei Li and Xiaochen Bo. They carried out and completed all the research experiments.

References

Barnard, C. J., Collins, S. A., Daisley, J. N., & Behnke, J. M. (2009). Immunodepression reduces learning performance in male laboratory mice (Mus musculus). *Physiology & Behavior, 96*(2), 362–369.

Bellavance, M. A., & Rivest, S. (2012). The neuroendocrine control of the innate immune system in health and brain diseases. *Immunological Reviews, 248*(1), 36–55.

Bostanciklioglu, M. (2019). The role of gut microbiota in pathogenesis of Alzheimer's disease. *Journal of Applied Microbiology, 127*(4), 954–967.

Bowen, R. L., Perry, G., Xiong, C., Smith, M. A., & Atwood, C. S. (2015). A clinical study of lupron depot in the treatment of women with Alzheimer's disease: Preservation of cognitive function in patients taking an acetylcholinesterase inhibitor and treated with high dose lupron over 48 weeks. *Journal of Alzheimer's Disease, 44*(2), 549–560.

Brureau, A., Zussy, C., Delair, B., Ogier, C., Ixart, G., Maurice, T., et al. (2013). Deregulation of hypothalamic-pituitary-adrenal axis functions in an Alzheimer's disease rat model. *Neurobiology of Aging, 34*(5), 1426–1439.

Cashman, J. R., Ghirmai, S., Abel, K. J., & Fiala, M. (2008). Immune defects in Alzheimer's disease: New medications development. *BMC Neuroscience, 9*(Suppl 2), S13.

Cheng, X. R., Cui, X. L., Zheng, Y., Zhang, G. R., Li, P., Huang, H., et al. (2013). Nodes and biological processes identified on the basis of network analysis in the brain of the senescence accelerated mice as an Alzheimer's disease animal model. *Frontiers in Aging Neuroscience, 5*, 65.

Cheng, X. R., Cui, X. L., Zheng, Y., Zhang, G. R., Li, P., Huang, H., et al. (2015). A co-module regulated by therapeutic drugs in a molecular subnetwork of Alzheimer's disease identified on the basis of traditional Chinese medicine and SAMP8 mice. *Current Alzheimer Research, 12*(9), 870–885.

Cheng, X. R., Qi, C. H., Wang, T. X., Zhou, W. X., & Zhang, Y. X. (2019). Characteristics of the traditional Liu-Wei-Di-Huang prescription reassessed in modern pharmacology. *Chinese Journal of Natural Medicines, 17*(2), 103–121.

Cheng, X. R., Zhou, W. X., & Zhang, Y. X. (2014). The behavioral, pathological and therapeutic features of the senescence-accelerated mouse prone 8 strain as an Alzheimer's disease animal model. *Ageing Research Reviews, 13*, 13–37.

Green, K. N., Billings, L. M., Roozendaal, B., McGaugh, J. L., & LaFerla, F. M. (2006). Glucocorticoids increase amyloid-beta and tau pathology in a mouse model of Alzheimer's disease. *Journal of Neuroscience, 26*(35), 9047–9056.

Green, R. C., Schneider, L. S., Amato, D. A., Beelen, A. P., Wilcock, G., Swabb, E. A., et al. (2009). Effect of tarenflurbil on cognitive decline and activities of daily living in patients with mild Alzheimer disease: A randomized controlled trial. *The Journal of the American Medical Association, 302*(23), 2557–2564.

Huang, Y., Hu, Z., Liu, G., Zhou, W., & Zhang, Y. (2012). The effect of Liuwei Dihuang decoction on long-term potentiation in BALB/c mice in vivo. *Pharmacology and Clinics of Chinese Materia Medica, 28*(5), 14–17.

Huang, Y., Li, D., Cheng, B., Liu, G., Zhang, Y. X., & Zhou, W. X. (2019). Active fraction combination from Liuwei Dihuang decoction (LW-AFC) ameliorates corticosterone-induced long-term potentiation (LTP) impairment in mice in vivo. *Journal of Ethnopharmacology, 236*, 147–154.

Huang, Y., Zhang, H., Yang, S., Qiao, H., Zhou, W., & Zhang, Y. (2012). Liuwei Dihuang decoction facilitates the induction of long-term potentiation (LTP) in senescence accelerated mouse/prone 8 (SAMP8) hippocampal slices by inhibiting voltage-dependent calcium channels (VDCCs) and promoting N-methyl-d-aspartate receptor (NMDA) receptors. *Journal of Ethnopharmacology, 140*(2), 384–390.

Jenkins, T. A., Nguyen, J. C., Polglaze, K. E., & Bertrand, P. P. (2016). Influence of tryptophan and serotonin on mood and cognition with a possible role of the gut-brain axis. *Nutrients, 8*(1), pii: E56. https://doi.org/10.3390/nu8010056.

Jiang, H., Liu, C. X., Feng, J. B., Wang, P., Zhao, C. P., Xie, Z. H., et al. (2010). Granulocyte colony-stimulating factor attenuates chronic neuroinflammation in the brain of amyloid precursor protein transgenic mice: An Alzheimer's disease mouse model. *Journal of International Medical Research, 38*(4), 1305–1312.

Kipnis, J., Cohen, H., Cardon, M., Ziv, Y., & Schwartz, M. (2004). T cell deficiency leads to cognitive dysfunction: Implications for therapeutic vaccination for schizophrenia and other psychiatric conditions. *Proceedings of the National Academy of Sciences of the United States of America, 101*(21), 8180–8185.

Kowalski, K., & Mulak, A. (2019). Brain-gut-microbiota axis in Alzheimer's disease. *Journal of Neurogastroenterology and Motility, 25*(1), 48–60.

Li, P., Chen, J., Zhang, W., Fu, B., & Wang, W. (2017). Transcriptome inference and systems approaches to polypharmacology and drug discovery in herbal medicine. *Journal of Ethnopharmacology*, *195*, 127–136.

Liu, Y. H., Zeng, F., Wang, Y. R., Zhou, H. D., Giunta, B., Tan, J., et al. (2013). Immunity and Alzheimer's disease: Immunological perspectives on the development of novel therapies. *Drug Discovery Today*, *18*(23–24), 1212–1220.

Masek, K., Slansky, J., Petrovicky, P., & Hadden, J. W. (2003). Neuroendocrine immune interactions in health and disease. *International Immunopharmacology*, *3*(8), 1235–1246.

Matsumoto, M., Kibe, R., Ooga, T., Aiba, Y., Sawaki, E., Koga, Y., et al. (2013). Cerebral low-molecular metabolites influenced by intestinal microbiota: A pilot study. *Frontiers in Systems Neuroscience*, *7*, 9.

Moalem, G., Gdalyahu, A., Shani, Y., Otten, U., Lazarovici, P., Cohen, I. R., et al. (2000). Production of neurotrophins by activated T cells: Implications for neuroprotective autoimmunity. *Journal of Autoimmunity*, *15*(3), 331–345.

Sanchez-Ramos, J., Song, S., Sava, V., Catlow, B., Lin, X., Mori, T., et al. (2009). Granulocyte colony stimulating factor decreases brain amyloid burden and reverses cognitive impairment in Alzheimer's mice. *Neuroscience*, *163*(1), 55–72.

Song, C., Vandewoude, M., Stevens, W., De Clerck, L., Van der Planken, M., Whelan, A., et al. (1999). Alterations in immune functions during normal aging and Alzheimer's disease. *Psychiatry Research*, *85*(1), 71–80.

Swanwick, G. R., Kirby, M., Bruce, I., Buggy, F., Coen, R. F., Coakley, D., et al. (1998). Hypothalamic-pituitary-adrenal axis dysfunction in Alzheimer's disease: Lack of association between longitudinal and cross-sectional findings. *The American Journal of Psychiatry*, *155*(2), 286–289.

Szablewski, L. (2018). Human gut microbiota in health and Alzheimer's disease. *Journal of Alzheimer's Disease*, *62*(2), 549–560.

Tan, M. S., Yu, J. T., Jiang, T., Zhu, X. C., Guan, H. S., & Tan, L. (2014). IL12/23 p40 inhibition ameliorates Alzheimer's disease-associated neuropathology and spatial memory in SAMP8 mice. *Journal of Alzheimer's Disease*, *38*(3), 633–646.

Tripathy, D., Thirumangalakudi, L., & Grammas, P. (2010). RANTES upregulation in the Alzheimer's disease brain: A possible neuroprotective role. *Neurobiology of Aging*, *31*(1), 8–16.

Verdile, G., Laws, S. M., Henley, D., Ames, D., Bush, A. I., Ellis, K. A., et al. (2014). Associations between gonadotropins, testosterone and beta amyloid in men at risk of Alzheimer's disease. *Molecular Psychiatry*, *19*(1), 69–75.

Verdu, E. F., Bercik, P., Verma-Gandhu, M., Huang, X. X., Blennerhassett, P., Jackson, W., et al. (2006). Specific probiotic therapy attenuates antibiotic induced visceral hypersensitivity in mice. *Gut*, *55*(2), 182–190.

Wang, Y. Y., Bai, H., Zhang, R. Z., Yan, H., Ning, K., & Zhao, X. M. (2017). Predicting new indications of compounds with a network pharmacology approach: Liuwei Dihuang Wan as a case study. *Oncotarget*, *8*(55), 93957–93968.

Wang, J., Cheng, X., Zeng, J., Yuan, J., Wang, Z., Zhou, W., et al. (2017). LW-AFC effects on N-glycan profile in senescence-accelerated mouse prone 8 strain, a mouse model of Alzheimer's disease. *Aging and Disease*, *8*(1), 101–114.

Wang, J., Cheng, X., Zhang, X., Cheng, J., Xu, Y., Zeng, J., et al. (2016). The anti-aging effects of LW-AFC via correcting immune dysfunctions in senescence accelerated mouse resistant 1 (SAMR1) strain. *Oncotarget*, *7*(19), 26949–26965.

Wang, J. H., Cheng, X. R., Zhang, X. R., Wang, T. X., Xu, W. J., Li, F., et al. (2016). Neuroendocrine immunomodulation network dysfunction in SAMP8 mice and PrP-hAbetaPPswe/PS1DeltaE9 mice: Potential mechanism underlying cognitive impairment. *Oncotarget*, *7*(17), 22988–23005.

Wang, T., Han, L., Zhang, X., Wu, R., Cheng, X., Zhou, W., et al. (2018). Knowledge-based neuroendocrine immunomodulation (NIM) molecular network construction and its application. *Molecules*, *23*(6), pii: E1312. https://doi.org/10.3390/molecules23061312.

Wang, J. H., Lei, X., Cheng, X. R., Zhang, X. R., Liu, G., Cheng, J. P., et al. (2016). LW-AFC, a new formula derived from Liuwei Dihuang decoction, ameliorates behavioral and pathological deterioration via modulating the neuroendocrine-immune system in PrP-hAbetaPPswe/PS1(DeltaE9) transgenic mice. *Alzheimer's Research & Therapy*, *8*(1), 57.

Wang, J., Liu, Y., Cheng, X., Zhang, X., Liu, F., Liu, G., et al. (2017). The effects of LW-AFC on the hippocampal transcriptome in senescence-accelerated mouse prone 8 strain, a mouse model of Alzheimer's disease. *Journal of Alzheimer's Disease*, *57*(1), 227–240.

Wang, J., Ye, F., Cheng, X., Zhang, X., Liu, F., Liu, G., et al. (2016). The effects of LW-AFC on intestinal microbiome in senescence-accelerated mouse prone 8 strain, a mouse model of Alzheimer's disease. *Journal of Alzheimer's Disease*, *53*(3), 907–919.

Wang, J., Zhang, X., Cheng, X., Cheng, J., Liu, F., Xu, Y., et al. (2017). LW-AFC, a new formula derived from Liuwei Dihuang decoction, ameliorates cognitive deterioration and modulates neuroendocrine-immune system in SAMP8 mouse. *Current Alzheimer Research*, *14*(2), 221–238.

Yang, S., Zhou, W., Zhang, Y., Yan, C., & Zhao, Y. (2006). Effects of Liuwei Dihuang decoction on ion channels and synaptic transmission in cultured hippocampal neuron of rat. *Journal of Ethnopharmacology*, *106*(2), 166–172.

Yano, J. M., Yu, K., Donaldson, G. P., Shastri, G. G., Ann, P., Ma, L., et al. (2015). Indigenous bacteria from the gut microbiota regulate host serotonin biosynthesis. *Cell*, *161*(2), 264–276.

Zhang, Y., Saito, H., & Nishiyama, N. (1994). Thymectomy-induced deterioration of learning and memory in mice. *Brain Research*, *658*(1–2), 127–134.

Zhang, R. Z., Yu, S. J., Bai, H., & Ning, K. (2017). TCM-Mesh: The database and analytical system for network pharmacology analysis for TCM preparations. *Scientific Reports*, 7(1), 2821.

Zhou, W., Cheng, X., & Zhang, Y. (2016). Effect of Liuwei Dihuang decoction, a traditional Chinese medicinal prescription, on the neuroendocrine immunomodulation network. *Pharmacology & Therapeutics*, *162*, 170–178.

Zhou, J. Z., Zhang, Y. X., Liu, C. H., & Zhou, J. H. (1999). Effect of Liuwei Dihuang decoction on long-term potentiation in hippocampal dentate gyrusin rats. *Chinese Journal of Integrative Medicine*, *19*, 209–213.

Zhou, J. Z., Zhang, Y. X., & Zhou, J. H. (1999). Cognition-enhancing effect of Liuwei Dihuang decoction on age-related deterioration of learning and memory in senescence-accelerated mouse (SAM). *Chinese Journal of Experimental Traditional Medical Formulae*, *5*(4), 29–33.

Ziv, Y., Ron, N., Butovsky, O., Landa, G., Sudai, E., Greenberg, N., et al. (2006). Immune cells contribute to the maintenance of neurogenesis and spatial learning abilities in adulthood. *Nature Neuroscience*, *9*(2), 268–275.

CHAPTER SEVEN

Pharmacological effects of icariin

Chunyang He[a,b,†], Ze Wang[b,†], Jingshan Shi[a,b,*]
[a]Key Laboratory of Basic Pharmacology of Ministry of Education and Joint International Research Laboratory of Ethnomedicine of Ministry of Education, Zunyi Medical University, Zunyi, Guizhou, P.R. China
[b]Generic Drug Research Center of Guizhou Province, School of Pharmacy, Zunyi Medical University, Zunyi, Guizhou, P.R. China
[*]Corresponding author: e-mail address: shijs@zmu.edu.cn

Contents

Abstract

Icariin (ICA) is a principal active component from traditional Chinese medicine *Epimedium* grandiflorum. To explain its traditional medical usages by modern science, a variety of pharmacological effects have been studied for ICA. In this review, we summarized the pharmacokinetics of ICA as well as its pharmacological mechanisms in neurodegenerative disease, cardiovascular disease, anti-osteoporosis, anti-inflammation, anti-oxidative stress, anti-depression and anti-tumors.

Abbreviations

Aβ amyloid β-protein
AD Alzheimer's disease
Bcl-2 B-cell lymphoma-2
CNS central nervous system

† Authors with equal contributions.

Advances in Pharmacology, Volume 87
ISSN 1054-3589
https://doi.org/10.1016/bs.apha.2019.10.004

ERK	extracellular regulated protein kinase
ICA	icariin
IL-6	interleukin 6
MAP	microtubule associated proteins
NF-κB	nuclear factor kappa-B
PD	Parkinson's disease
PI3K	phosphatidylinositol 3′ -kinase
PPAR	peroxisome proliferators-activated receptor
SOD	superoxide dismutase
SSRI	selective serotonin reuptake inhibitors
TCM	traditional Chinese medicine
TNF-α	tumor necrosis factor-α
6-OHDA	6-hydroxydopamine hydrochloride

1. Introduction

Epimedii (in Chinese: Yin Yang Huo) has been used for many centuries in the traditional Chinese medicine. The traditional use of *Epimedii* mixed with other herbs makes it difficult to explain its pharmacological effects in modern science. Actually, it was shown that even in a single *Epimedii* there exist at least 260 distinct compounds (Jiang, Jie, & Jia, 2015). The complexity and diversity in phytochemistry of *Epimedii* have hindered the investigation of the pharmacology of *Epimedii* for quite a long time.

With the development of separation science and ethnopharmacology, increasing evidence have proven that icarrin (ICA) is a main bioactive compound in *Epimedii*. ICA is a class of prenylated flavonoids which consists of a glucosyl group on C-3, a methoxyl group on C-4, a prenyl group on C-8 position and a rhamnosyl group on C-7 (Fig. 1). The substitution group on C-8 is a main active site for its pharmacological effect (Ma et al., 2011). In addition, the ICA could be transformed into glucuronide conjugates of isoflavonoids and flavonoid aglycones by metabolic enzymes (Qian et al., 2012).

According to the Chinese Pharmacopeia, ICA (molecular formula: $C_{33}H_{40}O_{15}$, molecular weight: 676.67 g/mol) is the main component of five *Epimedii* species (in Chinese Yinyanghuo), including *E. brevicornu* Maxim, *E. koreanum* Nakai, *E. sagittatim* Maxim, *E. pubescens* Maxim and *E. wushanense* T. S. Ying. In traditional Chinese medicine, *Epimedii* has been

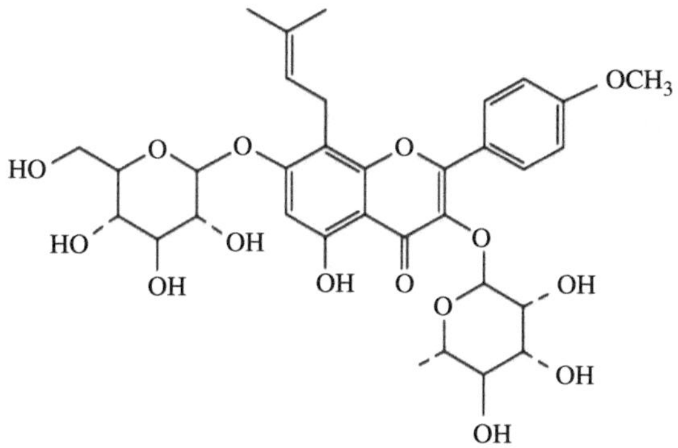

Fig. 1 Chemical structure of ICA.

used the treatment of different diseases, such as osteoporosis prevention, ameliorating sexual dysfunction, modulation of immune system, and improvement of cardiovascular function (Tang & Eisenbrand, 2011).

This review will outline the pharmacological effects of ICA including neuroprotective effect, protective effects of cardiovascular disease, anti-osteoporosis effect, anti-inflammation effect, improved effects of reproductive system, anti-oxidative stress effect, anti-depression, and anti-tumors effect. We will discuss the past and current discoveries of ICA in different pathological conditions.

2. Pharmacokinetics of ICA

Since the knowledge of pharmacokinetics is essential to fully understand the pharmacological effects of ICA, a number of studies have been performed to establish a global view of pharmacokinetics of ICA (Cheng, Qiu, Wang, & He, 2007; Liu & Lou, 2004; Qian et al., 2012; Wu, Zhang, et al., 2011; Zhao, Fan, Fan, Sun, & Guo, 2010). It is found that the pharmacokinetic properties of ICA strongly rely on its administration. Xu et al. have found that the half-life of ICA is 3.149 ± 2.364 h by oral administration, and a rapid decreasing of plasma concentration of ICA was found in intravenous administration with a half-life of 0.562 ± 0.200 h (Cheng et al., 2007; Xu et al., 2017). The low bioavailability of ICA is due to the chemical structure of ICA, which is a diglycoside and not readily to be absorbed and hence put additional constraints in its clinical application (Chen, Wang, Jia, Tan, & Hu, 2011; Li, Li, Mei, & Lu, 2015). The bioavailability of ICA could be improved by pharmaceutical methods such as inclusion with β-cyclodextrin and propyleneglycol (PG)-liposome

(Yang et al., 2012; Zhang, Wang, Cui, Meng, & Lin, 2012). Xu et al. have reported that ICA was distributed to the liver, lung, spleen, heart, kidney, brain, testicle, uterus, and ovary (Xu et al., 2017). The distribution is concentration- and sexual-dependent (Xu et al., 2017). In animals, for example, in rat, a moderate concentration of ICA was found in testicle of male rat, while a high concentration in both uterus and ovary of female rat. Ye et al. found that ICA is difficult to transmission across the blood-brain barrier (Ye, Chen, & Liu, 1999), However, Jin et al. and Li et al. had reported that ICA given peripheral has obvious central nervous system pharmacological activity (Jin et al., 2014; Li, Deng, et al., 2015; Li, Dong, et al., 2015; Li, Li, et al., 2015), While He et al. and Zhou et al. found that ICA metabolite, icariside II, the central pharmacological potency was much stronger than icariin administered by peripheral (He, Deng, Gao, Zeng, & Gong, 2018; Zhou et al., 2019). A possible explanation would be metabolites of ICA to the understanding of the widely neuropharmacological effects of ICA. It still needs to be explained by the detection and analysis of ICA and icariside II in the brain tissue after the administration of ICA. With the exception of icariside II, the major metabolites of ICA include may be desmethylicaritin, icaritin (Liu & Lou, 2004; Liu, Ye, & Lou, 2005; Wang et al., 2013; Wu, Wu, Xia, Li, & Dong, 2013; Yin et al., 2016), and monoglycoside (Chen et al., 2011).

3. Neuroprotective effects

Recent studies have shown that ICA exhibits a wide range of pharmacological activities in the prevention and therapeutics in various disorders in the nervous systems. Although many mechanisms of neuronal injury induced by ischemia have been identified, an effective therapeutic method is still lack for cerebral ischemia. In recent years, there are increasing interests in exploring novel drug candidates from traditional Chinese medicine. Li et al. used rat model to demonstrate that ICA can prevent neuronal damage and enhancing recognition ability after cerebral ischemia-reperfusion (Li, Zhou, & Shi, 2005). In addition, Zheng et al. have found that ICA can improve spatial recognition in a cerebral ischemia-reperfusion injury model (Zheng, Qu, & Lou, 2008). Xiong et al. have shown that ICA can protect the brain injury induced by ischemia/reperfusion, which is possibly due to a combination of the suppression of IκB-α degradation, pro-inflammatory cytokine production and NF-κB activation (Xiong et al., 2016). Clearly, the findings strongly supported both the neuroprotective effect and anti-neuroinflammatory effect of ICA.

Detailed mechanisms of the neuronal protective and anti-inflammative effects of ICA remain to be clarified. Derosa et al. proposed a hypothesis based on the protein family PPAR, including PPARα, PPARβ, PPARγ, and PPARδ (Derosa, Sahebkar, & Maffioli, 2018). PPAR is an important protein family involving in many physiological and pathological functions, especially in neuroinflammatory (Choi et al., 2017). Agonists of PPAR can significantly inhibit the overstimulation of microglia induced by ischemia-reperfusion (Xuan et al., 2015). In the experiment by Xiong and coworkers, it was shown that ICA can upregulate the expression level of PPAR in brain, which was evidence that the neuroprotective effect of ICA may due to the PPAR involving pathway.

Some recent studies have also indicated the anti-apoptotic mechanisms of ICA. Interestingly, Wang et al. have found that ICA can improve neuronal viability and alleviate neuronal death in their in vitro studies (Wang et al., 2009). They have demonstrated that the mechanism may through the activation of p38 and hence increasing SIRT1 activity (Wang et al., 2009). Similarly, Zhu et al. also discovered that ICA can reduce infarct size and brain edema, by possibly upregulating the expression of SIRT1 and PGC-1α, which is a target of PPAR protein (Zhu et al., 2010). Mo et al. reported that ICA can improve neuronal viability through the upregulating of Bcl-2 and down-regulating caspase-3, LC3-II, Beclin-1 and Bax (Mo, Li, Zhai, & Gong, 2016). The discoveries supported the hypothesis that anti-apoptotic effect of ICA is closely related to the Bcl-2 signaling pathway.

As a typical neurodegenerative disease, AD is accompanied with cognitive decline, as well as histopathological evidence of $A\beta$ plaques, tau protein accumulation, and synaptic loss. The $A\beta$ hypothesis considering the overproduction of $A\beta$ is the main theory for AD development (Selkoe & Hardy, 2016). In this model, $A\beta$ is formed from APP protein cleaved by BACE1, which is found to be upregulated in AD brains (Walker, Dixit, Saulsberry, May, & Harrison, 2017). Consequently, AD pathogenesis can be inhibited by interrupting the APP cleavage process catalyzed by BACE1. Studies have shown that ICA can significantly suppress various APP-related processes, including the accumulation of $A\beta$, down-regulating the expression of APP or BACE-1, reducing the level of SOD (Li, Dong, et al., 2015; Nie et al., 2010; Zhang, Shen, et al., 2014; Zhang, Li, et al., 2014).

A potential target in the treatment of AD is the inhibition of $A\beta$ assembly. Nie et al. have shown that ICA can enhance spatial cognition ability of $A\beta_{25-35}$-treated rats (Nie et al., 2010), indicating ICA is a potential therapeutic agent for AD. More importantly, recent studies have shown that ICA can reduce cognitive deficits and neuronal damages induced by chronic cerebral hypoperfusion (Li, Deng, et al., 2015; Xu et al., 2009). Since there is no candidate compound to the treatment of cognitive impairment in AD induced by chronic cerebral hypoperfusion (Ashok, Rai, Raza, Pandey, & Bandyopadhyay, 2016), their discoveries suggested that ICA may be a potential candidate for the treatment of cognitive disorder in AD (Li, Deng, et al., 2015; Xu et al., 2009). Luo et al. observed that a long-period treatment of ICA in spatial cognitive deficit mice model induced by aluminum can significantly protect brain injury, presumably by altering the activity of SOD and Aβ levels in the hippocampus (Luo et al., 2007). These findings definitely provide evidence that ICA may be a hopeful drug candidate for the therapeutics of Aβ toxicity-involved AD.

On the other hand, the tau hypothesis stated that microtubule associated proteins (MAPs) can promote the assembly process of tubulin and lead to the accumulation of tau protein in pathological neuronal inclusions in AD brains. It is believed that the tau inclusions are important in AD neurodegeneration (Laurent, Buée, & Blum, 2018; Mondragón-Rodríguez, Perry, Pena-Ortega, & Williams, 2017). Zeng et al. have reported that ICA can reduce cytotoxicity and cell apoptosis induced by Ab via the inhibition of PI3K/Akt activation (Zeng, Ko, Yang, & Wang, 2010). Song et al. have found that ICA can inhibit neuron cell apoptosis induced by formaldehyde, and the inhibition is closely related to phosphorylation of tau protein (Song, Miao, et al., 2016).

Besides the widely accepted model of AD, i.e., Aβ and tau hypothesis, it is discovered that the pharmacological effect of ICA may via other mechanisms, such as increasing NO synthase isoforms (Jin et al., 2014), increasing CART mRNA and protein expression (Sha, Li, Ye, Liu, & Xu, 2009), decreasing α-synuclein protein expression (Zhang et al., 2015), promoting neuronal activity (Chen et al., 2016) and enhancing neural stem cells (Fu et al., 2018).

Parkinson's disease (PD), characterized by the loss of midbrain substantia nigra dopaminergic neurons, is another important neurodegenerative disease. Since the mechanism of PD is still unknown, an effective therapy is not fully developed. Interests on herbal medicine have led to the discovery of the pharmacological effect of ICA on PD. Chen et al. have found that ICA can alleviate dopamine content in the SNpc (Chen et al., 2017).

More importantly, Chen et al. have demonstrated that ICA has neuroprotective effect by decreasing the expression of α-synuclein and inhibiting the PI3K/Akt and ERK1/2 signal pathways (Chen et al., 2017). Wang et al. have discovered that ICA can protect rat midbrain neuronal damage induced by 6-OHDA/LPS (Wang et al., 2018). Their experiment suggested that the neuroprotective effect of ICA may be associated with the reduction of inflammatory factors (Wang et al., 2018).

4. Protective effects of cardiovascular disease

Cardiovascular diseases, including atherosclerosis, ischemic heart disease, cardiomyopathy and congestive heart failure, are global health threatening diseases (Kessler, Vilne, & Schunkert, 2016). Although the exploration of the pathogenesis of cardiovascular diseases is significant, the detailed mechanisms and therapies are still lacking. Despite of the discovered neurohumoral factors such as angiotensin II, renin, endotheli, and transforming growth factor, an effective inhibition of the adaptive-hypertrophy-to-cardiac-negative-remodeling transition is not well developed. In recent years, researchers are searching for new therapeutics from traditional Chinese medicine.

Ding et al. have proven that ICA can promote the directional differentiation of murine stem cells into cardiomyocytes (Ding, Liang, Hu, Zhu, & Lou, 2008). Song et al. have showed that ICA can alleviate cardiac remodeling in rats with congestive heart failure (Song et al., 2011). In the later work, Song et al. used the oxidative stress injury model to clarify the mechanisms of the protective effect of ICA (Song, Cai, et al., 2016). They found that a pretreatment of ICA can protect the cells from the oxidative toxicity. In addition, ICA prevented the mitochondria membrane potential dissipation (Song, Cai, et al., 2016). In addition, ICA significantly suppressed the ROS generation and maintained Ca^{2+} homeostasis. Song et al. have found that ICA could also increase the phosphorylation of ERK (Song, Cai, et al., 2016).

In mitochondrial apoptotic pathway, the up-regulated expression of p53 protein can induce DNA damage and apoptosis through the increasing of mitochondrial membrane permeability. Studies have shown that the mitochondrial apoptotic pathway might play an important role in cardiac remodeling as well as cardiomyocyte apoptosis (Hamet et al., 1996; Zhang et al., 2016). Therefore, researchers are interested in exploring drug molecules target the mitochondrial apoptotic pathway. Heng et al. have demonstrated that ICA can significantly reduce cardiomyocyte apoptosis in the in vitro cardiomyocytes induced by angiotensin II (Zhou et al., 2014). Qian et al. have studied the in vivo potential of ICA in the protection of apoptosis in cardiomyocytes. They found that ICA can inhibit cardiomyocyte apoptosis and decrease blood pressure in rat model. The expression of Bcl-2 was up-regulated, and the expression of p53, Bax, Bok was down-regulated after oral administration of ICA.

5. Anti-osteoporosis

As one of global health problems in aging population, osteoporosis is a type of bone disorder resulted from an imbalance of bone formation and resorption. Features of osteoporosis include bone microstructure degeneration, bone mass reduction, and bone fractures. In cells, the balance of bone formation and resorption can be interrupted acids and enzymes, generating mineralized bone structure. Clinically, drugs used in bone therapy include inhibitors of bone resorption and promoters of bone formation. However, the adverse side effects, such as nasal irritation, acute phase response, musculoskeletal pain, and osteonecrosis of the jaw, have limited the clinical use of these traditional drugs (Papapetrou, 2009).

In recent years, researchers are searching new drug compounds from traditional Chinese medicine. Among the available TCMs, ICA from Herba Epimedii was reported to be safe, non-toxic, and osteoinductive (Zhao et al., 2009). Researchers have reported that ICA can effectively prevent estrogen deficiency-induced bone fractures, presumably by activating the estrogen receptors (Liu, Zhong, He, & Chen, 2012; Nian, Ma, Nian, & Xu, 2009). Mok et al. have found that ICA can alleviate bone mass loss and strengthen distal femur, which are associated with the up-regulation of mRNA of OPG/RANKL in tibia (Mok et al., 2010). Wei et al. observed a promotion of bone formation in mandibular distraction osteogenesis after oral administration of ICA (Wei et al., 2011). Nian et al. also discovered that the degree of mineralized bone and its strength was improved by taking ICA (Nian et al., 2009).

Chen et al. have found that ICA enhances the osteogenic differentiation of bone marrow stroma cells, and gene expression including alkaline phosphatase, osteocalcin, and cytokines (Chen, Ma, et al., 2007). Fan et al. have reported that the osteogenesis effect of ICA is dose-dependent, and ICA can promote osteogenic differentiation (Fan et al., 2011). Researchers also discovered that ICA promotes the proliferation of human osteoblast (Guo, Zhao, Wang, Xu, & Zhan, 2011). Xiao et al. found that the expression of collagen and OPN mRNA were greatly up-regulated in rat model, and the effect was in a dose-dependent manner with an optimized concentration of 10^{-5} mol/L (Qiangbing, Anmin, & Fengjin, 2005). On the other hand, it is found that ICA enhances the secretion of collagen I and mRNA of Cbfa1 and Osterix (Ming, Chen, Ge, Ma, & Zhou, 2011; Zhai et al., 2011), and up-regulates BMP2 and BMP4 significantly (He et al., 2009).

Besides, it was found that ICA can inhibit osteoclastic differentiation, reduce motility and bone resorption (Huang, Yuan, Wang, Zhang, & Wang, 2007). Chen et al. have concluded that ICA inhibits the bone formation and resorption of osteoclasts, suggesting that ICA is a potential bone strengthen component (Chen, Ge, et al., 2007). Wang et al. have found that after the treatment with ICA, the number and activity of osteoclast were suppressed, and the expression level of OPG/RANKL was up-regulated (Wang, Liu, Lin, Lu, & Xu, 2012). In the later studies, Hsieh et al. have demonstrated that ICA can inhibit osteoclasto genesis induced by LPS at low concentration even without a cell viability loss (Hsieh, Sheu, Sun, & Chen, 2011). It was found that pro-inflammatory cytokines induced by LPS was also suppressed by ICA. Hsieh et al. have identified that ICA can down-regulate the activation of IκB, JNK, ERK1/2, p38, and HIF-1α pathways, and therefore suppressed osteoclasts. In addition, they found that ICA suppressed IκB and ERK1/2 pathways in osteoblasts (Hsieh et al., 2011).

As reported by Wernike et al. vascularization is important in bone formation (Wernike et al., 2010). Chung et al. have shown that the endothelial cell proliferation and tubulogenesis was promoted by ICA (Chung et al., 2008). Some studies have shown that ICA can protect vascular endothelial cells through anti-apoptosis effect (Ji, Li, & Zhang, 2005; Wang & Huang, 2005). Liu et al. have reported that ICA can promote EGF-EGFR pathway and up-regulate the expression of endothelial NOS (Liu et al., 2011). More importantly, an enhancement of ERK, PI3K, Akt, endothelial NOS without influencing vascular endothelial growth factor implies that ICA can activate angiogenesis (Chung et al., 2008; Xu & Huang, 2007), which suggests ICA is a potential drug in angiogenic therapy.

Some studies have indicated that ICA is an effective compound for chondrogenesis (Liu, Sun, Tsai, Sheu, & Chen, 2010). Zhang et al. have found that a higher concentration of ICA can activate extracellular expression of chondrogenesis genes of chondrocytes (Zhang, Zhang, Fong, Yao, & Yang, 2012). It is discovered that ICA can promote the synthesis of

GAGs (glycosaminoglycans) and collagen of chondrocytes, which is presumably through the activation of collagen II Sox9 and suppression of collagen I gene of chondrocytes (Li et al., 2012). These findings suggest ICA would be a promising compound to promote chondrogenesis.

6. Anti-inflammation

Kong et al. have reported that ICA has anti-inflammatory potential in atopic dermatitis mouse (Kong et al., 2015). It is discovered that atopic dermatitis pathogenesis is due to an immune reaction in keratinocytes (Barker et al., 1991), which is closely related to the up-regulation of pro-inflammatory cytokines, including TNF-α, IFN-γ, IL-6, IL-1, and IL-8 (Seo, Youn, Choi, & Park, 2015). Kong et al. have evaluated the anti-inflammatory effect of ICA in the inflammatory response induced by TNF-α, IFN-γ. They found that ICA has a dose-dependent inhibition of the production of IL-6, IL-8, IL-1β, and MCP-1 induced by TNF-α/IFN-γ (Kong et al., 2015). The anti-inflammatory potential of ICA was a combination effect of the suppression of substance P, the p38-MAPK, TNF-α-R1 and IFN-γ-R1 signaling pathway (Kong et al., 2015).

Some studies have shown the anti-inflammatory effect of ICA by possibly regulating the activity of GR and NF-κB (Li et al., 2014; Xu et al., 2010). Sun et al. used inflammatory cell models of RAW 264.7 and HeLa cell induced by LPS to investigate the mechanism of the anti-inflammatory effect of ICA (Sun et al., 2018). They found that ICA can decrease the production of IL-6 and TNF-α induced by LPS, and up-regulate the amount of GRα, which in the nucleus will bound with excessive NF-κB, c-Jun, and Stat3. These findings suggest the anti-inflammatory effect of ICA may be due to an increased function of GR and suppression of pro-inflammatory transcription factors (Sun et al., 2018).

ICA also has anti-inflammatory effect in kidney inflammatory disease. Lupus nephritis is a serious systemic lupus erythematosus disease, which causes morbidity and mortality in patients (Bagavant & Fu, 2009). It was found that NF-κB activation and NLRP3 inflammasome activation are involved in lupus nephritis pathogenesis (Kahlenberg et al., 2011; Zhang & Sun, 2015). Therefore, researchers are searching for drug compound targeting these proteins. Su et al. have studied the anti-inflammatory effect of ICA by investigating MRL/lpr mouse model (Su et al., 2018). They have found that ICA treated group can significantly alleviate the renal disease, by decreasing anti-dsDNA antibody level and immune complex. Mechanistically, ICA suppressed the activation of NF-κBand the production of TNF-α, CCL2. The macrophage infiltration in MRL/lpr mouse model was also inhibited. In addition, ICA was shown to be an inhibitor to decrease the activation of NLRP3 inflammasome and the production of IL-1β.

The feature of chronic kidney disease is characterized by the pathology change of renal tubulointerstitial fibrosis. Some studies have demonstrated that in the development of renal fibrosis, there is frequently infiltration of inflammatory cells and the consecutive secretion of profibrotic factors (LeBleu, Sugimoto, Miller, Gattone Ii, & Kalluri, 2008; Sean Eardley & Cockwell, 2005; Zeisberg & Neilson, 2010). Also, researchers have shown that ICA has a potential to protect renal function (Huang et al., 2015; Liang, Tian, Han, &Xiong, 2014). Chen et al. have studied the mechanism of the protection effect of ICA on renal function (Chen et al., 2019). They found that ICA can significantly reverse the pathological changes, collagen deposition, and protein expressions of profibrotic factors in mouse model. The ICA treated group also suppressed the production of Smad2/3 and increased the expression level of E-cadherin. Pro-inflammatory factors such as NF-κB, COX-2 IL1β and NADPH oxidase-4 were alleviated by taking ICA (Chen et al., 2019). Their experiment indicated that ICA may be a therapeutic compound in renal fibrosis.

7. Improved effects of reproductive system

In traditional herbal formulations in Asian countries such as China, Japan, and Korea, *epimedium* usually used to treat erectile dysfunction. (Low & Tan, 2007) Animal experiments also showed that ICA administration improves erectile function in aged male rats. Therefore, the research on the principal bioactive compound in *epimedium* has drawn extensive interest (Makarova et al., 2007). For male reproductive system, experiments indicated that the treatment of ICA had virtually no effect on the body weight or organ coefficients of the testes or epididymides. However, 100 mg/kg ICA significantly increased epididymal sperm counts. In addition, 50 and 100 mg/kg ICA significantly increased testosterone levels. Real-time PCR suggests ICA may promote testosterone production by regulating mRNA expression of genes such as steroidogenic acute regulatory protein (StAR) and peripheral type benzodiazepine receptor (PBR). However, 50 and 100 mg/kg ICA treatment can improve anti-oxidative capacity, 200 mg/kg ICA treatment upregulated oxidative stress. These results suggest that ICA can benefit male reproductive functions within a certain dose range, meanwhile, higher doses of ICA may damage reproductive functions by increasing oxidative stress in the testes. (Chen, Hao, Yang, & Li, 2014). In another study, researchers found that ICA can improve the sexual function of male mice through the PI3K/AKT/eNOS/NO signaling pathway (Ding et al., 2018).

For female reproductive system, results indicated that ICA can enhance estrogen biosynthesis in human ovarian granulosa-like KGN cells by increasing the expression of aromatase (Yang et al., 2013). In another study, Treatment with ICA can significantly increase the duration of the estrus cycle. Ovary weight was also increased by the ICI treatments (Nie et al., 2019). The effects of ICA were also examined in a mouse model of D-galactose (D-gal)-induced ovarian aging. The experiments demonstrated that Ica can enhance follicular development, inhibit follicular atresia, decrease serum levels of luteinizing hormone (LH) and follicle-stimulating hormone (FSH), increase serum E2, and ovarian expression of AMH and the Bcl-2/Bax ratio in aging mice, therefore recover ovarian function in aging mice. Just like the previous reports, the optimal dosage of ICA was 100mg/kg (Wang, Liu, et al., 2019).

8. Antioxidant stress

Oxidative stress is essentially an imbalance between the production of free radicals and the ability of the body to counteract or detoxify their harmful effects through neutralization by antioxidants. Oxidative stress can lead to many pathophysiological conditions in the body, such as neurodegenerative diseases, gene mutations, cancers, heart and blood vessel disorders, fragile X syndrome, atherosclerosis, heart failure, heart attack, chronic fatigue syndrome, and inflammatory diseases (Aouache, Biquard, Vaiman, & Miralles, 2018; Farías et al., 2017; Reichmann, Voth, & Jakob, 2018). Therefore, the development inhibitors of oxidative stress provide valuable targets for treatment of the diseases mentioned above.

Experiments found ICA can protects vascular endothelial cells from oxidative stress through inhibiting endoplasmic reticulum stress. In human umbilical vein endothelial cells, ICA exhibit multiple effects, including improved cell viability and adhesion, reduced cell apoptosis, reduced H_2O_2 damage, and increased SOD and GSH-Px activity.

And that the mechanism underlying its protective effects may be the inhibition of ATF4 eIF2a and GRP78 protein expressions in the ERS, and then alleviation of oxidative stress damage (Wang, Jia, et al., 2019). In another experiment, ICA was found to protect the cardiac cells from oxidative stress injury through ROS scavenge and stimulation of ERK pathway (Song, Cai, et al., 2016).

9. Anti-depression

Depression is one of the most common psychiatric disorders which is hard to cure, hard to live with and hard to endure. According to the statistics of the World Health Organization (WHO), depression affects nearly 350 million people worldwide, and more than half of the suicides are accompanied by depression (Cavanagh, Carson, Sharpe, & Lawrie, 2003). The treatment techniques of depression can be divided into drug treatment and psychological treatment. Most of the widely clinically prescribed drugs for the depression therapy are selective serotonin reuptake inhibitors (SSRIs) and noradrenaline reuptake inhibitors. Besides the side effect of those drugs, SSRIs are fully effective in only approximately 40% of depressed patients (Berton & Nestler, 2006; Trivedi et al., 2006). Therefore, the discovery of a new and more effective therapy to treatment of depression is still of highly desirable.

Experiments have reported that ICA could suppress brain monoamine oxidase A and B activity and serum CRF levels, as well as increase brain monoamine neurotransmitter levels in FST in mice (Pan et al., 2005) and exhibit potent antidepressant-like effects in chronic mild stress (CMS) model of depression in rats via regulate the HPA axis hyperactivity and neuroinflammation (Liu et al., 2015; Pan et al., 2007; Pan, Zhang, Xia, & Kong, 2006). Moreover, ICA can exert an antidepressant-like activity in asocial defeat mouse model via up-regulation of glucocorticoid receptors (Wu, Du, et al., 2011). Further mechanism experiment investigate the effects of ICA on the depression-like behaviors in an unpredictable chronic mild stress (CMS) model. Rats exposed to CMS showed physical deficits and exhibited a significant increase in oxidative-nitrosative stress markers, inflammatory mediators, including TNF-α and IL-1β, activation of the NF-κB signaling pathway and increased inducible nitric oxide synthase (iNOS) mRNA expression in the hippocampus, which can be reversed by chronic treatment with ICA (20 or 40 mg/kg). In addition, ICA can also negatively regulate the activation of the nod-like receptor protein 3 (NLRP3) inflammasome/caspase-1/IL-1βaxis in the hippocampus of CMS rats (Liu et al., 2015). In another study, the therapeutic effect of

ICA in an animal model of glucocorticoid-induced depression was studied by using a combination of behavioral and biochemical assessments and NMR-based metabonomics. The results showed that ICA significantly increased sucrose intake and hippocampal BDNF level and decreased the immobility time in FST in CORT-induced depressive rats, suggesting its potent antidepressant activity. Mechanism investigation revealed that ICA reversed the pathological process of CORT-induced depression, partially via regulation of the disturbed metabolic pathways (Gong, Han, Wang, Liang, & Zou, 2016). Further studies on prenatally stressed male rats indicated that ICA ameliorates depression-like behavior via regulating abnormal expression of mGluR1, mGluR5 and EAAT2 in the hippocampus (Zhang et al., 2017).

10. Anti-tumors

Cancer treatment techniques include surgery, radiation therapy, chemotherapy, hormone therapy, and biological therapy (including immunotherapy and gene therapy). However, significant toxicity levels and the emergence of resistance toward anti-cancer drugs, making the process of treatment even more challenging. To solve the problem, scientific exploration of medicinal plants and herbs is now attracted great interest. In recent years, there has been a significant volume of research on the anti-cancer effect of ICA, the main active compounds from Herba Epimedii. In this section, an up-to-date of the anti-cancer mechanisms of ICA will be provided.

Studies revealed that the apoptotic effect of ICA has been associated with the activation of the intrinsic pathway of apoptosis (Li et al., 2010), which result in increase in Bax/Bcl2 ratio, release of cytochrome *c*, cleavage of poly (ADP-ribose) polymerase and activation of caspases in a wide range of cancer cells. Besides, endoplasmic reticulum stress (ERS) signaling in the anti-cancer activity of ICA has been studied on human adenocarcinoma and esophageal cancer cells (Di et al., 2015; Fan et al., 2016). ICA treatment upregulated ERS-related molecules such as p-PERK, ATF, GRP78, p-eIF2a, CHOP as well as apoptosis-related protein PUMA. At the same time, there was down-regulation of anti-apoptosis-related protein Bcl2. There result indicated that the apoptotic activity of ICA in cancer cells might be also closely related to the activation of ERS signaling.

The cell cycle consists of phases known as G0, G1, S, and G2M. Cyclin-dependent kinases (CDK) are the protein translating signals that push the cells through the cell cycle. When the normal regulation of cell cycle progression and division is disrupted, cancer might be triggered by the uncontrolled proliferation (Crespo-Ortiz & Wei, 2012). Experiments revealed that ICA can induce cell cycle arrest at G0/G1 and G2/M phases in colorectal cancer cells and gallbladder carcinoma cells respectively, which resulting in an anti-proliferative effect through down-regulation of cell cycle regulatory proteins (Jung et al., 2018; Zhu et al., 2015).

Angiogenesis is the formation of new blood vessels from preexisting ones, which is crucial for cancer development because blood vessels is required for supplying oxygen, nutrient, and growth factors to tumor growth and metastasis. Therefore, disruption of angiogenesis can cause inhibition of tumor invasion and metastasis. Experiments demonstrate that ICA was found to inhibit the proliferation, migration as well as tube formation of the cells. In a chick embryo chorioallantoic assay, the treatment of ICA can result in significant reduction in newly-formed blood vessels as well as reduced area and length of blood vessels. (Yang, Fichtner, Becker, Lemm, & Wang, 2009; Ye et al., 2015).

The outcome of cancer metastasis depends on multiple interactions between the malignant cell and the host environment. This process of invasion was initiated from the allowance of neoplastic cells to enter the lymphatic system and blood stream and reach other organs where secondary tumors may form, which is the major cause of treatment failure and death in cancer patients. ICA has also been investigated with reference to their anti-metastatic activity. Further experiment study revealed that the inhibition of human gastric cancer cell invasion by ICA was the suppression of expression of cell motility-related genes Rac1 and vasodilator-stimulated phosphoprotein (VASP) (Wang et al., 2010). A study on highly metastatic human lung main cancer cells also found a reduced ability of these cells to invade and migrate following treatment with ICA. In another experiment, ICA suppressed the adhesion of lung adenocarcinoma (Di et al., 2015). Recently, studies demonstrated that ICA could inhibit cell viability, migration, invasion, and induce apoptosis by down-regulation of miR-625-3p and inactive PI3K/AKT and MEK/ERK signaling pathways in thyroid cancer cells (Fang, Xu, & Kong, 2019).

Due to its excellent prospects in cancer therapy, tumor immunology has become a new focus for studies. Experiments indicated ICA can delay tumor progression and reduce the percentage of myeloid- derived suppressor cells (MDSCs), which possess immunosuppressive functions (Gabrilovich & Nagaraj, 2009). In another experiment, the results demonstrated that ICA could increase the cytotoxic T lymphocytes (CTL) response for P815AB peptide on the tumor-bearing DBA/2J mice. In addition, the percentage of CD4+CD8+/CD3+CD69+/CD69+NKG2D+ positive cells all increased after combined immunization with ICA and P815AB peptide. This indicated that ICA could enhance the immunogenicity of P815AB and improve the ability of T cells and CTLs in recognizing the tumor cells. In addition, ICA improved the function of peritoneal macrophages with effects of inhibition on tumor growth. Further mechanistic studies demonstrated that ICA has the potential to up-regulate LMP/TAP related molecules and induce the expression of MHC-I, which increase the immune surveillance and keep cancer in remission (Zhang et al., 2018). So, treatment with ICA not only kills tumor cells but can also involve anti-tumor immunity for tumor regression.

11. Conclusion

In this review, we have chosen ICA as an active component in the traditional Chinese herb to demonstrate its pharmacological effects by modern science. Since pharmacokinetics are essential to the understanding of drug pharmacology, we first reviewed a number of studies performed to establish a global view of the pharmacokinetics of ICA. We summarized recent advances in pharmacological studies of ICA, including neurodegenerative disease, cardiovascular disease, anti-osteoporosis, anti-inflammation, anti-oxidative stress, anti-depression and anti-tumors. As shown in this paper, ICA contains a broad spectrum of pharmacological effects, which we think will attract more interest for future studies.

Conflict of interest

The authors confirm that this article content has no conflict of interest.

Acknowledgments

The authors are grateful for the financial support by the National Science Foundation of China (NO. 81773739) and the first-class discipline projects of Pharmacy, and the Scientific Research Foundation for the Returned Overseas Chinese Scholars, Guizhou Province (2018)0013.

References

Aouache, R., Biquard, L., Vaiman, D., & Miralles, F. (2018). Oxidative stress in preeclampsia and placental diseases. *International Journal of Molecular Sciences*, *19*(5), 1496. https://doi.org/10.3390/ijms19051496.

Ashok, A., Rai, N. K., Raza, W., Pandey, R., & Bandyopadhyay, S. (2016). Chronic cerebral hypoperfusion-induced impairment of Abeta clearance requires HB-EGF-dependent sequential activation of HIF1alpha and MMP9. *Neurobiology of Disease*, *95*, 179–193. https://doi.org/10.1016/j.nbd.2016.07.013.

Bagavant, H., & Fu, S. M. (2009). Pathogenesis of kidney disease in systemic lupus erythematosus. *Current Opinion in Rheumatology*, *21*(5), 489–494. https://doi.org/10.1097/BOR.0b013e32832efff1.

Barker, J. N. W. N., Griffiths, C. E. M., Nickoloff, B. J., Mitra, R. S., Dixit, V. M., & Nickoloff, B. J. (1991). Keratinocytes as initiators of inflammation. *The Lancet*, *337*(8735), 211–214. https://doi.org/10.1016/0140-6736(91)92168-2.

Berton, O., & Nestler, E. J. (2006). New approaches to antidepressant drug discovery: Beyond monoamines. *Nature Reviews Neuroscience*, 7(2), 137–151. https://doi.org/10.1038/nrn1846.

Cavanagh, J. T. O., Carson, A. J., Sharpe, M., & Lawrie, S. M. (2003). Psychological autopsy studies of suicide: A systematic review. *Psychological Medicine*, *33*(3), 395–405. https://doi.org/10.1017/S0033291702006943.

Chen, H. A., Chen, C.-M., Guan, S.-S., Chiang, C.-K., Wu, C.-T., & Liu, S.-H. (2019). The antifibrotic and anti-inflammatory effects of icariin on the kidney in a unilateral ureteral obstruction mouse model. *Phytomedicine*, *59*, 152917. https://doi.org/10.1016/j.phymed.2019.152917.

Chen, K. M., Ge, B. F., Liu, X. Y., Ma, H. P., Lu, M. B., Bai, M. H., et al. (2007). Icariin inhibits the osteoclast formation induced by RANKL and macrophage-colony stimulating factor in mouse bone marrow culture. *Die Pharmazie—An International Journal of Pharmaceutical Sciences*, *62*(5), 388–391. https://doi.org/10.1691/ph.2007.5.6682.

Chen, M., Hao, J., Yang, Q., & Li, G. (2014). Effects of icariin on reproductive functions in male rats. *Molecules*, *19*(7), 9502–9514. https://doi.org/10.3390/molecules19079502.

Chen, K. M., Ma, H. P., Ge, B. F., Liu, X. Y., Ma, L. P., Bai, M. H., et al. (2007). Icariin enhances the osteogenic differentiation of bone marrow stromal cells but has no effects on the differentiation of newborn calvarial osteoblasts of rats. *Die Pharmazie—An International Journal of Pharmaceutical Sciences*, *62*(10), 785–789. https://doi.org/10.1691/ph.2007.10.7504.

Chen, Y., Wang, J., Jia, X., Tan, X., & Hu, M. (2011). Role of intestinal hydrolase in the absorption of prenylated flavonoids present in Yinyanghuo. *Molecules*, *16*(2), 1336–1348. https://doi.org/10.3390/molecules16021336.

Chen, W.-F., Wu, L., Du, Z.-R., Chen, L., Xu, A.-L., Chen, X.-H., et al. (2017). Neuroprotective properties of icariin in MPTP-induced mouse model of Parkinson's disease: Involvement of PI3K/Akt and MEK/ERK signaling pathways. *Phytomedicine*, *25*, 93–99. https://doi.org/10.1016/j.phymed.2016.12.017.

Chen, Y.-J., Zheng, H.-Y., Huang, X.-X., Han, S.-X., Zhang, D.-S., Ni, J.-Z., et al. (2016). Neuroprotective effects of icariin on brain metabolism, mitochondrial functions, and cognition in triple-transgenic Alzheimer's disease mice. *CNS Neuroscience & Therapeutics*, *22*(1), 63–73. https://doi.org/10.1111/cns.12473.

Cheng, S., Qiu, F., Wang, S., & He, J. (2007). HPLC analysis and pharmacokinetics of icariin in rats. *Journal of Separation Science*, *30*(9), 1307–1312. https://doi.org/10.1002/jssc.200600313.

Choi, M.-J., Lee, E.-J., Park, J.-S., Kim, S.-N., Park, E.-M., & Kim, H.-S. (2017). Anti-inflammatory mechanism of galangin in lipopolysaccharide-stimulated microglia: Critical role of PPAR-γ signaling pathway. *Biochemical Pharmacology*, *144*, 120–131. https://doi.org/10.1016/j.bcp.2017.07.021.

Chung, B.-H., Kim, J.-D., Kim, C.-K., Kim, J. H., Won, M.-H., Lee, H.-S., et al. (2008). Icariin stimulates angiogenesis by activating the MEK/ERK- and PI3K/Akt/eNOS-dependent signal pathways in human endothelial cells. *Biochemical and Biophysical Research Communications*, *376*(2), 404–408. https://doi.org/10.1016/j.bbrc.2008.09.001.

Crespo-Ortiz, M. P., & Wei, M. Q. (2012). Antitumor activity of artemisinin and its derivatives: From a well-known antimalarial agent to a potential anticancer drug. *Journal of Biomedicine & Biotechnology, 2012*, 247597. https://doi.org/10.1155/2012/247597.

Derosa, G., Sahebkar, A., & Maffioli, P. (2018). The role of various peroxisome proliferator-activated receptors and their ligands in clinical practice. *Journal of Cellular Physiology, 233*(1), 153–161. https://doi.org/10.1002/jcp.25804.

Di, S., Fan, C., Yang, Y., Jiang, S., Liang, M., Wu, G., et al. (2015). Activation of endoplasmic reticulum stress is involved in the activity of icariin against human lung adenocarcinoma cells. *Apoptosis, 20*(9), 1229–1241. https://doi.org/10.1007/s10495-015-1142-0.

Ding, L., Liang, X.-G., Hu, Y., Zhu, D.-Y., & Lou, Y.-J. (2008). Involvement of p38MAPK and reactive oxygen species in icariin-induced cardiomyocyte differentiation of murine embryonic stem cells in vitro. *Stem Cells and Development, 17*(4), 751–760. https://doi.org/10.1089/scd.2007.0206.

Ding, J., Tang, Y., Tang, Z., Zu, X., Qi, L., Zhang, X., et al. (2018). Icariin improves the sexual function of male mice through the PI3K/AKT/eNOS/NO signalling pathway. *Andrologia, 50*(1), e12802. https://doi.org/10.1111/and.12802.

Fan, J.-J., Cao, L.-G., Wu, T., Wang, D.-X., Jin, D., Jiang, S., et al. (2011). The dose-effect of icariin on the proliferation and osteogenic differentiation of human bone mesenchymal stem cells. *Molecules, 16*(12), 10123–10133. https://doi.org/10.3390/molecules161210123.

Fan, C., Yang, Y., Liu, Y., Jiang, S., Di, S., Hu, W., et al. (2016). Icariin displays anticancer activity against human esophageal cancer cells via regulating endoplasmic reticulum stress-mediated apoptotic signaling. *Scientific Reports, 6*, 21145. https://doi.org/10.1038/srep21145. https://www.nature.com/articles/srep21145#supplementary-information.

Fang, L., Xu, W., & Kong, D. (2019). Icariin inhibits cell proliferation, migration and invasion by down-regulation of microRNA-625-3p in thyroid cancer cells. *Biomedicine & Pharmacotherapy, 109*, 2456–2463. https://doi.org/10.1016/j.biopha.2018.04.012.

Farías, G. J., Molina, M. V., Carrasco, A. R., Zepeda, B. A., Figueroa, E., Letelier, P., et al. (2017). Antioxidant therapeutic strategies for cardiovascular conditions associated with oxidative stress. *Nutrients, 9*(9), 966. https://doi.org/10.3390/nu9090966.

Fu, X., Li, S., Zhou, S., Wu, Q., Jin, F., & Shi, J. (2018). Stimulatory effect of icariin on the proliferation of neural stem cells from rat hippocampus. *BMC Complementary and Alternative Medicine, 18*(1), 34. https://doi.org/10.1186/s12906-018-2095-y.

Gabrilovich, D. I., & Nagaraj, S. (2009). Myeloid-derived suppressor cells as regulators of the immune system. *Nature Reviews Immunology, 9*, 162. https://doi.org/10.1038/nri2506.

Gong, M.-J., Han, B., Wang, S.-M., Liang, S.-W., & Zou, Z.-J. (2016). Icariin reverses corticosterone-induced depression-like behavior, decrease in hippocampal brain-derived neurotrophic factor (BDNF) and metabolic network disturbances revealed by NMR-based metabonomics in rats. *Journal of Pharmaceutical and Biomedical Analysis, 123*, 63–73. https://doi.org/10.1016/j.jpba.2016.02.001.

Guo, H.-L., Zhao, Y.-F., Wang, X., Xu, Y., & Zhan, H.-S. (2011). Experimental study on the mechanism of icariin improving human osteoblasts proliferation and the expression of OPG protein. *Zhongguo gu shang = China journal of orthopaedics and traumatology, 24*(7), 585–588.

Hamet, P., deBlois, D., Dam, T. V., Richard, L., Teiger, E., Tea, B. S., et al. (1996). Apoptosis and vascular wall remodeling in hypertension. *Canadian Journal of Physiology and Pharmacology, 74*(7), 850–861. https://doi.org/10.1139/y96-076.

He, L., Deng, Y., Gao, J., Zeng, L., & Gong, Q. (2018). Icariside II ameliorates ibotenic acid-induced cognitive impairment and apoptotic response via modulation of MAPK pathway in rats. *Phytomedicine, 41*, 74–81.

He, W., Li, Z.-L., Cui, Y.-L., Yi, B., Liang, C., Wang, X.-X., et al. (2009). Effect of icariin on the mRNA expressions of Cbfalpha1, BMP2, BMP4 in rat osteoblasts. *Beijing da xue xue bao Yi xue ban = Journal of Peking University Health sciences, 41*(6), 669–673.

Hsieh, T.-P., Sheu, S.-Y., Sun, J.-S., & Chen, M.-H. (2011). Icariin inhibits osteoclast differentiation and bone resorption by suppression of MAPKs/NF-κB regulated HIF-1α and PGE2 synthesis. *Phytomedicine, 18*(2), 176–185. https://doi.org/10.1016/j.phymed.2010.04.003.

Huang, K.-T., Wu, C.-T., Huang, K.-H., Lin, W.-C., Chen, C.-M., Guan, S.-S., et al. (2015). Titanium nanoparticle inhalation induces renal fibrosis in mice via an oxidative stress upregulated transforming growth factor-β pathway. *Chemical Research in Toxicology, 28*(3), 354–364. https://doi.org/10.1021/tx500287f.

Huang, J., Yuan, L., Wang, X., Zhang, T.-L., & Wang, K. (2007). Icaritin and its glycosides enhance osteoblastic, but suppress osteoclastic, differentiation and activity in vitro. *Life Sciences, 81*(10), 832–840. https://doi.org/10.1016/j.lfs.2007.07.015.

Ji, R.-R., Li, F.-Y., & Zhang, X.-J. (2005). Effect of icariin on hypoxia induced vascular endothelial cells injury. *Zhongguo Zhong xi yi jie he za zhi Zhongguo Zhongxiyi jiehe zazhi = Chinese journal of integrated traditional and Western medicine, 25*(6), 525–530.

Jiang, J., Jie, S., & Jia, X. B. (2015). Phytochemistry and ethnopharmacology of epimedium L. species. *Chinese Herbal Medicines,* 7(3), 204–222.

Jin, F., Gong, Q.-H., Xu, Y.-S., Wang, L.-N., Jin, H., Li, F., et al. (2014). Icariin, a phoshphodiesterase-5 inhibitor, improves learning and memory in APP/PS1 transgenic mice by stimulation of NO/cGMP signalling. *International Journal of Neuropsychopharmacology, 17*(6), 871–881. https://doi.org/10.1017/S1461145713001533.

Jung, Y. Y., Lee, J. H., Nam, D., Narula, A. S., Namjoshi, O. A., Blough, B. E., et al. (2018). Anti-myeloma effects of icariin are mediated through the attenuation of JAK/STAT3-dependent signaling cascade. *Frontiers in Pharmacology, 9,* 531. https://doi.org/10.3389/fphar.2018.00531.

Kahlenberg, J. M., Thacker, S. G., Berthier, C. C., Cohen, C. D., Kretzler, M., & Kaplan, M. J. (2011). Inflammasome activation of IL-18 results in endothelial progenitor cell dysfunction in systemic lupus erythematosus. *The Journal of Immunology, 187*(11), 6143. https://doi.org/10.4049/jimmunol.1101284.

Kessler, T., Vilne, B., & Schunkert, H. (2016). The impact of genome-wide association studies on the pathophysiology and therapy of cardiovascular disease. *EMBO Molecular Medicine, 8*(7), 688–701. https://doi.org/10.15252/emmm.201506174.

Kong, L., Liu, J., Wang, J., Luo, Q., Zhang, H., Liu, B., et al. (2015). Icariin inhibits TNF-α/IFN-γ induced inflammatory response via inhibition of the substance P and p38-MAPK signaling pathway in human keratinocytes. *International Immunopharmacology, 29*(2), 401–407. https://doi.org/10.1016/j.intimp.2015.10.023.

Laurent, C., Buée, L., & Blum, D. (2018). Tau and neuroinflammation: What impact for Alzheimer's disease and tauopathies? *Biomedical Journal, 41*(1), 21–33. https://doi.org/10.1016/j.bj.2018.01.003.

LeBleu, V. S., Sugimoto, H., Miller, C. A., Gattone Ii, V. H., & Kalluri, R. (2008). Lymphocytes are dispensable for glomerulonephritis but required for renal interstitial fibrosis in matrix defect-induced Alport renal disease. *Laboratory Investigation, 88,* 284. https://doi.org/10.1038/labinvest.3700715.

Li, W.-X., Deng, Y.-Y., Li, F., Liu, B., Liu, H.-Y., Shi, J.-S., et al. (2015). Icariin, a major constituent of flavonoids from Epimedium brevicornum, protects against cognitive deficits induced by chronic brain hypoperfusion via its anti-amyloidogenic effect in rats. *Pharmacology Biochemistry and Behavior, 138,* 40–48. https://doi.org/10.1016/j.pbb.2015.09.001.

Li, F., Dong, H. X., Gong, Q. H., Wu, Q., Jin, F., & Shi, J. S. (2015). Icariin decreases both APP and Aβ levels and increases neurogenesis in the brain of Tg2576 mice. *Neuroscience, 304,* 29–35. https://doi.org/10.1016/j.neuroscience.2015.06.010.

Li, S., Dong, P., Wang, J., Zhang, J., Gu, J., Wu, X., et al. (2010). Icariin, a natural flavonol glycoside, induces apoptosis in human hepatoma SMMC-7721 cells via a

ROS/JNK-dependent mitochondrial pathway. *Cancer Letters, 298*(2), 222–230. https://doi.org/10.1016/j.canlet.2010.07.009.

Li, C., Li, Q., Mei, Q., & Lu, T. (2015). Pharmacological effects and pharmacokinetic properties of icariin, the major bioactive component in Herba Epimedii. *Life Sciences, 126*, 57–68. https://doi.org/10.1016/j.lfs.2015.01.006.

Li, L.-L., Sun, J., Xu, C.-Q., Zhang, H.-Y., Wu, J.-F., Liu, B.-J., et al. (2014). Icariin ameliorates cigarette smoke induced inflammatory responses via suppression of NF-κB and modulation of GR in vivo and in vitro. *PLoS One, 9*(8), e102345. https://doi.org/10.1371/journal.pone.0102345.

Li, D., Yuan, T., Zhang, X., Xiao, Y., Wang, R., Fan, Y., et al. (2012). Icariin: A potential promoting compound for cartilage tissue engineering. *Osteoarthritis and Cartilage, 20*(12), 1647–1656. https://doi.org/10.1016/j.joca.2012.08.009.

Li, L., Zhou, Q.-X., & Shi, J.-S. (2005). Protective effects of icariin on neurons injured by cerebral ischemia/reperfusion. *Chinese Medical Journal, 118*(19), 1637–1643.

Liang, J., Tian, S., Han, J., & Xiong, P. (2014). Resveratrol as a therapeutic agent for renal fibrosis induced by unilateral ureteral obstruction. *Renal Failure, 36*(2), 285–291. https://doi.org/10.3109/0886022X.2013.844644.

Liu, J., & Lou, Y.-J. (2004). Determination of icariin and metabolites in rat serum by capillary zone electrophoresis: Rat pharmacokinetic studies after administration of icariin. *Journal of Pharmaceutical and Biomedical Analysis, 36*(2), 365–370. https://doi.org/10.1016/j.jpba.2004.06.021.

Liu, T., Qin, X.-C., Li, W.-R., Zhou, F., Li, G.-Y., Xin, H., et al. (2011). Effects of icariin and icariside II on eNOS expression and NOS activity in porcine aorta endothelial cells. *Beijing da xue xue bao. Yi xue ban = Journal of Peking University. Health sciences, 43*(4), 500–504.

Liu, M.-H., Sun, J.-S., Tsai, S.-W., Sheu, S.-Y., & Chen, M.-H. (2010). Icariin protects murine chondrocytes from lipopolysaccharide-induced inflammatory responses and extracellular matrix degradation. *Nutrition Research, 30*(1), 57–65. https://doi.org/10.1016/j.nutres.2009.10.020.

Liu, B., Xu, C., Wu, X., Liu, F., Du, Y., Sun, J., et al. (2015). Icariin exerts an antidepressant effect in an unpredictable chronic mild stress model of depression in rats and is associated with the regulation of hippocampal neuroinflammation. *Neuroscience, 294*, 193–205. https://doi.org/10.1016/j.neuroscience.2015.02.053.

Liu, J., Ye, H., & Lou, Y. (2005). Determination of rat urinary metabolites of icariin in vivo and estrogenic activities of its metabolites on MCF-7 cells. *Pharmazie, 60*(2), 120–125.

Liu, M., Zhong, C., He, R.-X., & Chen, L.-F. (2012). Icariin associated with exercise therapy is an effective treatment for postmenopausal osteoporosis. *Chinese Medical Journal, 125*(10), 1784–1789. https://doi.org/10.3760/cma.j.issn.0366-6999.2012.10.018.

Low, W.-Y., & Tan, H.-M. (2007). Asian traditional medicine for erectile dysfunction. *The Journal of Men's Health and Gender, 4*(3), 245–250. https://doi.org/10.1016/j.jmhg.2007.05.010.

Luo, Y., Nie, J., Gong, Q.-H., Lu, Y.-F., Wu, Q., & Shi, J.-S. (2007). Protective effects of icariin against learning and memory deficits induced by aluminium in rats. *Clinical and Experimental Pharmacology and Physiology, 34*(8), 792–795. https://doi.org/10.1111/j.1440-1681.2007.04647.x.

Ma, H.-P., Ming, L.-G., Ge, B.-F., Zhai, Y.-K., Song, P., Xian, C. J., et al. (2011). Icariin is more potent than genistein in promoting osteoblast differentiation and mineralization in vitro. *Journal of Cellular Biochemistry, 112*(3), 916–923. https://doi.org/10.1002/jcb.23007.

Makarova, M. N., Pozharitskaya, O. N., Shikov, A. N., Tesakova, S. V., Makarov, V. G., & Tikhonov, V. P. (2007). Effect of lipid-based suspension of Epimedium koreanum Nakai extract on sexual behavior in rats. *Journal of Ethnopharmacology, 114*(3), 412–416. https://doi.org/10.1016/j.jep.2007.08.021.

Ming, L., Chen, K., Ge, B., Ma, H., & Zhou, J. (2011). Comparative study on effect of icariin and genistein on proliferation and mineralization of osteoblasts in vitro. *Zhongguo Zhong yao za zhi = Zhongguo zhongyao zazhi = China journal of Chinese materia medica*, *36*(16), 2240–2245.

Mo, Z.-T., Li, W.-T., Zhai, Y.-R., & Gong, Q.-H. (2016). Icariin attenuates OGD/R-induced autophagy via Bcl-2-dependent cross talk between apoptosis and autophagy in PC12 cells. *Evidence-based Complementary and Alternative Medicine*, *2016*, 6. https://doi.org/10.1155/2016/4343084.

Mok, S.-K., Chen, W.-F., Lai, W.-P., Leung, P.-C., Wang, X.-L., Yao, X.-S., et al. (2010). Icariin protects against bone loss induced by oestrogen deficiency and activates oestrogen receptor-dependent osteoblastic functions in UMR 106 cells. *British Journal of Pharmacology*, *159*(4), 939–949. https://doi.org/10.1111/j.1476-5381.2009.00593.x.

Mondragón-Rodríguez, S., Perry, G., Pena-Ortega, F., & Williams, S. (2017). Tau, amyloid beta and deep brain stimulation: Aiming to restore cognitive deficit in Alzheimer's disease. *Current Alzheimer Research*, *14*(1), 40–46.

Nian, H., Ma, M. H., Nian, S. S., & Xu, L. L. (2009). Antiosteoporotic activity of icariin in ovariectomized rats. *Phytomedicine*, *16*(4), 320–326. https://doi.org/10.1016/j.phymed.2008.12.006.

Nie, J., Luo, Y., Huang, X.-N., Gong, Q.-H., Wu, Q., & Shi, J.-S. (2010). Icariin inhibits beta-amyloid peptide segment 25–35 induced expression of β-secretase in rat hippocampus. *European Journal of Pharmacology*, *626*(2), 213–218. https://doi.org/10.1016/j.ejphar.2009.09.039.

Nie, X., Sheng, W., Hou, D., Liu, Q., Wang, R., & Tan, Y. (2019). Effect of Hyperin and Icariin on steroid hormone secretion in rat ovarian granulosa cells. *Clinica Chimica Acta*, *495*, 646–651. https://doi.org/10.1016/j.cca.2018.05.004.

Pan, Y., Kong, L.-D., Li, Y.-C., Xia, X., Kung, H.-F., & Jiang, F.-X. (2007). Icariin from Epimedium brevicornum attenuates chronic mild stress-induced behavioral and neuroendocrinological alterations in male Wistar rats. *Pharmacology Biochemistry and Behavior*, *87*(1), 130–140. https://doi.org/10.1016/j.pbb.2007.04.009.

Pan, Y., Kong, L., Xia, X., Zhang, W., Xia, Z., & Jiang, F. (2005). Antidepressant-like effect of icariin and its possible mechanism in mice. *Pharmacology Biochemistry and Behavior*, *82*(4), 686–694. https://doi.org/10.1016/j.pbb.2005.11.010.

Pan, Y., Zhang, W.-Y., Xia, X., & Kong, L.-D. (2006). Effects of icariin on hypothalamic-pituitary-adrenal axis action and cytokine levels in stressed sprague-dawley rats. *Biological and Pharmaceutical Bulletin*, *29*(12), 2399–2403. https://doi.org/10.1248/bpb.29.2399.

Papapetrou, P. D. (2009). Bisphosphonate-associated adverse events. *Hormones*, *8*(2), 96–110. https://doi.org/10.14310/horm.2002.1226.

Qian, Q., Li, S.-L., Sun, E., Zhang, K.-R., Tan, X.-B., Wei, Y.-J., et al. (2012). Metabolite profiles of icariin in rat plasma by ultra-fast liquid chromatography coupled to triple-quadrupole/time-of-flight mass spectrometry. *Journal of Pharmaceutical and Biomedical Analysis*, *66*, 392–398. https://doi.org/10.1016/j.jpba.2012.03.053.

Qiangbing, X., Anmin, C., & Fengjin, G. (2005). Effects of icariin on expression of OPN mRNA and type I collegen in rat osteoblastsin vitro. *Journal of Huazhong University of Science and Technology [Medical Sciences]*, *25*(6), 690–692. https://doi.org/10.1007/BF02896172.

Reichmann, D., Voth, W., & Jakob, U. (2018). Maintaining a healthy proteome during oxidative stress. *Molecular Cell*, *69*(2), 203–213. https://doi.org/10.1016/j.molcel.2017.12.021.

Sean Eardley, K., & Cockwell, P. (2005). Macrophages and progressive tubulointerstitial disease. *Kidney International*, *68*(2), 437–455. https://doi.org/10.1111/j.1523-1755.2005.00422.x.

Selkoe, D. J., & Hardy, J. (2016). The amyloid hypothesis of Alzheimer's disease at 25 years. *EMBO Molecular Medicine*, *8*(6), 595–608. https://doi.org/10.15252/emmm.201606210.
Seo, W. Y., Youn, G. S., Choi, S. Y., & Park, J. (2015). Butein, a tetrahydroxychalcone, suppresses pro-inflammatory responses in HaCaT keratinocytes. *BMB Reports*, *48*(9), 495–500. https://doi.org/10.5483/BMBRep.2015.48.9.259.
Sha, D., Li, L., Ye, L., Liu, R., & Xu, Y. (2009). Icariin inhibits neurotoxicity of β-amyloid by upregulating cocaine-regulated and amphetamine-regulated transcripts. *Neuroreport*, *20*(17), 1564–1567. https://doi.org/10.1097/WNR.0b013e328332d345.
Song, Y.-H., Cai, H., Gu, N., Qian, C.-F., Cao, S.-P., & Zhao, Z.-M. (2011). Icariin attenuates cardiac remodelling through down-regulating myocardial apoptosis and matrix metalloproteinase activity in rats with congestive heart failure. *Journal of Pharmacy and Pharmacology*, *63*(4), 541–549. https://doi.org/10.1111/j.2042-7158.2010.01241.x.
Song, Y.-H., Cai, H., Zhao, Z.-M., Chang, W.-J., Gu, N., Cao, S.-P., et al. (2016). Icariin attenuated oxidative stress induced-cardiac apoptosis by mitochondria protection and ERK activation. *Biomedicine & Pharmacotherapy*, *83*, 1089–1094. https://doi.org/10.1016/j.biopha.2016.08.016.
Song, Y.-X., Miao, J.-Y., Qiang, M., He, R.-Q., Wang, X.-M., & Li, W.-W. (2016). Icariin protects SH-SY5Y cells from formaldehyde-induced injury through suppression of Tau phosphorylation. *Chinese Journal of Integrative Medicine*, *22*(6), 430–437. https://doi.org/10.1007/s11655-015-2116-3.
Su, B., Ye, H., You, X., Ni, H., Chen, X., & Li, L. (2018). Icariin alleviates murine lupus nephritis via inhibiting NF-κB activation pathway and NLRP3 inflammasome. *Life Sciences*, *208*, 26–32. https://doi.org/10.1016/j.lfs.2018.07.009.
Sun, X., Deng, X., Cai, W., Li, W., Shen, Z., Jiang, T., et al. (2018). Icariin inhibits LPS-induced cell inflammatory response by promoting GRα nuclear translocation and upregulating GRα expression. *Life Sciences*, *195*, 33–43. https://doi.org/10.1016/j.lfs.2018.01.006.
Tang, W., & Eisenbrand, G. (2011). *Handbook of Chinese medicinal plants*. John Wiley.
Trivedi, M. H., Rush, A. J., Wisniewski, S. R., Nierenberg, A. A., Warden, D., Ritz, L., et al. (2006). Evaluation of outcomes with citalopram for depression using measurement-based care in STAR*D: Implications for clinical practice. *American Journal of Psychiatry*, *163*(1), 28–40. https://doi.org/10.1176/appi.ajp.163.1.28.
Walker, J. M., Dixit, S., Saulsberry, A. C., May, J. M., & Harrison, F. E. (2017). Reversal of high fat diet-induced obesity improves glucose tolerance, inflammatory response, β-amyloid accumulation and cognitive decline in the APP/PSEN1 mouse model of Alzheimer's disease. *Neurobiology of Disease*, *100*, 87–98. https://doi.org/10.1016/j.nbd.2017.01.004.
Wang, Y., Dong, H., Zhu, M., Ou, Y., Zhang, J., Luo, H., et al. (2010). Icariin exterts negative effects on human gastric cancer cell invasion and migration by vasodilator-stimulated phosphoprotein via Rac1 pathway. *European Journal of Pharmacology*, *635*(1), 40–48. https://doi.org/10.1016/j.ejphar.2010.03.017.
Wang, Y.-K., & Huang, Z.-Q. (2005). Protective effects of icariin on human umbilical vein endothelial cell injury induced by H_2O_2 in vitro. *Pharmacological Research*, *52*(2), 174–182. https://doi.org/10.1016/j.phrs.2005.02.023.
Wang, F.-Y., Jia, J., Song, H.-H., Jia, C.-M., Chen, C.-B., & Ma, J. (2019). Icariin protects vascular endothelial cells from oxidative stress through inhibiting endoplasmic reticulum stress. *Journal of Integrative Medicine*, *17*(3), 205–212. https://doi.org/10.1016/j.joim.2019.01.011.
Wang, G.-Q., Li, D.-D., Huang, C., Lu, D.-S., Zhang, C., Zhou, S.-Y., et al. (2018). Icariin reduces dopaminergic neuronal loss and microglia-mediated inflammation in vivo and in vitro. *Frontiers in Molecular Neuroscience*, *10*, 441. https://doi.org/10.3389/fnmol.2017.00441.

Wang, F., Liu, Z., Lin, S., Lu, H., & Xu, J. (2012). Icariin enhances the healing of rapid palatal expansion induced root resorption in rats. *Phytomedicine, 19*(11), 1035–1041. https://doi.org/10.1016/j.phymed.2012.06.001.

Wang, J.-L., Liu, B., Zhang, C., Wang, X.-M., Zhen, D., Huang, X.-M., et al. (2019). Effects of icariin on ovarian function in d-galactose-induced aging mice. *Theriogenology, 125*, 157–167. https://doi.org/10.1016/j.theriogenology.2018.10.028.

Wang, X.-L., Wang, N., Zheng, L.-Z., Xie, X.-H., Yao, D., Liu, M.-Y., et al. (2013). Phytoestrogenic molecule desmethylicaritin suppressed adipogenesis via Wnt/β-catenin signaling pathway. *European Journal of Pharmacology, 714*(1), 254–260. https://doi.org/10.1016/j.ejphar.2013.06.008.

Wang, L., Zhang, L., Chen, Z.-B., Wu, J.-Y., Zhang, X., & Xu, Y. (2009). Icariin enhances neuronal survival after oxygen and glucose deprivation by increasing SIRT1. *European Journal of Pharmacology, 609*(1), 40–44. https://doi.org/10.1016/j.ejphar.2009.03.033.

Wei, H., Zili, L., Yuanlu, C., Biao, Y., Cheng, L., Xiaoxia, W., et al. (2011). Effect of icariin on bone formation during distraction osteogenesis in the rabbit mandible. *International Journal of Oral and Maxillofacial Surgery, 40*(4), 413–418. https://doi.org/10.1016/j.ijom.2010.10.015.

Wernike, E., Montjovent, M. O., Liu, Y., Wismeijer, D., Hunziker, E. B., Siebenrock, K. A., et al. (2010). VEGF incorporated into calcium phosphate ceramics promotes vascularisation and bone formation in vivo. *European Cells & Materials, 19*, 30–40.

Wu, J., Du, J., Xu, C., Le, J., Xu, Y., Liu, B., et al. (2011). Icariin attenuates social defeat-induced down-regulation of glucocorticoid receptor in mice. *Pharmacology Biochemistry and Behavior, 98*(2), 273–278. https://doi.org/10.1016/j.pbb.2011.01.008.

Wu, X., Wu, J., Xia, S., Li, B., & Dong, J. (2013). Icaritin opposes the development of social aversion after defeat stress via increases of GR mRNA and BDNF mRNA in mice. *Behavioural Brain Research, 256*, 602–608. https://doi.org/10.1016/j.bbr.2013.09.034.

Wu, C., Zhang, J., Zhou, T., Guo, B., Wang, Y., & Hou, J. (2011). Simultaneous determination of seven flavonoids in dog plasma by ultra-performance liquid chromatography–tandem mass spectrometry and its application to a bioequivalence study of bioactive components in Herba Epimedii and Er-Xian Decoction. *Journal of Pharmaceutical and Biomedical Analysis, 54*(1), 186–191. https://doi.org/10.1016/j.jpba.2010.07.010.

Xiong, D., Deng, Y., Huang, B., Yin, C., Liu, B., Shi, J., et al. (2016). Icariin attenuates cerebral ischemia–reperfusion injury through inhibition of inflammatory response mediated by NF-κB, PPARα and PPARγ in rats. *International Immunopharmacology, 30*, 157–162. https://doi.org/10.1016/j.intimp.2015.11.035.

Xu, H.-B., & Huang, Z.-Q. (2007). Icariin enhances endothelial nitric-oxide synthase expression on human endothelial cells in vitro. *Vascular Pharmacology, 47*(1), 18–24. https://doi.org/10.1016/j.vph.2007.03.002.

Xu, C.-Q., Liu, B.-J., Wu, J.-F., Xu, Y.-C., Duan, X.-H., Cao, Y.-X., et al. (2010). Icariin attenuates LPS-induced acute inflammatory responses: Involvement of PI3K/Akt and NF-κB signaling pathway. *European Journal of Pharmacology, 642*(1), 146–153. https://doi.org/10.1016/j.ejphar.2010.05.012.

Xu, R.-X., Wu, Q., Luo, Y., Gong, Q.-H., Yu, L.-M., Huang, X.-N., et al. (2009). Protective effects of icariin on cognitive deficits induced by chronic cerebral hypoperfusion in rats. *Clinical and Experimental Pharmacology and Physiology, 36*(8), 810–815. https://doi.org/10.1111/j.1440-1681.2009.05149.x.

Xu, S., Yu, J., Zhan, J., Yang, L., Guo, L., & Xu, Y. (2017). Pharmacokinetics, tissue distribution, and metabolism study of icariin in rat. *BioMed Research International, 2017*, 17. https://doi.org/10.1155/2017/4684962.

Xuan, A.-G., Chen, Y., Long, D.-H., Zhang, M., Ji, W.-D., Zhang, W.-J., et al. (2015). PPARα agonist fenofibrate ameliorates learning and memory deficits in rats following global cerebral ischemia. *Molecular Neurobiology*, *52*(1), 601–609. https://doi.org/10.1007/s12035-014-8882-7.

Yang, J.-X., Fichtner, I., Becker, M., Lemm, M., & Wang, X.-M. (2009). Anti-proliferative efficacy of icariin on HepG2 hepatoma and its possible mechanism of action. *The American Journal of Chinese Medicine*, *37*(06), 1153–1165. https://doi.org/10.1142/S0192415X09007569.

Yang, L., Lu, D., Guo, J., Meng, X., Zhang, G., & Wang, F. (2013). Icariin from Epimedium brevicornum Maxim promotes the biosynthesis of estrogen by aromatase (CYP19). *Journal of Ethnopharmacology*, *145*(3), 715–721. https://doi.org/10.1016/j.jep.2012.11.031.

Yang, W., Yu, X.-C., Chen, X.-Y., Zhang, L., Lu, C.-T., & Zhao, Y.-Z. (2012). Pharmacokinetics and tissue distribution profile of icariin propylene glycol-liposome intraperitoneal injection in mice. *Journal of Pharmacy and Pharmacology*, *64*(2), 190–198. https://doi.org/10.1111/j.2042-7158.2011.01388.x.

Ye, L. K., Chen, J. M., & Liu, S. H. (1999). Pharmacokinetics of icariin in rats. *Chinese Pharmaceutical Journal*, *34*(1), 33–36.

Ye, Y. H., Hu, F. H., Zou, J. P., Zhan, Y., Wang, S. Q., & Liu, J. Y. (2015). Vivo and in vitro inhibitory effects of icariin on angiogenesis. *Zhongguo Yi Xue Ke Xue Yuan Xue Bao*, *37*(3), 264–268. https://doi.org/10.3881/j.issn.1000-503X.2015.03.003.

Yin, C., Deng, Y., Gao, J., Li, X., Liu, Y., & Gong, Q. (2016). Icariside II, a novel phosphodiesterase-5 inhibitor, attenuates streptozotocin-induced cognitive deficits in rats. *Neuroscience*, *328*, 69–79. https://doi.org/10.1016/j.neuroscience.2016.04.022.

Zeisberg, M., & Neilson, E. G. (2010). Mechanisms of tubulointerstitial fibrosis. *Journal of the American Society of Nephrology*, *21*(11), 1819. https://doi.org/10.1681/ASN.2010080793.

Zeng, K.-W., Ko, H., Yang, H. O., & Wang, X.-M. (2010). Icariin attenuates β-amyloid-induced neurotoxicity by inhibition of tau protein hyperphosphorylation in PC12 cells. *Neuropharmacology*, *59*(6), 542–550. https://doi.org/10.1016/j.neuropharm.2010.07.020.

Zhai, Y.-K., Li, Z.-Z., Chen, K.-M., Zhang, N., Cheng, G.-Z., & Zhu, R.-Q. (2011). Effects of icariin on the proliferation, differentiation and maturation of rat calvarial osteoblasts in vitro. *Zhong yao cai = Zhongyaocai = Journal of Chinese medicinal materials*, *34*(6), 917–922.

Zhang, X.-D., Kang, Z.-C., Li, Q.-J., Zhang, J., Cheng, S., Chang, H., et al. (2018). Antigen-adjuvant effects of icariin in enhancing tumor-specific immunity in mastocytoma-bearing DBA/2J mice. *Biomedicine & Pharmacotherapy*, *99*, 810–816. https://doi.org/10.1016/j.biopha.2018.01.139.

Zhang, Z.-Y., Li, C., Zug, C., & Schluesener, H. J. (2014). Icariin ameliorates neuropathological changes, TGF-β1 accumulation and behavioral deficits in a mouse model of cerebral amyloidosis. *PLoS One*, *9*(8), e104616. https://doi.org/10.1371/journal.pone.0104616.

Zhang, L., Shen, C., Chu, J., Liu, Y., Li, Y., Zhang, L., et al. (2015). Icariin reduces α-synuclein over-expression by promoting α-synuclein degradation. *Age*, *37*(4), 72. https://doi.org/10.1007/s11357-015-9811-z.

Zhang, L., Shen, C., Chu, J., Zhang, R., Li, Y., & Li, L. (2014). Icariin decreases the expression of APP and BACE-1 and reduces the β-amyloid burden in an APP transgenic mouse model of Alzheimer's disease. *International Journal of Biological Sciences*, *10*(2), 181–191. https://doi.org/10.7150/ijbs.6232.

Zhang, H., & Sun, S.-C. (2015). NF-κB in inflammation and renal diseases. *Cell & Bioscience*, *5*(1), 63. https://doi.org/10.1186/s13578-015-0056-4.

Zhang, X., Sun, H., Su, Q., Lin, T., Zhang, H., Zhang, J., et al. (2017). Antidepressant-like activity of icariin mediated by group I mGluRs in prenatally stressed offspring. *Brain and Development*, *39*(7), 593–600. https://doi.org/10.1016/j.braindev.2017.03.021.

Zhang, Y., Wang, Q.-S., Cui, Y.-L., Meng, F.-C., & Lin, K.-M. (2012). Changes in the intestinal absorption mechanism of icariin in the nanocavities of cyclodextrins. *International Journal of Nanomedicine*, 7, 4239–4249. https://doi.org/10.2147/IJN.S33014.

Zhang, C., Wang, F., Zhang, Y., Kang, Y., Wang, H., Si, M., et al. (2016). Celecoxib prevents pressure overload-induced cardiac hypertrophy and dysfunction by inhibiting inflammation, apoptosis and oxidative stress. *Journal of Cellular and Molecular Medicine*, *20*(1), 116–127. https://doi.org/10.1111/jcmm.12709.

Zhang, D., Zhang, J., Fong, C., Yao, X., & Yang, M. (2012). Herba epimedii flavonoids suppress osteoclastic differentiation and bone resorption by inducing G2/M arrest and apoptosis. *Biochimie*, *94*(12), 2514–2522. https://doi.org/10.1016/j.biochi.2012.06.033.

Zhao, H., Fan, M., Fan, L., Sun, J., & Guo, D. (2010). Liquid chromatography–tandem mass spectrometry analysis of metabolites in rats after administration of prenylflavonoids from Epimediums. *Journal of Chromatography B*, *878*(15), 1113–1124. https://doi.org/10.1016/j.jchromb.2010.03.023.

Zhao, J., Ohba, S., Komiyama, Y., Shinkai, M., Chung, U.-i., & Nagamune, T. (2009). Icariin: A potential osteoinductive compound for bone tissue engineering. *Tissue Engineering Part A*, *16*(1), 233–243. https://doi.org/10.1089/ten.tea.2009.0165.

Zheng, M., Qu, L., & Lou, Y. (2008). Effects of icariin combined with Panax notoginseng saponins on ischemia reperfusion-induced cognitive impairments related with oxidative stress and CA1 of hippocampal neurons in rat. *Phytotherapy Research*, *22*(5), 597–604. https://doi.org/10.1002/ptr.2276.

Zhou, J., Deng, Y., Li, F., Yin, C., Shi, J., & Gong, Q. (2019). Icariside II attenuates lipopolysaccharide-induced neuroinflammation through inhibiting TLR4/My D88/NF-KB pathway in rats. *Biomedicine & Pharmacotherapy*, *111*, 315–324.

Zhou, H., Yuan, Y., Liu, Y., Deng, W., Zong, J., Bian, Z. Y., et al. (2014). Icariin attenuates angiotensin II-induced hypertrophy and apoptosis in H9c2 cardiomyocytes by inhibiting reactive oxygen species-dependent JNK and p38 pathways. *Experimental and Therapeutic Medicine*, 7(5), 1116–1122. https://doi.org/10.3892/etm.2014.1598.

Zhu, S., Wang, Z., Li, Z., Peng, H., Luo, Y., Deng, M., et al. (2015). Icaritin suppresses multiple myeloma, by inhibiting IL-6/JAK2/STAT3. *Oncotarget*, *6*(12), 10460–10472. https://doi.org/10.18632/oncotarget.3399.

Zhu, H.-R., Wang, Z.-Y., Zhu, X.-L., Wu, X.-X., Li, E.-G., & Xu, Y. (2010). Icariin protects against brain injury by enhancing SIRT1-dependent PGC-1α expression in experimental stroke. *Neuropharmacology*, *59*(1), 70–76. https://doi.org/10.1016/j.neuropharm.2010.03.017.

CHAPTER EIGHT

Seaweed-derived bioactives as potential energy regulators in obesity and type 2 diabetes

Giovanna Bermano[a,†], Teodora Stoyanova[a], Franck Hennequart[b], Cherry L. Wainwright[a,*,†]
[a]Centre for Natural Products in Health, School of Pharmacy & Life Sciences, Robert Gordon University, Aberdeen, United Kingdom
[b]R&D Department, Algaia, Saint-Lô, France
*Corresponding author: e-mail address: c.wainwright@rgu.ac.uk

Contents

Abstract

There is epidemiological evidence that dietary intake of seaweeds is associated with a lower prevalence of chronic diseases. While seaweeds are of high nutritious value, due to their high content of fiber, polyunsaturated fatty acids and minerals, they also contain an abundance of bioactive compounds. There is a growing body of scientific data that these bioactive moieties exert effects that could correct the metabolic dysregulation that is present in obesity and Type 2 diabetes (T2D). In this review we describe how

† These authors share co-senior authorship.

Advances in Pharmacology, Volume 87
ISSN 1054-3589
https://doi.org/10.1016/bs.apha.2019.10.002

the molecular mechanisms, specific to different tissues, that underly obesity and T2D are influenced by both seaweed extracts and seaweed-derived bioactive molecules. In obesity, modulation of antioxidant capacity and reduction of intracellular ROS levels within tissues, and regulation of signaling pathways involved in enhancing browning of white adipose tissue, have been highlighted as key mechanism and identified as a potential target for optimal energy metabolism. In T2D, management of post-prandial blood glucose by modulating α-glucosidase or α-amylase activities, modulation of the AMPK signaling pathway, and similarly to obesity, reduction of ROS and NO production with subsequent increased expression of antioxidant enzymes have been shown to play a key role in glucose metabolism and insulin signaling. Future studies aimed at discovering new therapeutic drugs from marine natural products should, therefore, focus on bioactive compounds from seaweed that exert antioxidant activity and regulate the expression of key signaling pathways involved in glucose homeostasis, mechanisms that are common to both obesity and T2D management. In addition, more data is required to provide evidence of clinical benefit.

Abbreviations

3T3-LI	adipocyte cell line
ACC	acyl-coA carboxylase
AGE's	advanced glycation end-products
Akt/PKB	protein kinase B
AMPK	AMP-activated protein kinase
BAT	brown adipose tissue
BMI	body mass index
C/EBP-α/β	CCAAT/enhancer-binding proteins α/β
cAMP	cyclic adenine monophosphate
CCK	cholecystokinin
COX-2	cyclooxygenase-2
CPT1a	carnitine palmitoyltransferase-1a
DPP-4	dipeptidyl peptidase-4
EER	energy efficiency ratio
ERK	extracellular signal-regulated kinases
FABP4	fatty acid binding protein 4
FAS	fatty acid synthase
G6PDH	glucose-6-phosphate dehydrogenase
GAE	gallic acid equivalents
GLP-1	glucagon-like peptide-1
GLUT-4	glucose transporter type 4
GSH	glutathione
IL-6	interleukin-6
iNOS	inducible nitric oxide synthase
IRS-1	insulin receptor substrate
JNK	Jun N-terminal kinase
K_{ATP}	ATP-sensitive potassium channels

MAPK	mitogen activated protein kinase
MCP-1	monocyte chemoattractant protein-1
Nox4	nicotinamide adenine dinucleotide phosphate hydrogen (NADPH) oxidase 4
NQO1	NAD(P)H quinone oxidoreductase1
PAI-1	plasminogen activator inhibitor-1
PEPCK	phosphoenolpyruvate carboxykinase
PI3K	phosphatidylinositol 3-kinases
PPAR-γ	peroxisome proliferator-activated receptor-γ
PTP1B	protein-tyrosine phosphatase 1B
PYY	peptide YY
ROS	reactive oxygen species
SCD1	stearoyl-coenzyme A desaturase-1
SREBP-1C	sterol regulatory element binding protein 1c
SUR1	subunit sulfonylurea receptor 1
T2D	type 2 diabetes
TBARS	thiobarbituric acid reactive substances
TNFα	tumor necrosis factor alpha
UCP2	uncoupling protein 2
WAT	white adipose tissue

1. Introduction

Globally, obesity has reached epidemic proportions and it is contributing significantly to the problem of chronic diseases such as insulin resistance, type 2 diabetes mellitus, heart-related diseases, certain cancers, osteoarthritis, and sleep apnoea (Barness, Opitz, & Gilbert-Barness, 2007; Berrington de Gonzalez et al., 2010). It results from an imbalance between caloric intake and expenditure and is characterized by a disproportionate accumulation of adipose tissue that is commonly accompanied by systemic inflammation (Gonzalez-Muniesa et al., 2017). As obesity possesses different etiological and pathological origins, no single treatment or drug can effectively control the condition (Bakhai & Tirgar, 2013).

One of the major metabolic consequences of obesity is the development of Type 2 diabetes (T2D). In contrast to Type 1 diabetes, in which the destruction of pancreatic β-cells results in failure of insulin secretion and can only be treated by insulin replacement therapy, T2D results from reduced insulin secretion and/or insulin resistance and is open to therapeutic management by pharmacological means. A description of the physiological control of glucose and the development of insulin resistance is outside the scope of this review and has been well described elsewhere (e.g., Petersen & Shulman, 2018), but the main pharmacological approaches for the management of T2D involve the use of agents that target key events, from the point of entry of glucose into the circulation to the responsiveness to insulin at the cellular level. However, many of the drugs currently used for the management of T2D are associated with unpleasant side effects, and despite the variety of drugs available many do not achieve the appropriate glycemic control (Pramanik, Rathwa, Patel, Ramachandran, & Begum, 2018).

Seaweeds are of significant nutritious value due to their high content of fiber, polyunsaturated fatty acids and minerals, but they also contain an abundance of bioactive compounds. There is epidemiological evidence that in geographical regions (e.g., Japan and Korea) where the dietary intake of seaweeds is high, the prevalence of chronic diseases (e.g., hyperlipidemia, cardiovascular disease and cancer) is lower (Brown et al., 2014) and there is a growing body of scientific data that bioactive molecules present in seaweed (e.g., polyunsaturated fatty acids and phenolic compounds) exert effects that could correct the metabolic dysregulation that is present in obesity and T2D (Sharifuddin, Chin, Lim, & Phang, 2015; Wan-Loy & Siew-Moi, 2016). The cellular mechanisms underlying these biological effects, and the identity of the bioactive molecules responsible for the various pharmacological actions, are beginning to emerge. In this review we provide an up-to-date summary of how seaweed-derived bioactives may provide the basis for the development of novel therapeutics for the management of obesity and/or T2D.

2. Metabolic effects of seaweed in obesity

There are two main categories of anti-obesity drugs: ones that are able to reduce or limit energy absorption and those that aim to decrease fat mass by increasing energy expenditure or redistributing adipose tissue. Existing drugs have not been able to significantly and successfully reduce weight, and, as such, there is an urgent need for safe anti-obesity drugs that are therapeutically potent, and for research aimed at identifying their mechanism of action and at supporting the lack of side effects (Yun, 2010). One aspect of this research has focused on discovering extracts and/or bioactives with anti-obesity properties from the marine environment that might be readily available and have less adverse effects. Whole seaweed meal or seaweed extracts have been the focus of several studies; however, their mode of action in preventing fat accumulation and/or reducing weight is not totally understood; neither the classes of compounds nor the active ingredients responsible for seaweed anti-obesity properties have been fully characterized.

This section aims to provide a mechanistic evidence of the activity of whole seaweeds and extracts on metabolic physiology at the whole body level and highlight potential therapeutic targets at organ/tissue level. Scientific studies assessing the activity of whole seaweed, extracts or main bioactives via clinical trials, animal models or cell systems have been reviewed in the following sections and presented according to whole body or targeted tissues.

2.1 Activity of seaweed extracts and bioactive compounds at the whole-body level

Several animal studies have been undertaken over the years to test the anti-obesity properties of seaweeds and their extracts in mice or rats fed an obesogenic high-fat diet. Brown seaweeds have been widely studied, mainly because of their use as a food source in Far East Asian countries and Western Europe. Their high content in dietary fibers, minerals and vitamins, and low fat content, have made them interesting from a nutritional perspective, but they also offer a rich source of bioactive compounds, including complex polysaccharides (e.g., alginates, fucoidan and laminarin), polyphenols and phlorotannins, carotenoids such as fucoxanthin, and polyunsaturated fatty acids (Afonso, Catarino, Silva, & Cardoso, 2019), which can provide new sources of potential therapeutic drugs (Unnikrishnan & Jayasri, 2018).

2.1.1 Whole seaweed and seaweed extracts

The effect of the brown seaweed *Sargassum polycystum* on body weight and plasma biomarkers has been studied in rats fed a high fat diet supplemented with different doses of the seaweed powder for 8 weeks. The high-fat diet supplemented with 10% seaweed powder decreased the levels of plasma total cholesterol and triglycerides (35% and 45% vs high-fat control diet, respectively) and had a positive effect on the inhibition of weight gain (78% vs high-fat control diet) (Awang et al., 2014). Similarly, the effect of seamustard (*Undaria pinnatifida*) intake on body weight gain, blood glucose level and lipid profiles were studied in rats fed diets with different energy nutrient compositions (high fat vs high carbohydrate). Food intake, body weight gain and energy efficiency ratio (EER) were reduced in the high fat diet supplemented with 10% seamustard group (HFM10) compared with animals fed a high carbohydrate diet with 5% seamustard (HCM5). Fecal cholesterol excretion and serum LDL-cholesterol concentration in HFM10 group were the highest, while serum HDL-cholesterol level was the lowest among groups. Interestingly, HDL-cholesterol concentration was the highest in HCM5 group among groups. From these results, it was suggested that seamustard intake might be more effective for body weight control, more so with a high-fat diet than a high carbohydrate diet, but not for improving blood lipid profiles (Shin, 2009). Seaweed extract of *Ascophyllum nodosum*, ID-alG™, administered for 9 weeks to high-fat-fed Sprague-Dawley rats at a concentration of 40 and 400 mg/kg/day improved significantly the mean body weight gains and decreased significantly the percentage of body fat mass of rats (−9.8% and −19.0%), in comparison to high-fat diet fed rats. In the same way, triglyceride blood level was also significantly improved for the dose of 400 mg/kg/day (−30.6% vs +49.9% for the positive control); whereas total cholesterol, LDL and HDL blood levels were not modified (Terpend, Bisson, Le Gall, & Linares, 2012).

Fewer studies have investigated the response to green seaweeds in animal models of obesity and/or metabolic syndrome. Food supplementation with 5% dried *Ulva ohnoi* (UO) and *Derbesia tenuissima* (DT) for 8 weeks showed that UO lowered total final body fat mass by 24%, systolic blood pressure by 29 mmHg, and improved glucose utilization and insulin sensitivity. In contrast, DT did not change total body fat mass but decreased plasma triglycerides by 38% and total cholesterol by 17%. The different composition of the two seaweeds especially in relation to soluble fiber (UO contained 18.1% soluble fiber as part of 40.9% total fiber, while DT contained 23.4% total fiber, essentially as insoluble fiber) may justify why UO was more effective in reducing metabolic syndrome than DT (Kumar, Magnusson, Ward, Paul, & Brown, 2015).

2.1.2 Complex polysaccharides

Bioactive compounds extracted from brown seaweed have also been shown to exert anti-obesity properties. In particular, the hypolipidemic activity of a fucoidan extracted from the brown seaweed *Sargassum henslowianum* was tested in a mouse model of obesity: oral administration of the fucoidan at 100 mg/kg/day decreased blood cholesterol, triglyceride and LDL-cholesterol levels by 20% compared to obese mice administered water instead of seaweed extracts (Cuong, Thuy, Huong, Ly, & Van, 2015). Laminarin, a type of β-glucan isolated from brown seaweeds, affected energy homeostasis in obese mice orally administrated with laminarin. Chronic intragastric administration of laminarin (1 g/kg) every 2 days for 4 weeks decreased high fat-diet-induced body weight gain and fat deposition, and reduced blood glucose level and glucose tolerance; whereas acute laminarin administration (one single dose of 1 g/kg) enhanced serum glucagon-like peptide-1 (GLP-1) content, and suppressed food intake of mice after 3 h (Yang et al., 2017). The anti-obesity effects of enzymatic-digested alginate oligomers (E-AO) obtained from IL-6M and ULV-L3 (trade name of alginate products prepared from *Durvillaea* species and *Lessonia nigrescens*, respectively) were investigated at a 10% concentration in male mice fed a high-fat diet. E-AO showed strong anti-obesity effects judged by the reduction in body and adipose tissue weights (23% decrease in body weight gain and 40% decrease in epididymal fat weigh compared to mice fed high-fat diet). In addition, they suppressed plasma leptin level in females (Nakazono et al., 2016). Extracts from *Gelidium amansii* (GA) obtained by ethanol extraction were administered to male C57BL/6 mice in addition to a high fat diet, for 12 weeks. *G. amansii* extract (GAE) had protective effects: body weight was greatly decreased in mice fed a high-fat diet and supplemented with 1% or 3% GAE; blood glucose and serum insulin levels were also reduced by GAE treatment, suggesting improvement in glucose metabolism. GAE supplementation also led to a significant decrease in total cholesterol and triglyceride levels. Furthermore H&E staining confirmed smaller adipocytes size in mice fed a high-fat diet supplemented with GAE and reduced levels of steatosis in the liver (Kang et al., 2016).

From the studies highlighted above and summarized in Table 1, it is evident that, at least in animal models of obesity, whole seaweed or bioactive compounds prevent body weight gain and ameliorate plasma lipid profile and glucose metabolism; however the mechanisms by which they do so have not been fully defined. Changes in lipid absorption at the gastro-intestinal level, in glucose homeostasis and/or in leptin secretion/action may be partly responsible for the anti-obesity effects.

2.1.3 Human studies

Despite the number of studies carried out in animals, clinical studies are limited and do not encompass the assessment of potential mechanisms of action. Few studies have assessed alginates for their potential role in energy regulation through the inhibition of energy intake and/or an increase in the feeling of satiety. Postprandial satiety, energy intake, and gastric emptying rate (GER) were studied in normal-weight subjects via a four-way placebo-controlled, double-blind, crossover trial, who were randomly assigned to receive a 3% preload concentration of either low volume (LV; 9.9 g alginate in 330 mL)

Table 1 Summary of the anti-obesity effects of seaweed bioactives.

Seaweed color	Seaweed species	Country of origin	Extracts/specific compounds (concentration)	Biological model	Action	Reference source
Whole body						
Brown	*Ascophyllum nodosum*		Extract—ID-alG™—Bioserae (40, 400 mg/kg/day)	Female Sprague-Dawley rats fed high-fat diet	↓ Weight gain, body fat mass, plasma triglycerides	Terpend et al. (2012)
Brown	*Durvillaea* species *Lessonia nigrescens*	South Korea	Alginates oligomers enzymatically digested (IL-6M and ULV-L3 trade name) (10% w/w)	Male and female ddY mice fed high-fat diet	↓ Body weight gain, adipose tissue weight ↓ Plasma leptin levels in female mice	Nakazono et al. (2016)
Red	*Gelidium amansii*	South Korea	Ethanol extract (1%, 3% w/w)	Male C57BL/6 mice fed high-fat diet	= Body weight gain, adipose tissue weight with 1% ↓ Body weight gain, adipose tissue weight, serum total cholesterol, triglyceride with 3% ↓ Adipocytes size, steatosis in liver	Kang et al. (2016)
Brown	*Laminaria digitata*		Alginate (CM3 from Mayo Research Pharmacy)	Male and female healthy overweight/obese American adult volunteers	= Gastric functions, satiation, appetite, and gut hormones (ghrelin, CCK, GLP-1, PYY)	Odunsi et al. (2010)
Brown	*Laminaria hyperborea Lessonia trabeculata*		Alginate (Algogel DPG JO; Cargill) (low volume (LV) = 9.9 g sodium alginate/330 mL water; high volume (HV) = 15 g sodium alginate/500 mL water)	Male and female healthy young Danish subjects	↓ Energy intake with LV = Satiety feelings with LV ↑ Satiety feelings with HV ↓ Hunger, feeling of prospective food consumption with HV	Georg Jensen, Kristensen, Belza, Knudsen, and Astrup (2012)
Brown	*Sargassum henslowianum*	Vietnam	Fucoidan (100 mg/kg/day)	BALB/c strain mice fed high-fat diet	↓ Body weight, cholesterol, triglyceride, LDL-cholesterol	Cuong et al. (2015)

Brown	*Sargassum polycystum*	Malaysia	Whole seaweed powder (10% w/w)	Male Sprague-Dawley rats fed high-fat diet	↓ Weight gain, plasma total cholesterol, triglycerides	Awang et al. (2014)
Brown	*Undaria pinnatifida* (Seamustard)	Korea	Whole seaweed powder (5%, 10% w/w)	Male Sprague-Dawley rats fed high-fat diet or high carbohydrate diet	↓ Food intake, body weight gain, EER in HFM10 vs HCM5 ↑ Fecal cholesterol excretion, serum LDL-cholesterol in HFM10 ↓ Serum HDL-cholesterol level in HFM10	Shin (2009)
Brown			Fucoxanthin (1 and 3 mg/day)	Male and female healthy Japanese obese subjects	↓ Relative (ratio versus before treatment) body weight, BMI, visceral fat area in 3 mg/day group ↓ Relative total fat mass, subcutaneous fat area, waist circumference = Blood pressure, pulse rate, blood parameters, urinalysis	Hitoe and Shimoda (2017)
Brown			Laminarin (1 g/kg)	C57/BL6 mice fed high-fat diet	↓ Body weight, body weight gain, feeding efficiency = Food intake ↑ Serum GLP-1, in acute administration	Yang et al. (2017)
Green	*Derbesia tenuissima*	Australia	Dried seaweed (5% w/w)	Wistar rats fed a high carbohydrate/high-fat diet	= Total body fat mass ↓ Plasma triglycerides	Kumar et al. (2015)
Green	*Ulva ohnoi*	Australia	Dried seaweed (5% w/w)	Wistar rats fed a high carbohydrate/high-fat diet	↓ Total body fat mass, systolic blood pressure	Kumar et al. (2015)

BMI, body mass index; *CCK*, cholecystokinin, *EER*, energy efficiency ratio; *GLP-1*, glucagon-like peptide-1; *HCM5*, a high carbohydrate diet with 5% seamustard; *HFM10*, high-fat diet supplemented with 10% seamustard; *PYY*, peptide YY.

or high volume (HV; 15.0g alginate in 500mL) alginate-based beverage (Algogel DPG JO; Cargill, Minneapolis, MN, a combination of extracts from brown seaweeds *Laminaria hyperborea* and *Lessonia trabeculata*), or an iso-volume placebo beverage, 30min before a fixed breakfast and again before an ad libitum lunch. Consumption of LV-alginate preload induced an 8.0% reduction in energy intake compared to the placebo beverage at the following lunch meal, without differences in satiety. The HV alginate significantly increased satiety, reduced hunger and the feeling of prospective food consumption compared to the placebo, suggesting that alginate consumption does affect satiety and energy intake (Georg Jensen et al., 2012). On the contrary, a study evaluating the effects of 10 days treatment with alginate (CM3 alginate-based on brown seaweed *Laminaria digitate*) or placebo on gastric functions, satiation, appetite, and gut hormones (ghrelin, cholecystokinin (CCK), GLP-1, peptide YY (PYY)), showed no effect on any of the variable measured questioning the potential use of short-term alginate treatment for weight loss (Odunsi et al., 2010).

In another study in which the effect of fucoxanthin (Fx) (1 or 3mg daily) was tested in Japanese obese subjects, in a double-blind placebo-controlled study, administration of capsules containing Fx or placebo for 4 weeks induced a significant reduction of the relative (ratio versus before treatment) body-weight, BMI, and visceral fat area in the 3mg/day Fx group compared to the placebo group. Relative values of total fat mass, subcutaneous fat area and waist circumference were also significantly lower in the 1mg/day Fx group than the placebo group. No abnormalities in blood pressure, pulse rate, blood parameters, and urinalysis parameters were observed, thereby suggesting no adverse effects and supporting its potential use to improve a moderate overweight state by acting on both visceral and subcutaneous fat (Hitoe & Shimoda, 2017).

2.2 Activity of seaweed extracts and bioactive compounds in adipose tissue

The development of obesity is characterized by an increase in the number (hyperplasia) and size (hypertrophy) of adipocytes due to the processes of mitogenesis and differentiation, which are regulated by several factors, including genetic, endocrine, metabolic, environmental, and nutritional ones. Adipocyte function is associated with lipid homeostasis and energy balance: storing energy in the form of fatty acids, playing a central role in lipid and glucose metabolism and producing several hormones and cytokines (Rasouli & Kern, 2008). Targeting both adipogenesis and triglycerides synthesis may have, therefore, promising outcomes in controlling adipose tissue growth and numerous metabolic disorders in obesity. Several anti-obesity medications, such as orlistat (Xenical), lorcaserin, and topiramate have been developed to combat adipose tissue growth and expansion; however, these medications are associated with various adverse effects and so suitable and safe alternatives are needed. Seaweed extracts and/or bioactive compounds from seaweed may thus play a role in modulating such processes and energy metabolism and several studies aimed to identify their efficacy, molecular mechanisms and molecular targets, have been carried out (summarized in Table 2), using the murine 3T3-L1 preadipocyte cell line to investigate adipogenesis and to study the differentiation processes of preadipocytes into adipocytes.

2.2.1 Whole seaweed and seaweed extracts

Extracts obtained by macerating brown seaweed *Sargassum oligocystum* (SE) and *Padina australis* (PE) using acetone, were applied to 3T3-L1 cells during the differentiation stage and during the mature stage of the adipocyte life cycle to assess the effects of extracts on adipogenesis and adipolysis. Application of SE at 12.5 and 50 μg/mL decreased adipogenesis by 71.7%, and 84.8%, respectively, while cells treated with 12.5 and 50 μg/mL PE showed 85.7%, and 89.0% adipogenesis, respectively, compared to control. Application of SE and PE to mature lipid cells stimulated adipolysis and the release of glycerol by up to 88.6% and 93.0%, respectively, with 12.5 and 50 μg/mL SE, while PE increased glycerol release up to 92.9% and 95.6% respectively, compared to isoproterenol, used as positive control (Jaswir et al., 2017). Fermentation of *Laminaria japonica* (LJF) was performed to increase its physiological activity, before screening its anti-obesity potential using 3T3-L1 adipocyte cells: LJF inhibited adipocyte differentiation by significantly reducing the expression levels of CCAAT/enhancer-binding proteins α/β (C/EBP-α/β) and peroxisome proliferator-activated receptor-γ (PPAR-γ), involved in the early and late stages of adipocyte differentiation, and by decreasing the concentration of the adipocytokine adiponectin (Kim & Jang, 2018). Seaweed extracts from 49 species were firstly tested for free radical scavenging properties and the 3 species containing the highest levels of polyphenols were tested on adipocyte differentiation and reactive oxygen species (ROS) production during adipogenesis in 3T3-L1 cells. High total phenol contents were observed in the extracts of *Ecklonia cava* (681.1 μg gallic acid equivalents (GAE)/g), *Dictyopteris undulata* (641.3 μg GAE/g), and *Laurencia intermedia* (560.9 μg GAE/g); whereas *Sargassum*

Table 2 Summary of the effects of seaweed bioactives on adipose tissue.

Seaweed color	Seaweed species	Country of origin	Extracts/specific compounds (concentration)	Biological model	Action	Reference source
Adipose tissue						
Green	*Caulerpa okamurae*	South Korea	Ethanol extract (25–500 μg/mL)	3T3-L1 Male C57BL/6 mice fed a high-fat diet	↓ Lipid accumulation (ORO staining) ↓ C/EBP-α, PPAR-γ, SREBP-1c proteins	Sharma, Kim, Kim, Park, and Rhyu (2017)
Green	*Caulerpa okamurae*	South Korea	Ethanol extract (250 mg/kg)	Male C57BL/6 mice fed a high-fat diet	↓ Weight gain markers such as free fatty acid, triglycerides, total cholesterol, glucose in plasma ↓ PPAR-γ, C/EBP-α, FAS, SRBP1c, acetyl-CoA synthetase proteins	Sharma et al. (2017)
Brown	*Ecklonia cava*	South Korea	Methanol extract (100 μg/mL) Dieckol (phlorotannin) (100 μM)	3T3-L1	↓ Adipogenesis (ORO staining) ↓ Adipogenesis (ORO staining) ↓ PPAR-γ, C/EBP-α, SREBP1, FABP4 mRNA and protein ↑ AMPK activation	
Brown	*Eisenia bicyclis*	South Korea	6,6′-bieckol, 6,8′-bieckol, 8,8′-bieckol, dieckol, phlorofucofuroeckol A (phlorotannin) (10, 25 and 50 μg/mL) 6,6′-bieckol (50 μg/mL)	3T3-L1	↓ Lipid accumulation (ORO staining)—all phlorotannins ↓ PPAR-γ, C/EBP-α, SREBP-1c mRNA and protein—6,6′-bieckol ↓ FAS, ACC mRNA-6,6′-bieckol	Kwon et al. (2015)

Brown	*Fucus vesiculosus*	Brazil	Fucoidan rich fractions (different ratios fucose/glucuronic acid/galactose/xylose/sulfate—F0.5, F0.9, F1.1 and F2.0) (200 μg/mL)	3T3-L1	↑ Lipolysis (Glycerol release)—all fractions ↓ Adipogenesis (ORO staining)—F1.1, F2.0 ↑ Adipogenesis (ORO staining)—F0.5 ↓ C/EBP-α, C/EBP-β, PPAR-γ—F1.1, F2.0	Oliveira et al. (2018)
Brown	*Laminaria japonica*	South Korea	Extract from fermented seaweed	3T3-L1	↓ Adipocyte differentiation (C/EBP-α/β, PPAR-γ proteins) ↓ Adiponectin levels	Kim et al. (2018)
Brown	*Padina australis* *Sargassum oligocystum*	Malaysia	Acetone extract (12.5, 50 μg/mL)	3T3-L1	↓ Adipogenesis (ORO staining) ↑ Adipolysis (glycerol release)	Jaswir, Ahmad, Susanti, Bakhtiar, and Octavianti (2017)
Green Brown Brown Red	*Ulva* species *Palmaria palmata* *Undaria pinnatifida* *Himanthalia elongata*	Spain	Methanolic extracts (0.1 mg/mL)	3T3-L1	↓ Triacylglycerol levels	Rico et al. (2018)
Brown	*Sargassum echinocarpum*	Indonesia	Fucoxanthin	Pre-adipocyte cell from viscera tissue of wistar rats	↑ Adiponectin levels ↓ TNF-α expression	Firdaus, Nurdiani, and Prihanto (2015)

Continued

Table 2 Summary of the effects of seaweed bioactives on adipose tissue.—cont'd

Seaweed color	Seaweed species	Country of origin	Extracts/specific compounds (concentration)	Biological model	Action	Reference source
Brown	*Sargassum thunbergii*	Korea	Six indole derivatives (STCs) STC1: indole-2-carboxaldehyde STC-2: indole-3-carboxaldehyde STC-3: indole-4-carboxaldehyde STC-4: indole-5-carboxaldehyde STC-5: indole-6-carboxaldehyde STC-6: indole-7-carboxaldehyde (25, 50, 100 μM)	3T3-L1	↓ Adipocytes differentiation, lipid accumulation (ORO staining)—all STCs ↓ PPAR-γ, C/EBP-α, and SREBP-1c Protein—STC-1 and STC-5 ↓ AMPK activation and AMPK—STC-1 and STC-5	Kang et al. (2017)
Brown	*Undaria pinnatifida*	South Korea	Fucoidan (100 μg/mL)	3T3-L1	↓ Lipid accumulation (ORO staining) ↓ PPAR-γ, C/EBP-α, aP2 mRNA ↓ TNFα, MCP-1, PAI-1 ↓ ROS production	Kim and Lee (2012)
Brown	*Undaria pinnatifida*	Japan	Fucoxanthin (acetone extract) Fucoxanthinol (metabolite in white adipose tissue) (2.5 μM)	3T3-F442A adipocytes	↓ MCP-1 and IL-6 mRNA	Hosokawa et al. (2010)

Brown	*Undaria pinnatifida*	Japan	Fucoxanthin (acetone extract) (0.2% w/w)	C57Bl/6 and KK-A(y) mice	↓ WAT weight gain and hyperglycemia in KK-A(y) not C57Bl/6 mice ↓ MCP-1, TNF-α in MCP-1 in KK-A(y) not C57Bl/6 mice ↓ IL-6, PAI-1 mRNA in KK-A(y) mice	Hosokawa et al. (2010)
Brown	*Undaria pinnatifida*	South Korea	Fucoxanthin (ethanol extract) (0.2% w/w)	C57BL/6J mice fed high-fat diet	↓ WAT weights ↓ FA synthesis, ↓ UCP1 mRNA expression in epididymal WAT	Jeon et al. (2010), Maeda, Hosokawa, Sashima, Funayama, and Miyashita (2005), Maeda, Tsukui, Sashima, Hosokawa, and Miyashita (2008), Maeda, Hosokawa, Sashima, Murakami-Funayama, and Miyashita (2009)
Brown	*Undaria pinnatifida*	Japan	Fucoxanthin (acetone extract) (0.2% w/w)	KK-A(y) mice	↓ WAT weight gain ↑ UCP1 mRNA ↓ Leptin, TNF-α mRNA	Maeda et al. (2005), Maeda, Hosokawa, Sashima, and Miyashita (2007), Okada, Mizuno, Sibayama, Hosokawa, and Miyashita (2011)
Brown			Fucoidan (50, 100, and 200 μg/mL)	3T3-L1	↓ Lipid accumulation (ORO staining) ↓ C/EBP-α; PPAR-γ, aP2 mRNA ↓ p38 MAPKs, ERK, JNK activation factors	Kim, Lee, and Lee (2010)

Continued

Table 2 Summary of the effects of seaweed bioactives on adipose tissue.—cont'd

Seaweed color	Seaweed species	Country of origin	Extracts/specific compounds (concentration)	Biological model	Action	Reference source
Brown			Fucoidan (2% w/w)	Male C57BL/6 mice fed a high-fat diet	↓ Body-weight gain and epididymal fat mass ↓ PPAR-γ, aP2, ACC mRNA	Kim, Jeon, and Lee (2014), Kim, Rioux, and Turgeon (2014)
Red	*Gracilaria vermiculophylla papenfuss*	Korea	Ethanol extract/ethyl acetate fraction	3T3-L1	↓ Triglycerides accumulation (ORO staining) ↓ PPARγ, C/EBP-α, aP2 protein ↑ AMPK, LKB1 activation in mature adipocytes ↑ Intracellular ROS ↑ CPT1a, UCP2 mRNA	Kim et al. (2012)
Red	*Grateloupia lanceolata*	Korea	Ethanol extract (10 and 50 μg/mL)	3T3-L1	↓ Lipid accumulation (ORO staining) ↓ ROS production ↓ PPAR-γ and C/EBP-α mRNA, and aP2 protein ↓ Nox4, G6PDH mRNA ↑ SOD, glutathione peroxidase, catalase, adiponectin mRNA	Seo, Choi, Lee, and Lee (2013)
Red	*Plocamium telfairia*	South Korea	Ethanol extract (25, 50, 100 μg/mL)	3T3-L1	↓ Lipogenesis (ORO staining) ↓ PPAR-γ, C/EBP-α, SREBP1, FABP4 protein	Kang et al. (2016)

ACC, acyl-coA carboxylase; *aP2*, adipocytes protein 2; *C/EBP-α/β*, CCAAT/enhancer-binding proteins α/β; *CPT1a*, carnitine palmitoyltransferase-1a; *ERK*, extracellular signal-regulated kinases; *FA*, fatty acids; *FABP4*, fatty acid-binding protein 4; *FAS*, fatty acid synthase; *G6PDH*, NADPH-producing glucose-6-phosphate dehydrogenase; *JNK*, Jun N-terminal kinase; *IL-6*, interleukin-6; *LKB1*, liver kinase B1; *MCP-1*, monocyte chemoattractant protein-1; *Nox4*, nicotinamide adenine dinucleotide phosphate hydrogen (NADPH) oxidase 4; *ORO*, oil red O; *PAI-1*, plasminogen activator inhibitor-1; *PPAR-γ*, peroxisome proliferator-activated receptor-γ; *ROS*, reactive oxygen species; *SOD*, superoxide dismutase; *SREBP-1c*, sterol regulatory element binding protein 1c; *UCP1*, uncoupling protein 1; *UCP2*, uncoupling protein 2; *TNFα*, tumor necrosis factor alpha; *WAT*, white adipose tissue.

macrocarpum (60.2%), *Polysiphonia morrowii* (55.0%), and *Ishige okamurae* (52.9%) had highest DPPH radical scavenging activities. Among the 49 species tested, extracts from *D. undulata, S. micracanthum, C. ocellatus, G. amansii, G. verrucosa,* and *G. lanceolate* (100 μg/mL) significantly decreased cellular fat accumulation, which was paralleled by inhibition of ROS production during the differentiation of 3T3-L1 preadipocytes (Lee, Yoon, Kim, You, & Lee, 2011). The ethanolic extract of *Caulerpa okamurae* (COE), at a concentration of 25–500 μg/mL, significantly inhibited lipid accumulation and reduced the expression of adipogenesis master regulators: C/EBP-α, PPAR-γ, and sterol regulatory element binding protein 1c (SREBP-1C) in 3T3-L1 adipocytes (Sharma et al., 2017). Extracts from *Ulva* spp., *Palmaria palmata, Undaria pinnatifida* and *Himanthalia elongata* at a concentration of 0.1 mg/mL were similarly shown to significantly inhibit triacylglycerol accumulation in mature 3T3-L1 adipocytes (43–52% inhibition) (Rico et al., 2018).

Extracts from red algae have also been studied for their anti-obesity properties. In particular, an ethanol extract from *Grateloupia lanceolata* (Okamura), a red seaweed native to coastal areas of East Asia, was shown to inhibit lipid accumulation (25% and 50% at 10 and 50 μg/mL concentrations, respectively) and ROS production (18% at 50 μg/mL) during adipogenesis in 3T3-L1 cells. Treatment with the *G. lanceolata* extract led to a reduction in the mRNA levels of the transcription factors PPAR-γ and C/EBP-α, and, at the protein level, for the target protein, fatty acid binding protein 2 (aP2). Moreover, ROS-producing nicotinamide adenine dinucleotide phosphate hydrogen (NADPH) oxidase 4 (Nox4) and NADPH-producing glucose-6-phosphate dehydrogenase (G6PDH) mRNAs were decreased following *G. lanceolata* extract treatment, whereas mRNA levels of ROS scavenging enzymes, including superoxide dismutase (SOD), glutathione peroxidase, and catalase, were increased in the extract-treated group in addition to enhanced mRNA levels of adiponectin. These finding suggest that *G. lanceolata* extract inhibited lipid accumulation and ROS production by controlling adipogenic signals and ROS regulating genes (Seo et al., 2013). Similarly, an ethanol extract from the red seaweed *Plocamium telfairiae* (PTE) showed an inhibitory effect on lipogenesis in adipocytes (42.08%, 26.41%, and 17.86% at the concentrations of 25, 50, and 100 μg/mL, respectively) indicating that PTE reduced the accumulation of triglycerides in adipocytes. PTE treatment significantly decreased the expression (~50%) of adipogenic-specific proteins such as PPAR-γ, C/EBP-α, SREBP1, and fatty acid binding protein 4 (FABP4) compared with untreated 3T3-L1 cells, indicating that PTE inhibits adipogenic differentiation through down-regulation of adipogenic-specific proteins (Kang et al., 2016). In a different study, the ethyl acetate fraction of a komulkosiraegi (*Gracilaria vermiculophylla* (Ohmi) *Papenfuss*) ethanol extract (GEFr) was found to potently inhibit adipogenesis of 3T3-L1 preadipocytes, decreasing triglycerides accumulation and the expression of PPAR-γ, C/EPB-α, and aP2 at concentrations between 1 and 50 μg/mL. In mature adipocytes, GEFr was found to significantly activate AMP-activated protein kinase (AMPK) by activating liver kinase B1 (LKB1) and stimulating intracellular ROS. The mRNA levels of genes involved in lipid catabolism such as carnitine palmitoyltransferase-1a (CPT1a), and uncoupling protein 2 (UCP2) were also up-regulated (Kim et al., 2012).

2.2.2 Phlorotannins

The potential inhibitory effect of five species of brown seaweeds (*Sargassum thunbergii, Ishige okamurae, Ecklonia cava, Padina arborescens* and *Undaria wrightii*) on adipogenesis and differentiation of 3T3-L1 pre-adipocytes into mature adipocytes was assessed by Ko et al. (2013). The *Ecklonia cava* extract (100 μg/mL) showed profound adipogenesis inhibitory effect (40% reduction), compared to the other four brown seaweed extracts, and was then selected for isolation of active compounds including the three polyphenol compounds of phlorotannins, dieckol, 6,6′, bieckol and phlorofucofuroeckol A. Dieckol, at a concentration of 100 μM, exhibited greatest potential adipogenesis inhibition and down-regulated the expression of PPAR-γ, C/EBP-α, SREBP1 and fatty acid binding protein 4 (FABP4) in a dose-dependent manner by activating AMPK (Ko et al., 2013). The anti-obesity effects of 6,6′-bieckol, 6,8′-bieckol, 8,8′-bieckol, dieckol and phlorofucofuroeckol A isolated from *Eisenia bicyclis* were also tested by Kwon et al. (2015), by examining the inhibition of differentiation of 3T3-L1 adipocytes and the expression of PPAR-γ, C/EBP-α and SREBP-1c at mRNA and protein level. Differentiated 3T3-L1 cells were treated with the purified phlorotannins at concentrations of 10, 25 and 50 μg/mL for 8 days. All the purified phlorotannins suppressed the differentiation of 3T3-L1 adipocytes in a dose-dependent manner, without toxic effects, however 6,6′-bieckol markedly decreased lipid accumulation and expression levels of PPAR-γ, C/EBP-α, SREBP-1c (mRNA and protein), and fatty acid synthase (FAS) and acyl-coA carboxylase (ACC) (mRNA), suggesting an effect of *E. bicyclis* through downregulation of adipogenesis and lipogenesis (Kwon et al., 2015).

Six indole derivatives (STCs)-indole-2-carboxaldehyde (STC-1), indole-3-carboxaldehyde (STC-2), indole-4-carboxaldehyde (STC-3), indole-5-carboxaldehyde (STC-4), indole-6-carboxaldehyde (STC-5), and indole-7-carboxaldehyde (STC-6) were extracted from *Sargassum thunbergii* and their inhibitory effects on adipocyte differentiation evaluated in 3T3-L1 cells at 25–100 μM. STC-1 and STC-5 resulted in non-toxic inhibition of 3T3-L1 adipocytes differentiation and significantly inhibited lipid accumulation and downregulated the protein expression of PPAR-γ, C/EBP-α, and SREBP-1c in a dose-dependent manner. The specific mechanism by which STC-1 and STC-5 inhibit lipid accumulation and adipogenesis in adipocytes involved AMPK activation and AMPK signaling pathway (Kang et al., 2017) Two bioactive subfractions from the brown alga *Fucus distichus*, a monoglycosyldiacylglycerol subfraction and a phlorotannin subfraction, decreased lipid accumulation up to 55% and increased free glycerol concentrations by 28–45% at a concentration of 50 μg/mL, paralleled by increases in adiponectin and uncoupling protein 1 (UCP-1) and decreases in leptin mRNA expression (Kellogg, Esposito, Grace, Komarnytsky, & Lila, 2015).

2.2.3 Complex polysaccharides

The sulfated polysaccharide fucoidan has been reported to affect the development of adipocytes, although its role in adipogenesis is not fully understood. Incubation of 3T3-L1 preadipocytes with 50, 100, and 200 μg/mL of fucoidan during differentiation induced a decrease in lipid accumulation of 29.1%, 50.5% and 52.4%, respectively. Furthermore, 200 μg/mL fucoidan induced down regulation in gene expression of both early (22% reduction for C/EBP-α and 17.6% for PPAR-γ) and late (73.9% reduction for activating protein 2 (aP2)) adipogenic markers, which have a crucial role in adipocyte development. Early activation of p38 MAPKs, extracellular signal-regulated kinases (ERK) and Jun N-terminal kinase (JNK) was also inhibited by fucoidan suggesting a potential role of fucoidan in inhibiting adipogenesis in 3T3-L1 preadipocytes, by affecting the MAPK signaling pathway that involves adipogenic transcription factors (Kim et al., 2010). Similarly, fucoidan extracted from the sporophyll of *U. pinnatifida* (100 μg/mL) exerted anti-obesity effects via suppressing the expression of PPAR-γ (36%), C/EBP-α (44%), and aP2 (71%), which decreased expression of the inflammation-related genes such as tumor necrosis factor alpha (TNFα, 35%), monocyte chemoattractant protein-1 (MCP-1, 66%) and plasminogen activator inhibitor-1 (PAI-1, 29%) during adipogenesis.

Moreover, fucoidan reduced lipid accumulation and ROS production in adipocytes, demonstrating that fucoidan from the sporophyll of *U. pinnatifida* may suppress adipogenesis through inhibition of major adipogenesis markers and inflammation-related cytokines in adipocytes (Kim & Lee, 2012). Four fucoidan-rich fractions (F0.5, F0.9, F1.1 and F2.0) obtained by differential precipitation with acetone from a commercial source of fucoidan from *Fucus vesiculosus* and containing different proportions of fucose:glucuronic acid:galactose:xylose:sulfate, were tested in 3T3-L1 cells for their lipolytic and anti-adipogenic activity at a concentration of 200 μg/mL. All samples had lipolytic action, especially F2.0, which tripled the amount of glycerol released in the cellular medium, whereas antiadipogenic activity was limited to F1.1 and F2.0 with F0.5 inducing adipogenesis, as determined by oil red O staining. The effect of the different fractions on adipogenesis was matched by the expression of key proteins of adipogenic differentiation (C/EBP-α, C/EBP-β, and PPAR-γ) with F2.0 decreasing their levels by 55%. Not all the fractions had similar effects, suggesting that the relative amount of fucose:glucuronic acid:galactose: xylose:sulfate affects differently their potential as anti-obesity compounds (Oliveira et al., 2018).

2.2.4 Carotenoids—Fucoxanthin

Fucoxanthin (Fx) is a marine carotenoid found in edible brown seaweeds and has been associated with lipid metabolism. Fx isolated from *Sargassum echinocarpum* was added to pre-adipocyte cell obtained from viscera tissue of Wistar rats and was able to increase adiponectin levels and decrease of TNF-α expression suggesting its ability to enhance β-oxidation in adipocyte cells (Firdaus et al., 2015). In differentiating 3T3-F442A adipocytes, fucoxanthinol, which is a fucoxanthin metabolite found in white adipose tissue (WAT), attenuated TNF-α-induced monocyte chemotactic protein-1 (MCP-1) and interleukin-6 (IL-6) mRNA overexpression and protein secretion into the culture medium. In addition, fucoxanthinol decreased TNF-α, inducible nitric oxide synthase (iNOS), and cyclooxygenase-2 (COX-2) mRNA expression in RAW264.7 macrophage-like cells stimulated by palmitic acid (Hosokawa et al., 2010).

2.2.5 Animal studies

Some of the molecular mechanisms identified to be affected by seaweed extracts or bioactive compounds treatment in cell models of obesity have also been the focus of studies in adipose tissue from animal model of obesity. For example, supplementation of a high-fat diet with an ethanol extract of

Caulerpa okamurae (COE) (250 m/kg) significantly reduced PPAR-γ, C/EBP-α, FAS, SRBP1c, cluster of differentiation 36, and acetyl-CoA synthetase in the adipose tissue of COE-treated HFD-fed mice in addition to a reduction in markers of weight gain. These included free fatty acids, triglycerides, total cholesterol, glucose and insulin in the plasma and free fatty acids, triglycerides, total cholesterol and total lipid in the liver (Sharma et al., 2017). Fucoidan (2%) administered to mice fed either a standard diet or high fat diet (HFD) for 5 weeks significantly decreased body-weight gain (47.3%), food efficiency ratio and relative liver and epididymal fat mass (16.1% and 32% reduction, respectively), compared with the HFD group. Furthermore, fucoidan affected adipogenesis in epididymal adipose tissue, by decreasing the expression of adipogenic genes, such as PPAR-γ, aP2 and ACC by 34.0%, 36.4% and 28.4%, respectively, in the 2% supplemented group compared with the HFD group (Kim, Jeon, & Lee, 2014).

Fucoxanthin (Fx), extracted from the commercial *Undaria pinnatifida* seaweed powder using acetone and further purified by silica gel column chromatography with n-hexane/acetone (8:2, v/v), was administered to diabetic/obese KK-A(y) mice as part of their diet (0.2% Fx), and attenuated WAT weight gain and hyperglycemia, although it did not affect these parameters in lean C57BL/6J mice. In perigonadal and mesenteric WAT of KK-A(y) mice fed Fx, mRNA expression levels of MCP-1 and TNF-α were markedly reduced compared to control mice. In contrast to KK-A(y) mice, Fx did not alter MCP-1 and TNF-α mRNA expression levels in the WAT of lean C57BL/6J mice. Moreover interleukin-6 (IL-6) and PAI-1 mRNA expression levels in WAT were also decreased by Fx in KK-A(y) mice, suggesting that Fx regulates mRNA expression of inflammatory adipocytokines in WAT and has specific effects on diabetic/obese KK-A(y) mice (Hosokawa et al., 2010). Similar findings were obtained by Maeda et al. (2007) in a study that evaluated the anti-obesity and antidiabetic effects of Fx (0.2%, obtained from commercial *Undaria pinnatifida* dried seaweed after acetone extraction and purification by silica gel column chromatography with n-hexane/acetone (7:3, v/v)) in KK-A (y) mice. After 4 weeks of feeding, 0.2% Fx in the diet markedly attenuated the gain of WAT weight in KK-A(y) mice with increasing UCP1 expression compared with the control mice. Leptin and TNF-α mRNA expression in WAT were significantly down-regulated by 0.2% Fx, suggesting that Fx might influence inflammation and energy metabolism (Maeda et al., 2007). An additional study by Jeon et al. (2010) examined the effectiveness of an ethanol extract of Fx-rich seaweed as a nutraceutical for body fat-lowering agent and for an anti-obesity effect based on mode of actions in

C57BL/6J mice. Animals were randomized to receive a semi-purified high fat diet supplemented with 0.2% conjugated linoleic acid (CLA) as positive control, and 1.43% or 5.72% Fx-rich seaweed ethanol extract (Fx-SEE), equivalent to 0.05% or 0.2% dietary Fx for 6 weeks. Fx-SEE significantly reduced body and abdominal WAT weights, plasma and hepatic triglyceride (TG), and/or cholesterol concentrations compared to the high fat control group. Activities of adipocytic fatty acid (FA) synthesis, hepatic FA and TG synthesis, and cholesterol-regulating enzyme were also lowered by Fx-SEE supplement. Concentrations of plasma HDL-cholesterol, fecal TG and cholesterol, as well as FA oxidation enzyme activity and UCP1 mRNA expression in epididymal WAT were significantly higher in the Fx-SEE groups than in the high fat control group, indicating that Fx-SEE affects the plasma and hepatic lipid profile, fecal lipids and body fat mass, and alters hepatic cholesterol metabolism, FA synthesis and lipid absorption (Jeon et al., 2010). Several other studies have focused their attention on the effect of Fx rich extracts on UCP1 expression: a key molecule for metabolic thermogenesis to avoid fat accumulation excess is usually expressed only in brown adipose tissue (BAT), and, therefore, its expression in tissues other than BAT is expected to reduce abdominal fat. Fx rich lipid fractions from *Undaria pinnatifida* (Maeda et al., 2005, 2008, 2009; Okada et al., 2011) fed to mice in addition to a high-fat diet significantly suppressed body weight and WAT weight gain induced by the HF diet by upregulating the expression of UCP1 in WAT, which may contribute to reducing WAT weight and ameliorate alterations in lipid metabolism.

The above studies provide a good starting point to identify therapeutic targets that link metabolic disorders with altered adipocyte function. Adipocyte hyperplasia and hypertrophy are key processes in metabolic dysfunction; a "critical" adipocyte size exists that triggers the recruitment of preadipocytes that will differentiate into mature adipocytes and induce changes in levels of ROS and inflammatory molecules and their subsequent deleterious effects at cellular/tissue level. Targeting some of the key proteins involved in such tightly regulated processes or adipocyte-derived secretory proteins and their receptors with seaweed extracts and bioactive compounds may, therefore, provide promising pharmacological targets.

2.3 Activity of seaweed extracts and bioactive compounds in liver

The liver has long been recognized to be an essential metabolic organ and plays a crucial role in whole-body energy homeostasis by regulating the metabolism of nutrients. When carbohydrates are abundant, during the postprandial phase, the liver converts glucose into glycogen and lipids, which provide metabolic fuels during fasting. In the fasted state, the liver produces and secretes glucose through both glycogenolysis and gluconeogenesis. The metabolic switch between fasted and fed states in the liver is tightly controlled by neuronal and hormonal systems and, in obesity, such switches are affected: adipose tissue regulates liver energy metabolism directly by secreting a variety of adipokines including adiponectin and cytokines, and, indirectly, by secreting leptin which acts on the brain to regulate liver metabolism. The liver also regulates the metabolic activity of adipose tissue. Bioactive compounds that affect liver energy metabolism may have beneficial effects as potential anti-obesity drugs: examples of the effect of seaweed extracts or their bioactive compounds are reported below, and the findings summarized in Table 3.

2.3.1 *Whole seaweed and seaweed extracts*

Studies have assessed the effect of feeding a diet containing the brown seaweed *Undaria pinnatifida* (wakame) (0, 0.1, or 1.0 g/100 g diet of dried wakame powder) to rats for 28 days. Administration of 1% wakame significantly decreased serum total cholesterol levels, and in the liver suppressed the lipogenic pathway by downregulating SREBF-1. Moreover, gluconeogenesis was promoted by upregulation of the PPAR signaling pathway, which leads to a reduction in the accumulation of cholesterol and promotion of β-oxidation, suggesting that wakame ingestion affects glucose and lipid metabolism by altering the expression of SREBP-1 and PPAR signal-related genes (Yoshinaga et al., 2018).

2.3.2 *Carotenoids—Fucoxanthin*

The effect of Fx on hepatic stearoyl-coenzyme A desaturase-1 (SCD1), a rate-limiting enzyme that catalyzes the biosynthesis of monounsaturated fatty acids from saturated fatty acids, has been studied in obese mouse models of hyperleptinemia (KK-A(y)) and leptin-deficiency (ob/ob). In KK-A(y) mice fed a diet containing 0.2% Fx for 2 weeks, SCD1 mRNA and protein expression were reduced in the liver with a concomitant decrease in serum leptin levels. In contrast, the suppressive effects of Fx on hepatic SCD1 and body weight gain were not observed in leptin-deficient ob/ob mice. These findings support the hypothesis that Fx down-regulates SCD1 expression and alters fatty acid composition of the liver through regulation of leptin signaling (Beppu et al., 2013).

Table 3 Summary of the metabolic effects of seaweed extracts on the liver.

Seaweed color	Seaweed species	Country of origin	Extracts/specific compounds (concentration)	Biological model	Action	Reference source
Liver						
Brown	*Phaeodactylum tricornutum*		Fucoxanthin (acetone extract) (0.2% w/w)	Male C57BL/6J mice fed high-fat diet	↑ SOD, catalase, glutathione peroxidase activity ↓ TBARS, glutathione levels	Kang, Kim, et al. (2013), Kang, Wijesinghe, et al. (2013)
Brown	*Undaria pinnatifida*	Japan	Dried seaweed (0.1, 1.0 g/100 g diet)	Male Sprague-Dawley fed high-fat diet	↓ Lipogenic pathway by downregulating SREBF-1 ↑ Gluconeogenesis ↑ PPAR signaling pathway	Yoshinaga, Maruya, Koikeda, and Nakano (2018)
Brown	*Undaria pinnatifida*	Japan	Fucoxanthin (acetone extract) (0.2% w/w)	KK-A(y) and ob/ob mice	↓ SCD1 mRNA and protein in KK-A(y) not in ob/ob	Beppu, Hosokawa, Yim, Shinoda, and Miyashita (2013)
Brown			Fucoxanthin (0.2% w/w)	Male Sprague-Dawley fed high-fat diet	↑ Catalase and GSH-Px activity ↑ Nrf2, NQO1 mRNA	Ha, Na, and Kim (2013)

GSH-Px, glutathione peroxidase; *Nrf2*, nuclear erythroid factor like 2; *NQO1*, NAD(P)H quinone oxidoreductase1 (NQO1); *PPAR-γ*, peroxisome proliferator-activated receptor-γ; *SCD1*, stearoyl-coenzyme A desaturase; *SOD*, superoxide dismutase; *SREBP-1c*, sterol regulatory element binding protein 1c; *TBARS*, thiobarbituric acid reactive substances.

An alternative mechanism by which Fx may act as an anti-obesity compound is through modulation of liver antioxidant capacity to reduce intracellular ROS levels, which have been shown to mediate adipocyte differentiation (Kanda, Hinata, Kang, & Watanabe, 2011). Although not a seaweed, co-administration of the Fx-containing diatom *Phaeodactylum tricornutum* (0.7% lipid extract corresponding to 0.2% Fx) with a high-fat diet to mice for 8 weeks increased hepatic superoxide dismutase, catalase, and glutathione peroxidase activities and decreased thiobarbituric acid reactive substances (TBARS) and glutathione levels. Moreover, body weight and epididymal WAT was significantly decreased compared to mice fed the high-fat diet. Serum triglyceride, glucose, insulin, and leptin levels were also significantly lower in the *P. tricornutum* group than in the high-fat diet group (Kang, Kim, et al., 2013). Similar results were obtained in a different study: liver activities of catalase and GSH-Px were significantly higher in the high-fat diet + Fx group than those in the high-fat diet group and were increased by Fx by inducing higher mRNA expression of transcription factor, nuclear erythroid factor like 2 (Nrf2), and its target genes such as NAD(P)H quinone oxidoreductase1 (NQO1), suggesting that Fx supplementation improved liver antioxidant capacity, depleted by high-fat diet, by activating the Nrf2 pathway (Ha et al., 2013).

2.4 Activity of seaweed extracts and bioactive compounds on the gut microbiota

It is now recognized that modulating the diversity of gut microbiota, through dietary intervention, may significantly affect gut health as well as systemic health. Recent studies have implicated the gut microbiota as a critical determinant of nutrient uptake, energy regulation, and chronic metabolic disorders (Moreno-Indias, Cardona, Tinahones, & Queipo-Ortuno, 2014). The human gut contains a vast number and diversity of microorganisms that are shaped by natural selection and competition. Bioactive compounds able to modify the composition of the gut microbiota are gathering interest as changes they induced could improve nutrient utilization and increase microbial metabolite production, thus regulating lipid uptake and metabolism in the body in the case of obesity. Some of the very few studies that have looked at changes in gut microflora induced by seaweeds and/or their bioactive compounds are reported below and findings summarized in Table 4.

Table 4 Summary of the effects of seaweed extracts on the gut microbiota.

Seaweed color	Seaweed species	Country of origin	Extracts/specific compounds (concentration)	Biological model	Action	Reference source
Intestine—gut microflora						
Brown	*Ascophyllum nodosum* *Laminaria japonica*	China	Fucoidan (200 mg/kg)	Male C57BL/6 mice fed high-fat diet	↓ Body weight, fasting blood glucose, hepatic steatosis and systematic inflammation ↑ Benign microbes—*Akkermansia muciniphila* ↑ Short-chain fatty acid-producers—*Alloprevotella*, *Blautia*, *Bacteroides*	Shang et al. (2017)
Brown	*Laminaria japonica*	South Korea	Dried whole seaweed or heat treated dried whole seaweed (10% w/w)	Male Sprague-Dawley rats	↓ Body weight gain ↓ *Fimicutes* to *Bacteroidetes* ratio ↓ Obesity-associated bacterial genera—*Allobaculum*, *Turicibacter*, *Coprobacillus*, *Mollicute*, *Oscilibacter* ↓ Potential pathogenic genera—*Mollicute*, *Bacteroides*, *Clostridium*, *Escherichia*, *Prevotella* ↑ Leanness-associated genera—*Alistipes*, *Bacteroides*, and *Prevotella* ↑ Lactic acid bacterial genera—*Subdoligranulum*, *Streptococcus*, *Lactobacillus*, *Enterococcus*, *Bifidobacterium*	Kim et al. (2018)

Brown	*Laminaria japonica*	China	Alginates (pressurized hot water extraction) (0.25% w/w)	Male BALB/c mice fed high-fat diet	↓ Body weight, fat accumulation in liver and WAT = species richness of the gut microbiota ↑ *Rikenellaceae* and *Bacteroidales S24_7* = *Prevotellaceae* family	Duan et al. (2019)
Red Green	*Porphyra haitanensis* *Ulva prolifera*	China	Polysaccharides (hot water extraction) (250 mg/kg per day)	Male C57BL/6 mice	↑ *Bacteroidetes* contributing to fecal microbiota ↓ *Firmicutes* ↑ *Prevotellaceae UCG-001*, *Rikenellaceae RC9*	Zhang et al. (2018)
Brown	*Undaria pinnatifida*	Japan	Dried whole seaweed (4 g of dried wakame per day)	Healthy individuals suffering from low defecation frequency	↑ Defecation frequency and volume per week ↑ *Bifidobacteria* as a percentage of all fecal bacteria ↑ *Actinobacteria* relative abundance ↓ *Bacteroidetes* abundance	Yoshinaga et al. (2018)
Brown			Polymannuric acid (150 mg/kg body weight/day)	Male C57BL/6 mice fed high-fat diet	↓ Body weight gain ↑ Probiotic bacterium *Lactobacillus reuteri*	Liu et al. (2017)
Red	*Kappaphycus alvarezii*	Fiji	Dried whole seaweed (5% w/w)	Male Wistar rats fed a high/carbohydrate, high-fat diet	↓ Body weight and abdominal fat ↓ *Firmicutes* to *Bacteroidetes* ratio	Wanyonyi et al. (2017)

2.4.1 Whole seaweed and seaweed extracts

The prebiotic potential of the brown seaweed *Laminaria japonica* was tested by feeding a basal diet (control), basal diet supplemented with dried *L. japonica* (DLJ) or heat-treated dried *L. japonica* (HLJ), to rats for 16 weeks. The DLJ and HLJ groups had lower weight gain and serum triglyceride concentration compared to the control group and showed lower *Fimicutes* to *Bacteroidetes* ratio when compared with the control group. Moreover, obesity-associated bacterial genera (*Allobaculum, Turicibacter, Coprobacillus, Mollicute*, and *Oscilibacter*), and the genera with pathogenic potentials (*Mollicute, Bacteroides, Clostridium, Escherichia*, and *Prevotella*) decreased while leanness-associated genera (*Alistipes, Bacteroides*, and *Prevotella*), and lactic acid bacterial genera (*Subdoligranulum, Streptococcus, Lactobacillus, Enterococcus*, and *Bifidobacterium*) increased in all treatment groups, pointing to the potential of *L. japonica* as an effective prebiotic for promotion of host metabolism and reduction of obesity in humans (Kim et al., 2018). Relative to obese rats, animals treated with the red seaweed, *Kappaphycus alvarezii* (5% (w/w) dried and milled Kappaphycus) showed normalized body weight and adiposity, lower systolic blood pressure, improved heart and liver structure, and lower plasma lipids, even in presence of high-fat diet. *Kappaphycus* modulated the balance between *Firmicutes* and *Bacteroidetes* in the gut, which could serve as the potential mechanism for improved metabolic variables and was accompanied by no damage to the gut structure (Wanyonyi, Du Preez, Brown, Paul, & Panchal, 2017).

The ability of bioactive compounds from seaweed to affect gut microflora has also been tested in humans. The effect of a 2-week intake of the edible seaweed *Undaria pinnatifida* (wakame) on defecation frequency and intestinal microbiota was tested in 22 healthy individuals suffering from low defecation frequency. Supplementation of their diet with wakame significantly increased defecation frequency and volume per week in addition to increasing the fraction of *Bifidobacteria* as a percentage of all fecal bacteria and the relative abundance of *Actinobacteria*, while the abundance of *Bacteroidetes* decreased (Yoshinaga et al., 2018).

2.4.2 Polysaccharides

Polysaccharides from *Laminaria japonica* (LJPs) also prevented diet-induced obesity in a murine model, and improved obesity-related parameters (e.g., fat accumulation in the liver and adipose tissues, body composition, lipid profile) as well as the morphology of the intestine: such effects were associated with the modulation of the gut microbiota, involving some members of the *Bacteroidetes* phylum (Duan et al., 2019). Polysaccharides from two seaweeds, *Porphyra haitanensis* (PH) and *Ulva prolifera* (UP), also affected the intestinal microbiota in mice gavaged with 250 mg/kg per day: significant structural changes in the fecal microbiota were observed between the two treated groups and the control group, with changes evident at the phylum and genus levels. At the phylum level, the most predominant phylum was *Bacteroidetes* contributing 58.76%, 73.39% and 75.38% of the fecal microbiota in the control, PH and UP groups, respectively, followed by *Firmicutes*, contributing 37.61%, 23.99% and 21.87%. Many genera were significantly higher in the PH and UP group than in the control group, including *Prevotellaceae UCG-001* and *Rikenellaceae RC9* (Zhang, Wang, Han, Liu, & Liu, 2018). Similarly a 30-day treatment with polymannuric acid (PM), one of numerous alginates isolated from brown seaweeds, in mice fed a high-fat diet-induced a reduction in body weight gain and blood TAG levels (P2.0), but also had a profound impact on the microbial composition in the gut microbiome and resulted in a distinct microbiome structure and increased the abundance of a probiotic bacterium, *Lactobacillus reuteri* ($\log_{10}$ LDA score >2.0) (Liu et al., 2017). Two fucoidans from *Laminaria japonica* and *Ascophyllum nodosum* were also tested and found to significantly reduce body weight, fasting blood glucose, hepatic steatosis and systematic inflammation. As fucoidan is poorly absorbed after oral administration, in order to decipher the mechanism behind this therapeutic effect, the gut microbiota was analyzed: benign microbes, which conferred benefits upon host wellbeing including *Akkermansia muciniphila* and short-chain fatty acid-producers such as *Alloprevotella, Blautia* and *Bacteroides* were highly enriched by fucoidans (Shang et al., 2017).

2.5 Summary of the metabolic effects of seaweed in obesity

Obesity and overweight processes are determined not only by adipocyte hyperplasia and adipose tissues hypertrophy, but also by changes in liver energy metabolism and gut microbiota as a critical determinant of nutrients uptake and energy regulation. Pharmacological interventions focused on maintaining or improving adipose tissue health and liver energy metabolism, and modulating the diversity of gut microbiota, therefore forms the basis for therapeutic interventions in metabolic diseases. As described in the above sections, extracts from seaweeds and their bioactive compounds provide a good resource for discovering new therapeutic drugs for obesity management.

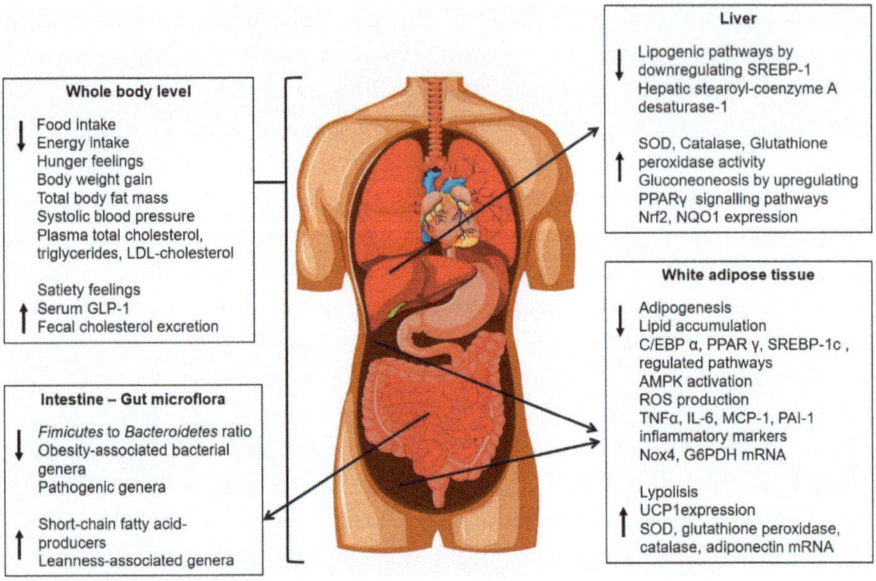

Fig. 1 Diagram summarizing the effects of seaweed extracts and bioactive compounds at whole body level, and on the adipose tissue, liver and gut microflora.

The molecular mechanisms affected by seaweed extracts and bioactive compounds are specific to different tissues (Fig. 1); however modulation of antioxidant capacity and reduction of intracellular ROS levels within tissues are the key mechanisms identified. At adipose tissue level, the programmed differentiation of preadipocytes into mature adipocytes is characterized by chronological changes in the expression of numerous genes and proteins, such as PPAR-γ, C/EBP family, SREBP-1c, and aP2, and is mediated by intracellular ROS levels. Seaweed extracts reduce the expression of Nox4 and G6PDH with subsequent increased activation of ROS scavenging enzymes, such as superoxide dismutase, glutathione peroxidase, and catalase. Moreover, modulation of adipogenesis also occurs via regulation of inflammation-related cytokines such as TNFα, MCP-1 and PAI-1: seaweed extracts affect such pathways in addition to induce the expression of the metabolic thermogenesis regulator UCP1. Similarly, in the liver suppression of lipogenic pathways and upregulation of gluconeogenesis and promotion of β-oxidation have been induced by seaweed extracts in addition to increasing activities of superoxide dismutase, catalase, and glutathione peroxidase by activating the Nrf2 pathway and improving liver antioxidant capacity.

Future studies aimed at discovering new therapeutic drugs from marine natural products should, therefore, focus on bioactive compounds from seaweeds that exert antioxidant properties and regulate the expression of key signaling pathways involved in enhancing browning of white adipose tissue, and reducing oxidative stress in adipose tissue and liver.

3. Metabolic effects of seaweed in type 2 diabetes

The main pharmacological approaches for the management of T2D involve the use of agents that target key events, from the point of entry of glucose into the circulation to the responsiveness to insulin at the cellular level (Fig. 2). For example, consumed dietary saccharides are hydrolyzed to absorbable glucose by the enzymes α-glucosidase and α-amylase in the gastrointestinal brush border, and so inhibitors of α-glucosidase (e.g., acarbose) are used to reduce the absorption and/or digestion of dietary saccharides to diminish post-prandial blood glucose. Glucagon-like peptide-1 (GLP-1), is released in response to ingestion of food and stimulates the release of insulin from pancreatic β-cells and GLP-1 agonists (e.g., exenatide) are used to mimic GLP-1, while inhibitors of dipeptidyl peptidase-4 (DPP-4), the enzyme responsible for the breakdown of GLP-1, are used to prolong its half-life (e.g., linagliptin), while the second generation sulfonylureas (e.g., glibenclamide) are used to directly stimulate pancreatic insulin secretion. At the cellular level, the metabolic actions of insulin can be enhanced by the biguanides (e.g., metformin) or the thiazolidinedione (e.g., pioglitazone)

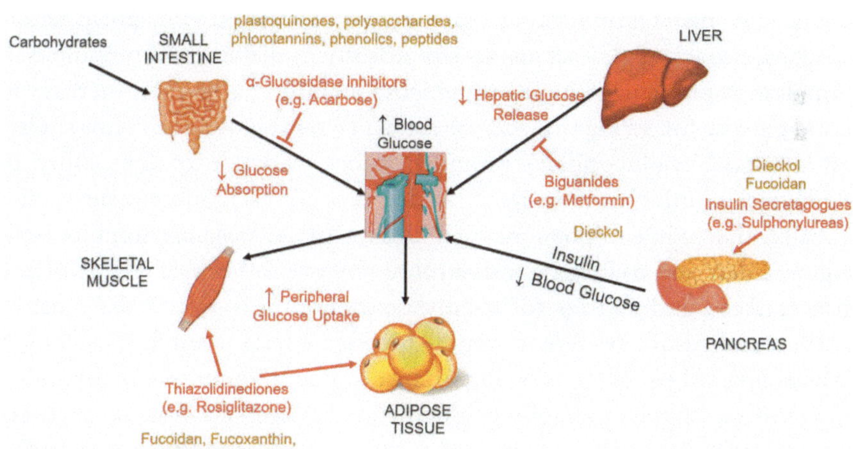

Fig. 2 Diagram illustrating sites of action of anti-diabetic drugs used in the management of T2D (red) and possible sites of action of bioactive molecules from seaweed (brown).

insulin sensitizers, the latter acting through PPAR-γ activation. Most of the studies to date into the anti-diabetic potential of seaweed/algae-based extracts, and pure compounds derived from them, have therefore focused on some of these pharmacological targets, but have also assessed their effectiveness at other potential targets.

3.1 α-Glucosidase and α-amylase inhibitory activity of algal extracts

Hyperglycemia can be suppressed using drugs that delay or prevent the absorption of glucose from the intestine, and the key digestive enzymes α-glucosidase and α-amylase, which are responsible for the breakdown of starch into glucose, represent an ideal target. The main clinically utilized drug to achieve this is acarbose, which inhibits both enzymes, however there are significant adverse effects associated with its use (abdominal discomfort, diarrhea and flatulence) that are believed to be due to inhibition of pancreatic amylase. Therefore, the optimum approach would be to inhibit α-glucosidase alone, and it is selective inhibition of this enzyme that has been the main focus for the exploration of the anti-diabetic potential of seaweed (Table 5).

3.1.1 *In vitro studies*

Most studies have focused on brown seaweed species, of which the *Ascophyllum nodosum* species is probably the most widely studied, and one of the very first reports found that oral administration of a polyphenol-enriched extract of *A. nodosum* to streptozotocin diabetic mice resulted in a modest improvement in fasting glucose alongside a blunted increase in blood glucose following oral sucrose tolerance testing, while in vitro studies (rat intestinal α-glucosidase) provided direct evidence of the ability of the extract to inhibit the enzyme (Zhang et al., 2007). Subsequent studies revealed that while a phenolic-rich extract of *A. nodosum* inhibits both α-glucosidase and α-amylase, it is a more potent inhibitor of α-glucosidase than acarbose and its IC_{50} for α-amylase inhibition is greater than that of acarbose, suggesting preference for α-glucosidase over α-amylase inhibition (Apostolidis & Lee, 2010). The importance of phenolic content in the ability of *A. nodosum* extract to inhibit α-glucosidase has been confirmed by studies on extracts of the seaweed harvested at different times of the year from the north eastern coastal waters of the United Sates, where seasonal variations in phenolic content (lowest in April and highest in July) revealed an inverse relationship between IC_{70} values for enzyme inhibition and total phenolic

Table 5 Summary of the α-glucosidase and α-amylase inhibitory effects of seaweed bioactives.

Seaweed species	Country of origin	Chemicals present	α-Glucosidase inhibition (IC_{50})		α-Amylase inhibition (IC_{50})		Reference source
			Extract/compound	Acarbose	Extract/compound	Acarbose	
Ascophyllum nodosum	Japan	Polyphenol-enriched	77 μg/mL	–	ND	–	Zhang et al. (2007)
	USA	Phenolic 4.2 mg/g ww	0.24 μg	0.37 μg	1.34 μg	0.68 μg	Apostolidis and Lee (2010)
	Ireland	Phenolic 44–56 (GAE/mg)	<1 μg/mL	150 μg/mL	44–53 μg/mL	ND	Lordan, Smyth, Soler-Vila, Stanton, and Ross (2013)
	Scotland	Phenolic 140–4550 (μg/gDW)	19 μg/mL	ND	0.1 μg/mL	ND	Nwosu et al. (2011)
	Scotland	Phenolic—171–363 μg GAE/mL Phlorotannin	10 μg GAE/mL 10 μg GAE/mL	40 μg/mL	0.05 μg GAE/mL 0.15 μg GAE/mL	1 μg/mL	Pantidos, Boath, Lund, Conner, and McDougall (2014)
	Canada	Fucoidan	13–47 μg/mL	1 mg/mL	0.12–4.64 mg/mL	1 mg/mL	Kim, Rioux, and Turgeon (2014)
Ecklonia cava	Korea	Dieckol	0.24 mM	1.05 mM	0.66 mM	1.09 mM	Lee et al. (2010)
Fucus distichus	USA	Phlorotannins comprising 3–18 fucophloroethol monomers	0.89 μg/mL	112 μg/mL	13.9 μg/mL	137.8 μg/mL	Kellogg, Grace, and Lila (2014)
Fucus vesiculosis	Canada China	Fucoidan Fucoidan	49 μg/mL 68 μg/mL	1 mg/mL ND	>10 mg/mL > 10 mg/mL	1 mg/mL ND	Kim, Jeon, and Lee (2014), Kim, Rioux, and Turgeon (2014)

Continued

Table 5 Summary of the α-glucosidase and α-amylase inhibitory effects of seaweed bioactives.—cont'd

Seaweed species	Country of origin	Chemicals present	α-Glucosidase inhibition (IC_{50})		α-Amylase inhibition (IC_{50})		Reference source
			Extract/compound	Acarbose	Extract/compound	Acarbose	
Ascophyllum nodosum and *Fucus vesiculosis*	Italy	Polysaccharides, polyphenols, fatty acids	1.5 μg/mL	130 μg/mL	0.6 μg/mL	207 μg/mL	Gabbia et al. (2017)
Hizikia fusiformis	South Korea	Fucoxanthin, fucosterol	40–60 μg/mL	231 μg/mL	ND	ND	Han, Ali, Woo, Jung, and Choi (2015)
Ishige okamurae	South Korea	Diphlorethohydroxycarmolol (DPHC)	0.16 mM	1.05 mM	0.53 mM	1.10 mM	Heo et al. (2009)
Laminaria digitata	Germany	Extract 2,5-dihydrobenzoic acid	750 μg/mL 46 μg/mL	1120 μg/mL	ND	ND	Zaharudin, Salmean, and Dragsted (2018)
Laminaria japonica	China	Polysaccharides	7500 μg/mL	ND	58 mg/mL	ND	Peng, Yuan, Wu, and Wang (2011)
Sargassum confusum	China	Polysaccharide hydrolysate (SCO)	9.9 mg/mL	3.0 mg/mL	ND	ND	Yang et al. (2017)
Sargassum hemiphyllum	Taiwan	Polyphenols 17–36 mg/g Fucoxanthin 8–15 mg/g	ND	ND	350 μg/mL	0.7 μg/mL	Hwang, Hung, Tsai, Chien, and Kong (2015)
Sargassum serratifolium	Korea	Sargachromenol Sargaquinoic acid	43 μM 96 μM	210 μM	ND	ND	Ali et al. (2017)

Sargassum wightii	India	Fucoidan	132 μg/mL	1 mg/mL	ND	ND	Kumar et al. (2015)
Turbinara conoides	India	Fucoidan	0.68 μM	3.5 μM	1.07 μM	5.3 μM	Lakshmana Senthil, Raghu, Arjun, and Anantharaman (2019)
Turbinaria ornata	India	Fucoidan	ND	ND	33.6 μg/mL	125 μg/mL	Lakshmana Senthil et al. (2014)
Undaria pinnatifida	N/K	Fucoxanthin	47 μg/mL	600 μg/mL	ND	ND	Zaharudin, Staerk, and Dragsted (2019)
Eucheuma denticulatum	Malaysia	Not determined, but known to contain polyphenols	ND	ND	67% Inhibition at 10 mg/mL	92% Inhibition at 1 mg/mL	Balasubramaniam et al. (2016)
Porphyra spp.	China	Gly-Gly-Ser-Lys Glu-Leu-Ser	ND ND ND	ND	1.86 mg/mL 2.6 mM 2.6 mM	ND	Admassu, Gasmalla, Yang, and Zhao (2018)
Halimeda macroloba	Malaysia	Not determined, but extracts in water	6.4 mg/mL	<1 mg/mL	ND	ND	Chin et al. (2015)
Codum fragile	Tunisia	Sulfated polysaccharides	ND	ND	~50% inhibition in vivo following 150 mg/kg p.o.	~50% inhibition following 5 mg/kg p.o.	Kolsi, Fakhfakh, Sassi, Elleuch, and Gargouri (2018)
Ulva fasciata	Malaysia	Terpenoids, flavonoids, glycosides and phenolics	ND	ND	69 μg/mL	49 μg/mL	Mohapatra, Bhattamisra, Panigrahy, and Parida (2018)

content (Apostolidis, Karayannakidis, Kwon, Lee, & Seeram, 2011). Other studies using both water- and ethanol-based extracts from *A. nodosum* have similarly shown a preference for α-glucosidase inhibition over α-amylase inhibition (Lordan et al., 2013) and superiority over acarbose at inhibiting α-glucosidase. In contrast, other studies have shown that the α-amylase inhibitory activity of *A. nodosum* extracts is greater than the α-glucosidase inhibitory activity (Nwosu et al., 2011), differences that can potentially be explained by variances in the extraction process. For example, the Sephadex fractionation process employed by Nwosu et al. (2011) resulted in a phenolic-rich fraction, while the water-based extraction employed by the Apostolidis group (Apostolidis et al., 2011) may have contained a greater amount of non-phenolic components that may have contributed to the greater inhibition of α-glucosidase. Subsequent comparison of the inhibitory activity of phenolic-enriched and phlorotannin-rich sub fractions of *A. nodosum* revealed that only the phenolic-enriched, but not the phlorotannin-rich, fractions exhibited α-amylase inhibitory activity, while both fractions inhibited α-glucosidase equally; interestingly, the presence of bovine serum albumin attenuated the inhibitory activity of the phlorotannin-rich fraction against α-amylase, suggestive of protein binding playing an important part in its mechanism of action (Pantidos et al., 2014). Moreover, co-incubation of the phlorotannin-rich fraction along with acarbose reduced the concentration of acarbose required to inhibit both enzymes, leading to the suggestion that a combination of acarbose with phlorotannin-rich seaweed extracts may be a suitable approach to the management of post-prandial glycemic control.

Findings from other brown seaweed species have found that α-amylase and α-glucosidase inhibitory activity is common to most (summarized in Table 5). Extracts from *Laminaria japonica* (Peng et al., 2011), *Laminaria digitata* (Zaharudin et al., 2018), *Undaria pinnatifida* (Zaharudin et al., 2018), *Sargassum serratifolium* (Ali et al., 2017) and *Saragassum heiphyllum* (Hwang et al., 2015), *Alaria marginata* (Kellogg et al., 2014) and *Fucus distichus* (Kellogg et al., 2014) to name a few, have all been shown to possess α-glucosidase and/or α-amylase inhibitory activities over concentration ranges similar to acarbose. Depending upon the extraction methods, the presence of a range of chemical groups including plastoquinones, polysaccharides, phlorotannins and phenolics have been aligned to the enzyme inhibitory effect. However, only a few studies have been able to provide more precise information as to potential candidate molecules present. Detailed chemical analysis of the most potent *F. distichus* extracts revealed that the dominant phytochemicals present were fucophloroethol structures of between 3 and 18 different phloroglucinol units (Kellogg et al., 2014), while 2,5-dihydroxybenzoic acid was identified as an important compound present in extracts from both *Laminaria digitata* and *Undaria pinnatifida* (Zaharudin et al., 2018) and the plastoquinones sargahydroquinoic acid, sargachromenol and sargaquinoic acid were identified as compounds of interest in *Sargassum serratifolium* (Ali et al., 2017). Perhaps the most studied pure compounds present in brown seaweed are the fucoxanthins, which have been found to be responsible for the α-glucosidase inhibitory activity in extracts from *Undaria pinnatifida* (Zaharudin et al., 2019), and the fucoidans, which have been isolated from several species including *Turbiniaria ornate* (Lakshmana Senthil et al., 2014), *Sargassum wightii* (Kumar et al., 2015) and *Turbinara conoides* (Lakshmana Senthil et al., 2019) and which inhibit both α-glucosidase and α-amylase.

As mentioned above, most seaweeds assessed for enzyme inhibitory activity have been brown seaweeds, however a small number of studies have determined activity in extracts from red and green seaweeds. Two peptides (Gly-Gly-Ser-Lys and Glu-Leu-Ser) were identified as the primary chemicals responsible for α-amylase inhibitory activity present in proteolytic enzyme hydrolysates from the red seaweed *Porphyris* spp. (laver; Admassu et al., 2018), while ethanolic extract from *Eucheuma denticulatum* similarly inhibits α-amylase activity (Balasubramaniam et al., 2016). To our knowledge, only one green seaweed species (*Halimeda macroloba*) has demonstrated inhibitory activity against α-amylase, although no chemical analysis was performed (Chin et al., 2015).

3.1.2 In vivo studies

Attempts to associate the ability of seaweed extracts to inhibit α-glucosidase and/or α-amylase in vitro with an in vivo reduction in post-prandial glucose and insulin levels have been made in a small number of animal studies, with mixed results. Acute administration of a commercially available combined water extract from *Fucus vesiculosis* and *Ascophyllum nodosum*, which was shown to be a more potent inhibitor of both α-glucosidase and α-amylase in vitro than acarbose, was found to blunt the initial increase in blood glucose, without influencing area under the curve, following starch ingestion in normal fed rats (Gabbia et al., 2017). Interestingly, when administered to high fat-fed rats the extract significantly reduced the area under the curve for both insulin and glucose, suggesting that the extract can slow down both the rate of carbohydrate digestion and assimilation. In contrast, while an ethyl extract of *Ulva fasciata* was found to inhibit α-amylase in vitro in micromolar concentrations, it induced only a moderate decrease in fasting glucose, and had no effect on the area under the curve of a glucose tolerance test, when given over several days to alloxan-induced diabetic mice (Mohapatra et al., 2018). Studies that have utilized purified seaweed-derived compounds (rather than crude extracts) have, however, tended to generate more consistent findings. Heo et al. (2009) studied diphlorethohydroxycarmolol (DPHC), isolated from *Ishige okamurae*, and found that in vitro enzyme (both α-glucosidase and α-amylase) inhibition was achieved at concentrations 2–10 times lower than acarbose, and was equipotent with acarbose at suppressing post-prandial blood glucose and area under the curve following starch ingestion in both normal and streptozotocin-induced diabetic mice. Similarly, dieckol, isolated from *Ecklonia cava*, preferentially inhibits α-glucosidase over α-amylase and reduces post-prandial blood glucose in streptozotocin-induced T2D mice (Lee et al., 2010). Sulfated polysaccharides from *Codium fragile* have been shown to reduce both fasting plasma glucose and the rise in glucose levels after an oral glucose tolerance test, an effect that was associated with a >50% reduction in both plasma and intestinal α-amylase (Kolsi et al., 2018). A study of fucoidan isolated from 11 different species of seaweed found that the enzyme inhibitory activity varied widely between species, and that only fucoidan from *Fucus vesiculosus* exhibited significant (>50%) α-glucosidase (but not α-amylase) inhibition and reduced fasting blood glucose levels in a dose-dependent manner after 3 weeks of administration to db/db mice (Shan et al., 2016). Structure-activity analysis of the different fucoidans revealed that the potency of each fucoidan was associated with the types of glycoside linkages within the molecules. In a direct comparison between fucoidan from *F. vesiculosus* and *A. nodosum*, Kim, Rioux, and Turgeon (2014) identified that enzyme inhibitory activity was not only determined by the time of harvest, but also that there were inter-species differences in both the molecular weight and the sulfate content of the fucoidans, leading to the proposition that fucoidan may exert its enzyme inhibitory activity through electrostatic interaction between the negatively charged sulfate groups of the fucoidan and the enzyme.

3.1.3 Human studies

Even fewer studies have explored the potential of α-amylase/α-glucosidase inhibition by seaweed extracts in humans. A polyphenol-rich (28% polyphenol/67% fucoidan) extract from *Fucus vesiculosus* did not have any effect on post-prandial glucose control when given acutely to either healthy volunteers (Murray, Dordevic, Ryan, & Bonham, 2018) or to subjects with high fasting glucose levels (Paradis, Couture, & Lamarche, 2011). However, in the latter group there was a decreased insulin response, suggesting that a beneficial effect is only seen when there is existing dysregulation of glucose handling. In contrast, chronic administration of algal-derived phenols have been shown to either have no effect on (Hernandez-Corona, Martinez-Abundis, & Gonzalez-Ortiz, 2014; Lee & Jeon, 2013) or to significantly reduce (Shin, Kim, Park, Lee, & Hwang, 2012) fasting blood glucose levels, although chronic administration of the phlorotannin dieckol did significantly reduced post-prandial glucose levels (Lee & Jeon, 2015). Taken together this suggests that prolonged consumption is required to see any beneficial effect, but, as highlighted in a recent systematic review into the potential anti-diabetic effects of marine algal polyphenols (Murray, Dordevic, Bonham, & Ryan, 2018), existing data is inconsistent and detailed randomized controlled trials are required to determine optimum doses, treatment regimens and, indeed, the preferred algal source and its post-harvest treatment.

From the above it is evident that there is significant potential for the use of seaweed components for management of post-prandial blood glucose. However, there is substantial variation in the selectivity (or lack thereof) for either α-glucosidase or α-amylase inhibition, not only among seaweed species, but also between extracts from the same species. There are multiple reasons for this variability: (i) the extraction process will determine the predominant chemical species within an extract, thus if extracts were to be used as a means of controlling post-prandial blood glucose in Type 2 diabetics, then close attention will be needed to define the precise extraction method to yield the required amounts of active components to achieve relevant in vivo concentrations; (ii) there is a clear seasonal (and probably geographic) influence over the compounds present within each seaweed species, which again would need to be given consideration when preparing extracts for this use; (iii) specific compounds (e.g., fucoidan) that exert inhibitory effects may vary in their chemical structure from species to species. Nevertheless, the research to date shows that progress is being made in terms of identifying extracts or pure compounds that possess inhibitory activity superior to that seen with acarbose (summarized in Table 5) and that also exhibit selective inhibition of α-glucosidase, which may pave the way for a replacement for acarbose to avoid the side effects associated with α-amylase inhibition.

3.2 Insulin-sensitizing activity of algal extracts

Improving insulin sensitivity is perhaps the "Holy Grail" of therapy for the management of T2D, with the two main classes of agents used clinically being the biguanides (e.g., metformin) and the thiazolidinediones ("glitazones" e.g., pioglitazone). Metformin increases insulin sensitivity in vivo, thus reducing plasma glucose concentrations, increasing glucose uptake, and decreasing gluconeogenesis. Although the precise mechanism of action of metformin is not fully elucidated, it has been shown to act via both AMP-activated protein kinase (AMPK)-dependent and AMPK-independent mechanisms although its pharmacology is likely to be more complex involving multi-organ actions and anti-inflammatory actions (Rena, Hardie, & Pearson, 2017). The glitazones on the other hand bind to the nuclear regulatory protein PPAR-γ which influences insulin-sensitive genes to enhance the production of insulin-dependent enzyme mRNAs and improve glucose utilization by the cells. The main targets (summarized in Fig. 2) that have been explored in the search for seaweed extracts with potential anti-diabetic actions include: Insulin Receptor Substrate (IRS-1), which ultimately results in translocation of GLUT4 to the plasma membrane to facilitate intracellular glucose uptake; AMPK, which, in skeletal muscle, induces fusion of GLUT4 vesicles with the plasma membrane (and thus stimulates glucose uptake), stimulates glycolysis by activating phosphorylation of glycogen phosphorylase, and it inhibits glycogen synthesis through inhibitory phosphorylation of glycogen synthase, while in the liver it inhibits gluconeogenesis; protein-tyrosine phosphatase 1B (PTP1B), which is a negative regulator of insulin through dephosphorylation of both the insulin receptor and the activated insulin receptor substrates.

Few studies have investigated the effects of crude algal extracts on insulin sensitivity but have rather focused more on specific compounds, or groups of compounds. Both ethanolic and water extracts from *Sargassum polycystum* were shown to reduce fasting blood glucose (~50% of the metformin response) without influencing plasma insulin levels in a rat model of T2D (high fat/high sugar diet combined with low dose streptozotocin), suggesting that the hypoglycemic effects were due to increased insulin sensitivity rather than an insulinotropic effect (Motshakeri, Ebrahimi, Goh, Matanjun, & Mohamed, 2013). These responses were attributed to antioxidant effects of fucoxanthin (which is abundant in this species), since a reduction in advanced glycation end-products (AGE's) was detected in the treated animals, reflecting a reduction in tissue damage induced by the diabetic state. In line with this, fucoidan has been shown in a model of non-alcoholic fatty liver disease (NAFLD) to similarly reduce fasting blood glucose and decrease insulin resistance, while at the same time protecting the liver against injury concomitant with a decrease in the expression of inflammatory markers (Heeba & Morsy, 2015). In a murine T2D model, both low molecular weight fucoidan and fucoxanthin independently decreased fasting blood glucose and increased hepatic glycogen, while fucoxanthin (but not fucoidan alone) was also seen to increase the expression of IRS-1, GLUT-4 and PPAR-γ in adipose tissue, representing an insulin-sensitizing action (Lin, Tsou, Chen, Lu, & Hwang, 2017); interestingly, a combination of fucoxanthin and fucoidan exhibited a synergistic effect in the increased expression of these markers of insulin sensitivity.

A dieckol extract from *Ecklonia cava* has also been shown in db/db mice to decrease fasting blood glucose and circulating insulin levels, effects that were associated with a reduction in hepatic glycogen production resulting from decreased G-6-phosphatase activity and a suppression of hepatic glucose regulating genes (e.g., phosphoenolpyruvate carboxykinase; PEPCK) that are known to be over-expressed in T2D (Lee et al., 2012). The extract also reduced both plasma and hepatic lipids, which again may contribute to the improved glucose profile since increased lipids are positively associated with the development of insulin resistance. The hypoglycemic effect of purified dieckol in db/db mice was subsequently shown to be associated with an increase in phosphorylation of AMPK/Akt in the skeletal muscle of these animals (Kang, Wijesinghe, et al., 2013). These findings are corroborated in a zebrafish model of alloxan-induced diabetes in which dieckol was shown to increase Akt activation in skeletal muscle and to improve regulation of hepatic glucose metabolism to a similar extant as that seen with metformin (Kim et al., 2016).

The AMPK/Akt pathway similarly appears to be the target for the insulin-sensitizing effects of other algal extracts, since extracts from both *Laminaria japonica* and *Hizikia fusiforme* increase glucose uptake in C2C12 myotubes (mouse-derived skeletal muscle) via phosphorylation of both PKB and AMPK, a finding that was mirrored in skeletal muscle from high fat/high sugar-fed mice (Kang, Kim, Kang, Lee, & Lee, 2018). Moreover, both ethanolic and water flavonoid-rich extracts from *Enteromorpha prolifera* improved glucose tolerance through alterations in the expression of insulin signal transduction genes, whereby IRSI (suppressed in T2D), phosphatidylinositol 3-kinase (PI3K) and AKT expression (gene and protein) was increased while gene expression of JNK (increased in T2D) was decreased (Yan et al., 2019). Taken together these findings support the suggestion that algal extracts rich in flavonoids improve glucose metabolism and hepatic glucose uptake via an increase in insulin signaling.

PTP1B overexpression may play a role in insulin resistance and therefore also presents as a potential therapeutic target although, as yet, there are no inhibitors available for clinical studies. Nevertheless, there is increasing interest in the search for novel PTP1B inhibitors from natural sources (Zhao et al., 2018). Several algal-derived bioactive molecules, such as fucoxanthin, sargahydroquinoic acid and sargachromenol, as well as crude algal extracts, have demonstrated activity as PTP1B inhibitors; the breadth of in vitro studies that have revealed this pharmacological action and determined the structural activity relationships of the various chemical groups contained within the extracts is beyond the scope of this review, however this was recently covered in depth in review by Ezzat et al. (2018). Despite the relative abundance of algal-derived PTP1B inhibitors, their potential for exploitation is compromised by the many pleiotropic actions they exhibit. For example, methanolic extract from the brown alga *Hizikia fusiformis* inhibits PTP1B in vitro, but it is also an α-glucosidase inhibitor, a powerful peroxynitrite scavenger and an inhibitor of inducible nitric oxide synthase (Han et al., 2015), which would make any association between PTP1B inhibition and a hypoglycemic effect difficult to make. Moreover, very few algal-derived PTP1B inhibitors have been assessed for their ability to exert an anti-diabetic effect in vivo and the only study we have identified showed that while an extract from *Rhodomelia confervoides* exhibited both in vitro inhibition of PTP1B and reduced fasting blood glucose in vivo in streptozotocin-induced Type 1 diabetic rats (Shi et al., 2008), a direct relationship between the two was not demonstrated. Therefore, while there may be great potential for bioactive molecules isolated from marine algae to be used as structural scaffolds for novel PTP1B inhibitors, a significant gap remains between demonstrating a cause/effect relationship between in vitro PTP1B inhibition and a hypoglycemic/insulin-sensitizing effect. Furthermore, randomized human clinical trials are also needed to determine whether findings from in vivo animal studies can be translated into a positive clinical outcome.

3.3 Stimulation/preservation of insulin secretion by algal extracts

Stimulation of insulin secretion from pancreatic islets or protecting insulin secreting cells from the damaging effects of hyperglycemia, is a further approach to improving glucose homeostasis in T2D although no currently used clinical agents appear to preserve pancreatic β-cell integrity. In the case of the former, the agent most widely used in the clinic is the sulfonylurea glibenclamide, which stimulates insulin release from pancreatic β-cells by inhibiting the ATP-sensitive potassium channels (K_{ATP}) inhibitory regulatory subunit sulfonylurea receptor 1 (SUR1), resulting in membrane depolarization and the opening of voltage-dependent calcium channels. However, the use of glibenclamide is limited by its potential to induce hypoglycemia and its efficacy in controlling glucose dysregulation is lower than that of metformin.

Extracts from *Sargassum polycystum* administered to rats with T2D induced by a combination of HF/HS and low dose streptozocin has been shown to decrease the extent of the resulting pathological changes in the islet cells, and perhaps more importantly to decrease the number of cells damaged by the induction of T2D (Motshakeri et al., 2014). Similarly, in models of Type 1 (alloxan or streptozotocin induced) diabetes, both *Laminaria japonica* (Long et al., 2012) and *Ecklonia cava* (Kim & Kim, 2012) extracts increased the pancreatic expression of superoxide dismutase, decreased the expression of inducible nitric oxide synthase and improved β-cell index (measure of cell structure) and mass, observations that were accompanied by an increase in serum insulin levels and a reduction in fasting blood glucose. Moreover, *Ecklonia cava* extract was also shown to increase insulin secretion from pancreatic islet cells. Some insight into the underlying mechanism of how the extract acts as a preserver of β-cells comes from studies with dieckol (present in high quantities in *E. cava*), where protection was observed against glucotoxicity in rat insulinoma cells (Lee et al., 2012). As with the in vivo studies with *E. cava* extract, dieckol reduced ROS and NO production by the cells, increased the expression of the antioxidant enzymes superoxide dismutase and catalase and reduced caspase-3 activation, indicating an anti-apoptotic effect. Fucoidan has also been demonstrated to reduce the histopathological changes in pancreatic islets in a rat strain that spontaneously develops non-insulin dependent diabetes and to act as an insulin secretagogue in RIN-SF rat insulin secreting cells. The latter effect appears to be through a cAMP signaling pathway, since phosphodiesterase inhibition abrogated the effects of fucoidan, rather than through a similar mechanism to glibenclamide, since amylin (a glibenclamide inhibitor) did not reverse its effects (Jiang, Yu, Ma, Zhang, & Xie, 2015). Interestingly, when fucoidan was applied in combination with glibenclamide an additive effect was seen, suggesting that a combination of K_{ATP} channel opening and activation of cAMP in pancreatic islets may be an approach to a greater insulin secretion response.

4. Conclusion

Extracts from seaweed and their bioactive compounds have been shown to provide a good source for discovering new therapeutic drugs for obesity and T2D management. Pharmacological interventions focused on maintaining/improving adipose tissue health and liver energy metabolism, modulating the diversity of gut microbiota, regulating glucose absorption from the intestine, and improving insulin sensitivity/secretion therefore form the basis for novel therapeutic interventions in obesity, T2D and metabolic diseases.

The molecular mechanisms affected by seaweed extracts and bioactive compounds are specific to different tissues and for obesity or T2D management, however key signaling pathways or targets have emerged. In obesity, modulation of antioxidant capacity and reduction of intracellular ROS levels within tissues, and regulation of signaling pathways involved in enhancing browning of white adipose tissue, have been highlighted as important mechanisms and potential targets for optimal energy metabolism. In T2D, management of post-prandial blood glucose by modulating α-glucosidase or α-amylase activities, modulation of AMPK signaling pathway, and similarly to obesity, reduction of ROS and NO production with subsequent increased expression of antioxidant enzymes have been shown to play a key role in glucose metabolism and insulin signaling.

Future studies aimed at discovering new therapeutics drug from marine natural products should, therefore, focus on bioactive compounds from seaweed that exert antioxidant properties and regulate the expression of key signaling pathways, which are common mechanisms to both obesity and T2D management. In addition, considering the paucity of data around the clinical benefits of seaweed-derived compounds in obesity and T2D, it is clear that a substantial effort, in the form of human clinical trials, is required.

Conflict of interest

C.W., G.B. and T.S. have no conflict of interest. F.H. is an employee of Algaia, which is a company that produces natural seaweed extracts and solutions.

References

Admassu, H., Gasmalla, M. A. A., Yang, R., & Zhao, W. (2018). Identification of bioactive peptides with alpha-amylase inhibitory potential from enzymatic protein hydrolysates of red seaweed (Porphyra spp.). *Journal of Agricultural and Food Chemistry*, *66*, 4872–4882. https://doi.org/10.1021/acs.jafc.8b00960.

Afonso, N. C., Catarino, M. D., Silva, A. M. S., & Cardoso, S. M. (2019). Brown macroalgae as valuable food ingredients. *Antioxidants (Basel)*, *8*, E365. https://doi.org/10.3390/antiox8090365.

Ali, M. Y., Kim, D. H., Seong, S. H., Kim, H., Jung, H. A., & Choi, J. S. (2017). Alpha-glucosidase and protein tyrosine phosphatase 1B inhibitory activity of plastoquinones from marine brown alga *Sargassum serratifolium*. *Marine Drugs*, *15*, 368. https://doi.org/10.3390/md15120368.

Apostolidis, E., Karayannakidis, P. D., Kwon, Y., Lee, C. M., & Seeram, N. P. (2011). Seasonal variation of phenolic antioxidant-mediated alpha-glucosidase inhibition of *Ascophyllum nodosum*. *Plant Foods for Human Nutrition*, *66*, 313–319. https://doi.org/10.1007/s11130-011-0250-4.

Apostolidis, E., & Lee, C. M. (2010). In vitro potential of *Ascophyllum nodosum* phenolic antioxidant-mediated alpha-glucosidase and alpha-amylase inhibition. *Journal of Food Science*, *75*, H97–H102. https://doi.org/10.1111/j.1750-3841.2010.01544.x.

Awang, A., Ng, J., Matanjun, P., Sulaiman, M., Tan, T., & Beng Houi Ooi, Y. (2014). Anti-obesity property of the brown seaweed, *Sargassum polycystum* using an in vivo animal model. *Journal of Applied Phycology*, *26*, 1043–1048.

Bakhai, M. N., & Tirgar, P. R. (2013). In-vivo investigation of antiobesity activity of polyherbal formulation. *International Journal of Research in Pharmaceutical and Biomedical Sciences*, *4*, 1095–1103.

Balasubramaniam, V., Lee, J. C., Noh, M. F. M., Ahmad, S., Brownlee, I. A., & Ismail, A. (2016). Alpha-amylase, antioxidant, and anti-inflammatory activities of *Eucheuma denticulatum* (NL Burman) FS Collins and Hervey. *Journal of Applied Phycology*, *28*, 1965–1974. https://doi.org/10.1007/s10811-015-0690-6.

Barness, L. A., Opitz, J. M., & Gilbert-Barness, E. (2007). Obesity: Genetic, molecular, and environmental aspects. *American Journal of Medical Genetics Part A*, *143A*, 3016–3034. https://doi.org/10.1002/ajmg.a.32035.

Beppu, F., Hosokawa, M., Yim, M. J., Shinoda, T., & Miyashita, K. (2013). Down-regulation of hepatic stearoyl-CoA desaturase-1 expression by fucoxanthin via leptin signaling in diabetic/obese KK-A(y) mice. *Lipids*, *48*, 449–455. https://doi.org/10.1007/s11745-013-3784-4.

Berrington de Gonzalez, A., Hartge, P., Cerhan, J. R., Flint, A. J., Hannan, L., MacInnis, R. J., et al. (2010). Body-mass index and mortality among 1.46 million white adults. *The New England Journal of Medicine*, *363*, 2211–2219. https://doi.org/10.1056/NEJMoa1000367.

Brown, E. S., Allsopp, P. J., Magee, P. J., Gill, C. I., Nitecki, S., Strain, C. R., et al. (2014). Seaweed and human health. *Nutrition Reviews*, *72*, 205–216.

Chin, Y. X., Lim, P. E., Maggs, C. A., Phang, S. M., Sharifuddin, Y., & Green, B. D. (2015). Anti-diabetic potential of selected Malaysian seaweeds. *Journal of Applied Phycology*, *27*, 2137–2148. https://doi.org/10.1007/s10811-014-0462-8.

Cuong, H. D., Thuy, T. T., Huong, T. T., Ly, B. M., & Van, T. T. (2015). Structure and hypolipidaemic activity of fucoidan extracted from brown seaweed *Sargassum henslowianum*. *Natural Product Research*, *29*, 411–415. https://doi.org/10.1080/14786419.2014.948436.

Duan, M., Sun, X., Ma, N., Liu, Y., Luo, T., Song, S., et al. (2019). Polysaccharides from Laminaria japonica alleviated metabolic syndrome in BALB/c mice by normalizing the gut microbiota. *International Journal of Biological Macromolecules*, *121*, 996–1004. S0141-8130(18)31205-4 [pii].

Ezzat, S. M., Bishbishy, M. H. E., Habtemariam, S., Salehi, B., Sharifi-Rad, M., Martins, N., et al. (2018). Looking at marine-derived bioactive molecules as upcoming anti-diabetic agents: A special emphasis on PTP1B inhibitors. *Molecules*, *23*, E3334. https://doi.org/10.3390/molecules23123334. [pii].

Firdaus, M., Nurdiani, R., & Prihanto, A. A. (2015). Antihyperglycemic of Sargassum sp. extract. In Anonymous (Ed.), *Marine algae extracts: Processes, products, and applications* (pp. 381–394).

Gabbia, D., Dall'Acqua, S., Di Gangi, I. M., Bogialli, S., Caputi, V., Albertoni, L., et al. (2017). The phytocomplex from *Fucus vesiculosus* and *Ascophyllum nodosum* controls postprandial plasma glucose levels: An in vitro and in vivo study in a mouse model of NASH. *Marine Drugs*, *15*, 41. https://doi.org/10.3390/md15020041.

Georg Jensen, M., Kristensen, M., Belza, A., Knudsen, J. C., & Astrup, A. (2012). Acute effect of alginate-based preload on satiety feelings, energy intake, and gastric emptying rate in healthy subjects. *Obesity (Silver Spring)*, *20*, 1851–1858. https://doi.org/10.1038/oby.2011.232.

Gonzalez-Muniesa, P., Martinez-Gonzalez, M. A., Hu, F. B., Despres, J. P., Matsuzawa, Y., Loos, R. J. F., et al. (2017). Obesity. *Nature Reviews Disease Primers*, *3*, 17034. https://doi.org/10.1038/nrdp.2017.34.

Ha, A. W., Na, S. J., & Kim, W. K. (2013). Antioxidant effects of fucoxanthin rich powder in rats fed with high fat diet. *Nutrition Research and Practice*, 7, 475–480. https://doi.org/10.4162/nrp.2013.7.6.475.

Han, Y. R., Ali, M. Y., Woo, M., Jung, H. A., & Choi, J. S. (2015). Anti-diabetic and anti-inflammatory potential of the edible brown alga Hizikia fusiformis. *Journal of Food Biochemistry*, *39*, 417–428. https://doi.org/10.1111/jfbc.12138.

Heeba, G. H., & Morsy, M. A. (2015). Fucoidan ameliorates steatohepatitis and insulin resistance by suppressing oxidative stress and inflammatory cytokines in experimental non-alcoholic fatty liver disease. *Environmental Toxicology and Pharmacology*, *40*, 907–914. https://doi.org/10.1016/j.etap.2015.10.003.

Heo, S. J., Hwang, J. Y., Choi, J. I., Han, J. S., Kim, H. J., & Jeon, Y. J. (2009). Diphlorethohydroxycarmalol isolated from Ishige okamurae, a brown algae, a potent alpha-glucosidase and alpha-amylase inhibitor, alleviates postprandial hyperglycemia in diabetic mice. *European Journal of Pharmacology*, *615*, 252–256. https://doi.org/10.1016/j.ejphar.2009.05.017.

Hernandez-Corona, D. M., Martinez-Abundis, E., & Gonzalez-Ortiz, M. (2014). Effect of fucoidan administration on insulin secretion and insulin resistance in overweight or obese adults. *Journal of Medicinal Food*, *17*, 830–832. https://doi.org/10.1089/jmf.2013.0053.

Hitoe, S., & Shimoda, H. (2017). Seaweed fucoxanthin supplementation improves obesity parameters in mild obese Japanese subjects. *Functional Foods in Health & Disease*, 7, 246–262.

Hosokawa, M., Miyashita, T., Nishikawa, S., Emi, S., Tsukui, T., Beppu, F., et al. (2010). Fucoxanthin regulates adipocytokine mRNA expression in white adipose tissue of diabetic/obese KK-Ay mice. *Archives of Biochemistry and Biophysics*, *504*, 17–25. https://doi.org/10.1016/j.abb.2010.05.031.

Hwang, P., Hung, Y., Tsai, Y., Chien, S., & Kong, Z. (2015). The brown seaweed Sargassum hemiphyllum exhibits alpha-amylase and alpha-glucosidase inhibitory activity and enhances insulin release in vitro. *Cytotechnology*, *67*, 653–660. https://doi.org/10.1007/s10616-014-9745-9.

Jaswir, I., Ahmad, H., Susanti, D., Bakhtiar, M. T., & Octavianti, F. (2017). Effects of *Sargassum oligocystum* and *Padina australis* extract on adipogenesis and adipolysis in 3T3-L1 cells. *International Food Research Journal*, *24*, S395–S401.

Jeon, S. M., Kim, H. J., Woo, M. N., Lee, M. K., Shin, Y. C., Park, Y. B., et al. (2010). Fucoxanthin-rich seaweed extract suppresses body weight gain and improves lipid metabolism in high-fat-fed C57BL/6J mice. *Biotechnology Journal*, *5*, 961–969. https://doi.org/10.1002/biot.201000215.

Jiang, X., Yu, J., Ma, Z., Zhang, H., & Xie, F. (2015). Effects of fucoidan on insulin stimulation and pancreatic protection via the cAMP signaling pathway in vivo and in vitro. *Molecular Medicine Reports*, *12*, 4501–4507. https://doi.org/10.3892/mmr.2015.3989.

Kanda, Y., Hinata, T., Kang, S. W., & Watanabe, Y. (2011). Reactive oxygen species mediate adipocyte differentiation in mesenchymal stem cells. *Life Sciences*, *89*, 250–258. https://doi.org/10.1016/j.lfs.2011.06.007.

Kang, M., Ding, Y., Kim, E., Choi, Y. K., de Araujo, T., Heo, S., et al. (2017). Indole derivatives isolated from brown alga Sargassum thunbergii inhibit adipogenesis through AMPK activation in 3T3-L1 preadipocytes. *Marine Drugs*, *15*, 119–128. https://doi.org/10.3390/md15040119.

Kang, M. C., Kang, N., Kim, S. Y., Lima, I. S., Ko, S. C., Kim, Y. T., et al. (2016). Popular edible seaweed, Gelidium amansii prevents against diet-induced obesity. *Food and Chemical Toxicology*, *90*, 181–187. https://doi.org/10.1016/j.fct.2016.02.014.

Kang, M., Kim, S., Jeong, S., Choi, H., Jang, Y., & Kim, J. (2013). Antioxidant effect of Phaeodactylum tricornutum in mice fed high-fat diet. *Food Science and Biotechnology*, *22*, 107–113.

Kang, S. Y., Kim, E., Kang, I., Lee, M., & Lee, Y. (2018). Anti-diabetic effects and anti-inflammatory effects of *Laminaria japonica* and *Hizikia fusiforme* in skeletal muscle: In vitro and in vivo model. *Nutrients*, *10*, E491. https://doi.org/10.3390/nu10040491 [pii].

Kang, M., Wijesinghe, W. A. J. P., Lee, S., Kang, S., Ko, S., Yang, X., et al. (2013). Dieckol isolated from brown seaweed Ecklonia cava attenuates type II diabetes in db/db mouse model. *Food and Chemical Toxicology*, *53*, 294–298. https://doi.org/10.1016/j.fct.2012.12.012.

Kellogg, J., Esposito, D., Grace, M., Komarnytsky, S., & Lila, M. (2015). Alaskan seaweeds lower inflammation in RAW 264.7 macrophages and decrease lipid accumulation in 3T3-L1 adipocytes. *Journal of Functional Foods*, *15*, 396–407.

Kellogg, J., Grace, M. H., & Lila, M. A. (2014). Phlorotannins from Alaskan seaweed inhibit carbolytic enzyme activity. *Marine Drugs*, *12*, 5277–5294. https://doi.org/10.3390/md12105277.

Kim, Y. M., & Jang, M. S. (2018). Anti-obesity effects of *Laminaria japonica* fermentation on 3T3-L1 adipocytes are mediated by the inhibition of C/EBP-alpha/beta and PPAR-gamma. *Cellular and Molecular Biology (Noisy-le-Grand, France)*, *64*, 71–77.

Kim, M. J., Jeon, J., & Lee, J. S. (2014). Fucoidan prevents high-fat diet-induced obesity in animals by suppression of fat accumulation. *Phytotherapy Research*, *28*, 137–143. https://doi.org/10.1002/ptr.4965.

Kim, H., Kang, S., Shin, H., Ko, H., Hong, Y., Kang, S., et al. (2012). Anti-obesity effect of Komulkosiraegi [Gracilaria vermiculophylla (Ohmi) Papenfuss] extract in 3T3-L1 cells. *Food Science and Biotechnology*, *21*, 83–89.

Kim, M., & Kim, H. K. (2012). Insulinotrophic and hypolipidemic effects of Ecklonia cava in streptozotocin-induced diabetic mice. *Asian Pacific Journal of Tropical Medicine*, *5*, 374–379. https://doi.org/10.1016/S1995-7645(12)60062-5.

Kim, J. Y., Kwon, Y. M., Kim, I. S., Kim, J. A., Yu, D. Y., Adhikari, B., et al. (2018). Effects of the brown seaweed *Laminaria japonica* supplementation on serum concentrations of IgG, triglycerides, and cholesterol, and intestinal microbiota composition in rats. *Frontiers in Nutrition*, *5*, 23. https://doi.org/10.3389/fnut.2018.00023.

Kim, K., & Lee, B. (2012). Fucoidan from the sporophyll of *Undaria pinnatifida* suppresses adipocyte differentiation by inhibition of inflammation-related cytokines in 3T3-L1 cells. *Nutrition Research*, *32*, 439–447. https://doi.org/10.1016/j.nutres.2012.04.003.

Kim, K. J., Lee, O. H., & Lee, B. Y. (2010). Fucoidan, a sulfated polysaccharide, inhibits adipogenesis through the mitogen-activated protein kinase pathway in 3T3-L1 preadipocytes. *Life Sciences*, *86*, 791–797. https://doi.org/10.1016/j.lfs.2010.03.010.

Kim, E., Lee, S., Lee, J., Kang, N., Oh, J., Seun-heui, et al. (2016). A marine algal polyphenol, dieckol, attenuates blood glucose levels by Akt pathway in alloxan induced hyperglycemia zebrafish model. *RSC Advances*, *6*, 78570–78575. https://doi.org/10.1039/c6ra12724j.

Kim, K., Rioux, L., & Turgeon, S. L. (2014). Alpha-amylase and alpha-glucosidase inhibition is differentially modulated by fucoidan obtained from *Fucus vesiculosus* and *Ascophyllum nodosum*. *Phytochemistry*, *98*, 27–33. https://doi.org/10.1016/j.phytochem.2013.12.003.

Ko, S. C., Lee, M., Lee, J. H., Lee, S. H., Lim, Y., & Jeon, Y. J. (2013). Dieckol, a phlorotannin isolated from a brown seaweed, Ecklonia cava, inhibits adipogenesis through AMP-activated protein kinase (AMPK) activation in 3T3-L1 preadipocytes. *Environmental Toxicology and Pharmacology*, *36*, 1253–1260. https://doi.org/10.1016/j.etap.2013.10.011.

Kolsi, R. B. A., Fakhfakh, J., Sassi, S., Elleuch, M., & Gargouri, L. (2018). Physico-chemical characterization and beneficial effects of seaweed sulfated polysaccharide against oxydatif and cellular damages caused by alloxan in diabetic rats. *International Journal of Biological Macromolecules*, *117*, 407–417. https://doi.org/10.1016/j.ijbiomac.2018.03.127.

Kumar, S. A., Magnusson, M., Ward, L. C., Paul, N. A., & Brown, L. (2015). Seaweed supplements normalise metabolic, cardiovascular and liver responses in high-carbohydrate, high-fat fed rats. *Marine Drugs*, *13*, 788–805. https://doi.org/10.3390/md13020788.

Kwon, T. H., Wu, Y. X., Kim, J. S., Woo, J. H., Park, K. T., Kwon, O. J., et al. (2015). 6,6'-Bieckol inhibits adipocyte differentiation through downregulation of adipogenesis and lipogenesis in 3T3-L1 cells. *Journal of the Science of Food and Agriculture*, *95*, 1830–1837. https://doi.org/10.1002/jsfa.6881.

Lakshmana Senthil, S., Raghu, C., Arjun, H. A., & Anantharaman, P. (2019). In vitro and in silico inhibition properties of fucoidan against alpha-amylase and alpha-D-glucosidase with relevance to type 2 diabetes mellitus. *Carbohydrate Polymers*, *209*, 350–355. S0144-8617(19)30052-9 [pii].

Lakshmana Senthil, S., Vinothkumar, T., Geetharamani, D., Marudhupandi, T., Suja, G., & Sindhu, N. S. (2014). Fucoidan-a novel α-amylase inhibitor from *Turbinaria ornata* with relevance to NIDDM therapy. *Biocatalysis and Agricultural Biotechnology*, *3*, 66–70. https://doi.org/10.1016/j.bcab.2014.02.003.

Lee, S. H., & Jeon, Y. J. (2013). Anti-diabetic effects of brown algae derived phlorotannins, marine polyphenols through diverse mechanisms. *Fitoterapia*, *86*, 129–136. https://doi.org/10.1016/j.fitote.2013.02.013.

Lee, S., & Jeon, Y. (2015). Efficacy and safety of a dieckol-rich extract (AG-dieckol) of brown algae, Ecklonia cava, in pre-diabetic individuals: A double-blind, randomized, placebo-controlled clinical trial. *Food & Function*, *6*, 853–858. https://doi.org/10.1039/c4fo00940a.

Lee, S. H., Min, K. H., Han, J. S., Lee, D. H., Park, D. B., Jung, W. K., et al. (2012). Effects of brown alga, Ecklonia cava on glucose and lipid metabolism in C57BL/KsJ-db/db mice, a model of type 2 diabetes mellitus. *Food and Chemical Toxicology*, *50*, 575–582. https://doi.org/10.1016/j.fct.2011.12.032.

Lee, S. H., Park, M. H., Heo, S. J., Kang, S. M., Ko, S. C., Han, J. S., et al. (2010). Dieckol isolated from Ecklonia cava inhibits alpha-glucosidase and alpha-amylase in vitro and alleviates postprandial hyperglycemia in streptozotocin-induced diabetic mice. *Food and Chemical Toxicology*, *48*, 2633–2637. https://doi.org/10.1016/j.fct.2010.06.032.

Lee, S. H., Park, M. H., Kang, S. M., Ko, S. C., Kang, M. C., Cho, S., et al. (2012). Dieckol isolated from Ecklonia cava protects against high-glucose induced damage to rat insulinoma cells by reducing oxidative stress and apoptosis. *Bioscience, Biotechnology, and Biochemistry*, *76*, 1445–1451. DN/JST.JSTAGE/bbb/120096 [pii].

Lee, O. H., Yoon, K. Y., Kim, K. J., You, S., & Lee, B. Y. (2011). Seaweed extracts as a potential tool for the attenuation of oxidative damage in obesity-related pathologies(1). *Journal of Phycology*, *47*, 548–556. https://doi.org/10.1111/j.1529-8817.2011.00974.x.

Lin, H.-T. V., Tsou, Y.-C., Chen, Y.-T., Lu, W.-J., & Hwang, P.-A. (2017). Effects of low-molecular-weight fucoidan and high stability fucoxanthin on glucose homeostasis, lipid metabolism, and liver function in a mouse model of type II diabetes. *Marine Drugs*, *15*, 113–127. https://doi.org/10.3390/md15040113. [doi].

Liu, F., Wang, X., Shi, H., Wang, Y., Xue, C., & Tang, Q. J. (2017). Polymannuronic acid ameliorated obesity and inflammation associated with a high-fat and high-sucrose diet by modulating the gut microbiome in a murine model. *The British Journal of Nutrition*, *117*, 1332–1342. https://doi.org/10.1017/S0007114517000964.

Long, S. H., Yu, Z. Q., Shuai, L., Guo, Y. L., Duan, D. L., Xu, X. Y., et al. (2012). The hypoglycemic effect of the kelp on diabetes mellitus model induced by alloxan in rats. *International Journal of Molecular Sciences*, *13*, 3354–3365. https://doi.org/10.3390/ijms13033354.

Lordan, S., Smyth, T. J., Soler-Vila, A., Stanton, C., & Ross, R. P. (2013). The α-amylase and α-glucosidase inhibitory effects of Irish seaweed extracts. *Food Chemistry*, *141*, 2170–2176. https://doi.org/10.1016/j.foodchem.2013.04.123.

Maeda, H., Hosokawa, M., Sashima, T., Funayama, K., & Miyashita, K. (2005). Fucoxanthin from edible seaweed, Undaria pinnatifida, shows antiobesity effect through UCP1 expression in white adipose tissues. *Biochemical and Biophysical Research Communications*, *332*, 392–397. S0006-291X(05)00957-5 [pii].

Maeda, H., Hosokawa, M., Sashima, T., & Miyashita, K. (2007). Dietary combination of fucoxanthin and fish oil attenuates the weight gain of white adipose tissue and decreases blood glucose in obese/diabetic KK-Ay mice. *Journal of Agricultural and Food Chemistry*, *55*, 7701–7706. https://doi.org/10.1021/jf071569n.

Maeda, H., Hosokawa, M., Sashima, T., Murakami-Funayama, K., & Miyashita, K. (2009). Anti-obesity and anti-diabetic effects of fucoxanthin on diet-induced obesity conditions in a murine model. *Molecular Medicine Reports*, *2*, 897–902.

Maeda, H., Tsukui, T., Sashima, T., Hosokawa, M., & Miyashita, K. (2008). Seaweed carotenoid, fucoxanthin, as a multi-functional nutrient. *Asia Pacific Journal of Clinical Nutrition*, *17*, 196–199.

Mohapatra, L., Bhattamisra, S. K., Panigrahy, R. C., & Parida, S. (2018). Evaluation of antioxidant, hypoglycaemic, antidiabetic and alpha amylase inhibiting activities of Sargassum wightii collected from the east coast of India. *Indian Drugs*, *55*, 61–69.

Moreno-Indias, I., Cardona, F., Tinahones, F. J., & Queipo-Ortuno, M. I. (2014). Impact of the gut microbiota on the development of obesity and type 2 diabetes mellitus. *Frontiers in Microbiology*, *5*, 190. https://doi.org/10.3389/fmicb.2014.00190.

Motshakeri, M., Ebrahimi, M., Goh, Y. M., Matanjun, P., & Mohamed, S. (2013). Sargassum polycystum reduces hyperglycaemia, dyslipidaemia and oxidative stress via increasing insulin sensitivity in a rat model of type 2 diabetes. *Journal of the Science of Food and Agriculture*, *93*, 1772–1778. https://doi.org/10.1002/jsfa.5971.

Motshakeri, M., Ebrahimi, M., Goh, Y. M., Othman, H. H., Hair-Bejo, M., & Mohamed, S. (2014). Effects of brown seaweed (*Sargassum polycystum*) extracts on kidney, liver, and pancreas of type 2 diabetic rat model. *Evidence-based Complementary and Alternative Medicine*, *2014*, 379407. https://doi.org/10.1155/2014/379407.

Murray, M., Dordevic, A. L., Bonham, M. P., & Ryan, L. (2018). Do marine algal polyphenols have antidiabetic, anti-hyperlipidemic or anti-inflammatory effects in humans? A systematic review. *Critical Reviews in Food Science and Nutrition*, *58*, 2039–2054. https://doi.org/10.1080/10408398.2017.1301876.

Murray, M., Dordevic, A. L., Ryan, L., & Bonham, M. P. (2018). The impact of a single dose of a polyphenol-rich seaweed extract on postprandial glycaemic control in healthy adults: A randomised cross-over trial. *Nutrients, 10,* 270. https://doi.org/10.3390/nu10030270.

Nakazono, S., Cho, K., Isaka, S., Abu, R., Yokose, T., Murata, M., et al. (2016). Anti-obesity effects of enzymatically-digested alginate oligomer in mice model fed a high-fat-diet. *Bioactive Carbohydrates and Dietary Fibre,* 7, 1–8.

Nwosu, F., Morris, J., Lund, V. A., Stewart, D., Ross, H. A., & McDougall, G. J. (2011). Anti-proliferative and potential anti-diabetic effects of phenolic-rich extracts from edible marine algae. *Food Chemistry, 126,* 1006–1012. https://doi.org/10.1016/j.foodchem.2010.11.111.

Odunsi, S. T., Vazquez-Roque, M. I., Camilleri, M., Papathanasopoulos, A., Clark, M. M., Wodrich, L., et al. (2010). Effect of alginate on satiation, appetite, gastric function, and selected gut satiety hormones in overweight and obesity. *Obesity (Silver Spring), 18,* 1579–1584. https://doi.org/10.1038/oby.2009.421.

Okada, T., Mizuno, Y., Sibayama, S., Hosokawa, M., & Miyashita, K. (2011). Antiobesity effects of Undaria lipid capsules prepared with scallop phospholipids. *Journal of Food Science, 76,* H2–H6. https://doi.org/10.1111/j.1750-3841.2010.01878.x.

Oliveira, R. M., Camara, R. B. G., Monte, J. F. S., Viana, R. L. S., Melo, K. R. T., Queiroz, M. F., et al. (2018). Commercial fucoidans from *Fucus vesiculosus* can be grouped into antiadipogenic and adipogenic agents. *Marine Drugs16.* , https://doi.org/10.3390/md16060193. E193 [pii].

Pantidos, N., Boath, A., Lund, V., Conner, S., & McDougall, G. J. (2014). Phenolic-rich extracts from the edible seaweed, *Ascophyllum nodosum*, inhibit alpha-amylase and alpha-glucosidase: Potential anti-hyperglycemic effects. *Journal of Functional Foods, 10,* 201–209. https://doi.org/10.1016/j.jff.2014.06.018.

Paradis, M. E., Couture, P., & Lamarche, B. (2011). A randomised crossover placebo-controlled trial investigating the effect of brown seaweed (*Ascophyllum nodosum* and *Fucus vesiculosus*) on postchallenge plasma glucose and insulin levels in men and women. *Applied Physiology, Nutrition, and Metabolism, 36,* 913–919. https://doi.org/10.1139/h11-115.

Peng, J., Yuan, J. P., Wu, C. F., & Wang, J. H. (2011). Fucoxanthin, a marine carotenoid present in brown seaweeds and diatoms: Metabolism and bioactivities relevant to human health. *Marine Drugs, 9,* 1806–1828. https://doi.org/10.3390/md9101806.

Petersen, M. C., & Shulman, G. I. (2018). Mechanisms of insulin action and insulin resistance. *Physiological Reviews, 98,* 2133–2223. https://doi.org/10.1152/physrev.00063.2017.

Pramanik, S., Rathwa, N., Patel, R., Ramachandran, A. V., & Begum, R. (2018). Treatment avenues for type 2 diabetes and current perspectives on adipokines. *Current Diabetes Reviews, 14,* 201–221. https://doi.org/10.2174/1573399813666170112142837.

Rasouli, N., & Kern, P. A. (2008). Adipocytokines and the metabolic complications of obesity. *The Journal of Clinical Endocrinology and Metabolism, 93,* S64–S73. https://doi.org/10.1210/jc.2008-1613.

Rena, G., Hardie, D. G., & Pearson, E. R. (2017). The mechanisms of action of metformin. *Diabetologia, 60,* 1577–1585. https://doi.org/10.1007/s00125-017-4342-z.

Rico, D., Diana, A., Milton-Laskibar, I., Fernández-Quintela, A., Silván, H., Rai, D., et al. (2018). Characterization and in vitro evaluation of seaweed species as potential functional ingredients to ameliorate metabolic syndrome. *Journal of Functional Foods, 46,* 185–194.

Seo, M. J., Choi, H. S., Lee, O. H., & Lee, B. Y. (2013). Grateloupia lanceolata (Okamura) Kawaguchi, the edible red seaweed, inhibits lipid accumulation and reactive oxygen species production during differentiation in 3T3-L1 cells. *Phytotherapy Research, 27,* 655–663. https://doi.org/10.1002/ptr.4765.

Shan, X., Liu, X., Hao, J., Cai, C., Fan, F., Dun, Y., et al. (2016). In vitro and in vivo hypoglycemic effects of brown algal fucoidans. *International Journal of Biological Macromolecules*, *82*, 249–255. https://doi.org/10.1016/j.ijbiomac.2015.11.036.

Shang, Q., Song, G., Zhang, M., Shi, J., Xu, C., Hao, J., et al. (2017). Dietary fucoidan improves metabolic syndrome in association with increased *Akkermansia* population in the gut microbiota of high-fat diet-fed mice. *Journal of Functional Foods*, *28*, 138–146.

Sharifuddin, Y., Chin, Y. X., Lim, P. E., & Phang, S. M. (2015). Potential bioactive compounds from seaweed for diabetes management. *Marine Drugs*, *21*, 5447–5491. https://doi.org/10.3390/md13085447.

Sharma, B. R., Kim, H. J., Kim, M. S., Park, C. M., & Rhyu, D. Y. (2017). Caulerpa okamurae extract inhibits adipogenesis in 3T3-L1 adipocytes and prevents high-fat diet-induced obesity in C57BL/6 mice. *Nutrition Research*, *47*, 44–52. S0271-5317(17)30531-6 [pii].

Shi, D. Y., Xu, F., He, J., Li, J., Fan, X., & Han, L. (2008). Inhibition of bromophenols against PTP1B and anti-hyperglycemic effect of *Rhodomela confervoides* extract in diabetic rats. *Chinese Science Bulletin*, *53*, 2476–2479.

Shin, D. (2009). The effect of seamustard on blood lipid profiles and glucose level of rats fed diet with different energy composition. *Nutrition Research and Practice*, *3*, 31–37. https://doi.org/10.4162/nrp.2009.3.1.31.

Shin, H. C., Kim, S. H., Park, Y., Lee, B. H., & Hwang, H. J. (2012). Effects of 12-week oral supplementation of Ecklonia cava polyphenols on anthropometric and blood lipid parameters in overweight Korean individuals: A double-blind randomized clinical trial. *Phytotherapy Research*, *26*, 363–368. https://doi.org/10.1002/ptr.3559.

Terpend, K., Bisson, J., Le Gall, C., & Linares, E. (2012). Effects of ID-alG™ on weight management and body fat mass in high-fat-fed rats. *Phytotherapy Research*, *26*, 727–733.

Unnikrishnan, P. S., & Jayasri, M. A. (2018). Marine algae as a prospective source for antidiabetic compounds—A brief review. *Current Diabetes Reviews*, *14*, 237–245. https://doi.org/10.2174/1573399812666161229151407.

Wan-Loy, C., & Siew-Moi, P. (2016). Marine algae as a potential source for anti-obesity agents. *Marine Drugs*, *14*, 222–241. https://doi.org/10.3390/md14120222.

Wanyonyi, S., Du Preez, R., Brown, L., Paul, N., & Panchal, S. (2017). Kappaphycus alvarezii as a food supplement prevents diet-induced metabolic syndrome in rats. *Nutrients*, *9*, 11.

Yan, X., Yang, C., Lin, G., Chen, Y., Miao, S., Liu, B., et al. (2019). Antidiabetic potential of green seaweed *Enteromorpha prolifera* flavonoids regulating insulin signaling pathway and gut microbiota in type 2 diabetic mice. *Journal of Food Science*, *84*, 165–173. https://doi.org/10.1111/1750-3841.14415.

Yang, L., Wang, L., Zhu, C., Wu, J., Yuan, Y., Yu, L., et al. (2017). Laminarin counteracts diet-induced obesity associated with glucagon-like peptide-1 secretion. *Oncotarget*, *8*, 99470–99481. https://doi.org/10.18632/oncotarget.19957.

Yoshinaga, K., Maruya, R., Koikeda, T., & Nakano, T. (2018). Effects of Undaria pinnatifida (wakame) on the human intestinal environment. *Functional Foods in Health & Disease*, *8*, 478–494.

Yun, J. W. (2010). Possible anti-obesity therapeutics from nature—A review. *Phytochemistry*, *71*, 1625–1641. https://doi.org/10.1016/j.phytochem.2010.07.011.

Zaharudin, N., Salmean, A. A., & Dragsted, L. O. (2018). Inhibitory effects of edible seaweeds, polyphenolics and alginates on the activities of porcine pancreatic alpha-amylase. *Food Chemistry*, *245*, 1196–1203. S0308-8146(17)31837-X [pii].

Zaharudin, N., Staerk, D., & Dragsted, L. O. (2019). Inhibition of alpha-glucosidase activity by selected edible seaweeds and fucoxanthin. *Food Chemistry*, *270*, 481–486. S0308-8146(18)31287-1 [pii].

Zhang, J., Tiller, C., Shen, J., Wang, C., Girouard, G. S., Dennis, D., et al. (2007). Antidiabetic properties of polysaccharide- and polyphenolic-enriched fractions from the brown seaweed *Ascophyllum nodosum*. *Canadian Journal of Physiology and Pharmacology*, *85*, 1116–1123. y07-105 [pii].
Zhang, Z., Wang, X., Han, S., Liu, C., & Liu, F. (2018). Effect of two seaweed polysaccharides on intestinal microbiota in mice evaluated by illumina PE250 sequencing. *International Journal of Biological Macromolecules*, *112*, 796–802. S0141-8130(17)33868-0 [pii].
Zhao, C., Yang, C., Chen, M., Lv, X., Liu, B., Yi, L., et al. (2018). Regulatory efficacy of brown seaweed *Lessonia nigrescens* extract on the gene expression profile and intestinal microflora in type 2 diabetic mice. *Molecular Nutrition & Food Research*, *62*. https://doi.org/10.1002/mnfr.201700730.

CHAPTER NINE

Preventive and therapeutic effect of *Ganoderma lucidum* on kidney injuries and diseases

Xiaoqiang Geng[a,b], Dandan Zhong[a,b], Limin Su[a,b], Zhibin Lin[a,b], Baoxue Yang[a,b,*]

[a]State Key Laboratory of Natural and Biomimetic Drugs, Department of Pharmacology, School of Basic Medical Sciences, Peking University, Beijing, China
[b]Key Laboratory of Molecular Cardiovascular Sciences, Ministry of Education, Beijing, China
[*]Corresponding author: e-mail address: baoxue@bjmu.edu.cn

Contents

Abstract

Ganoderma lucidum (*G. lucidum*, Lingzhi) is a well-known Chinese traditional medicine to improve health and to treat numerous diseases for over 2000 years in Asian countries. *G. lucidum* has the abundant chemical components such as triterpenes and polysaccharides, which have various biological activities including anti-oxidation, anti-inflammation, anti-liver disorders, anti-tumor growth and metastasis, *etc.* Recently, many lines of studies have elucidated the therapeutic effects of *G. lucidum* and its extractions on various acute kidney injury (AKI) and chronic kidney disease (CKD) pathogenesis, including autosomal dominant polycystic kidney disease, diabetic nephropathy, renal

Advances in Pharmacology, Volume 87
ISSN 1054-3589
https://doi.org/10.1016/bs.apha.2019.10.003

proximal tubular cell oxidative damage and fibrotic process, renal ischemia reperfusion injury, cisplatin-induced renal injury, adriamycin-induced nephropathy, chronic proteinuric renal diseases, *etc.* Clinical researches also showed potent anti-renal disease bioactivities of *G. lucidum*. In this chapter, we review experimental and clinical researches and provide comprehensive insights into the renoprotective effects of *G. lucidum*. In recent years, renal diseases have gradually aroused attention on account of their booming prevalence worldwide and lack of effective therapies. Although the complicated pathogenesis of kidney diseases, such as acute kidney injury (AKI) and chronic kidney diseases (CKD) have been intensively studied. The morbidity and mortality of AKI and CKD still rise continuously. Thanks to the conventional experience and the multi-target characteristics, natural products have been increasingly recognized as an alternative source for treating renal diseases.

Abbreviations

AD	Alzheimer's disease
ADPKD	autosomal dominant polycystic kidney disease
AKI	acute kidney injury
ALD	alcoholic liver disease
CAT	catalase
CKD	chronic kidney disease
CNS	central nervous system
CTL	cytotoxic T lymphocyte
CTLA-4	cytotoxic T lymphocyte antigen-4
DCs	dendritic cells
DM	diabetes mellitus
DN	diabetic nephropathy
FSGS	focal segmental glomerulosclerosis
FSK	forsklin
G	*Ganoderma*
GA	ganoderic acid
GLA	*Ganoderma lucidum* aqueos extract
GL-B	*Ganoderma lucidum* polysaccharides B
GLD	*Ganoderma lucidum* decoction
GLPP	*Ganoderma lucidum* polysaccharide peptide
GSH	glutathione
GSH-Px	glutathione peroxidase
GT	*Ganoderma* triterpenoid
GWA	*Ganoderma* hydroethanolic extract
HCC	hepatocellular carcinoma
HSCs	hepatic stellate cells.
IFN-γ	interferon-γ
IL-1β	interleukin-1β
IL-6	interleukin-6
MAPK	mitogen-activated protein kinase
MDA	malondialdehyde

MPO	myeloperoxidase
NAFLD	non-alcoholic fatty liver disease
Nrf2	nuclear factor erythroid 2-related factor 2
PD	Parkinson's disease
PD-1	programmed cell death protein-1
RIRI	renal ischemia reperfusion injury
ROS	reactive oxygen species
SOD	superoxide dismutase
STZ	streptozocin
T1DM	type 1 diabetes mellitus
TGF-β	transforming growth factor-β
TNF-α	tumor necrosis factor-α

1. Introduction

Ganoderma lucidum (*G. lucidum*) is a well-known Chinese traditional medicine to improve health and to treat numerous diseases for over 2000 years in Asian countries. In early Chinese history, *Shen Nong Ben Cao Jing* (*Shennong Materia Medica*) written in CA. 100 BC and other books documented the researches and scientific aspects of *Ganoderma* (Lingzhi) in respect to its categorization, habitat, bionomics, herbal nature, medication, *etc.* As is well known, *G. lucidum* has been historically viewed as a magic herb by Chinese.

Up to now, several hundreds of compounds such as triterpenes, meroterpenoids, nucleosides, alkaloids, and polysaccharides have been isolated and identified from the genus of *G. lucidum* (Niu, Li, Xiao, Sun, & Che, 2007; Qiu, Wang, & Song, 2016). Based the abundant components identified and isolated from *G. lucidum*, numerous pharmacological studies have been carried out for a long time. In the contemporary era, *G. lucidum* has been well studied for its various biological activities including anti-oxidation, anti-inflammation (Zhang et al., 2018), anti-liver disorders (Zhong et al., 2018), anti-tumor growth and metastasis (Chen et al., 2017; Lin & Zhang, 2004) *etc.*

Recently, many lines of studies have elucidated the therapeutic effects of *G. lucidum* and its extractions on various acute kidney injury (AKI) and chronic kidney disease (CKD) pathogenesis, including autosomal dominant polycystic kidney disease (Su et al., 2017), diabetic nephropathy (He, Li, Guo, Lin, & Lin, 2006; Pan et al., 2014), renal proximal tubular cell oxidative damage and fibrotic process (Dou et al., 2014; Yan et al., 2013), renal ischemia reperfusion injury (Zhong et al., 2015), cisplatin-induced renal injury (Pillai, John, & Sara Thomas, 2011), adriamycin-induced nephropathy (Yan et al., 2015), chronic proteinuric renal diseases (Lai, Chan, Tang, & Leung, 2006), *etc.* Clinical researches also showed potent anti-renal disease bioactivities of *G. lucidum* (Futrakul et al., 2004; Xiao, Liu, & Chen, 2003). This chapter mainly reviews the preventive and therapeutic effect of *G. lucidum* on kidney injuries and diseases based on experimental and clinical researches.

2. Effect of *Ganoderma* triterpenoid on autosomal dominant polycystic kidney disease

Autosomal dominant polycystic kidney disease (ADPKD) is a common monogenetic disease with a pretty high prevalence of 1/1000 to 1/400 worldwide (Harris & Torres, 2009). Progressively developed kidney cysts are the main pathological features and these enlarged cysts subsequently destruct and replace the normal kidney parenchyma leading to renal dysfunction. Nevertheless, there are very limited drugs effectively used in preventing or reversing ADPKD progression except hemodialysis or kidney transplantation (Ong, Devuyst, Knebelmann, Walz, & Diseases, 2015). On account of the common pathological physiology characters of ADPKD with solid tumors, many studies indicated that some anti-cancer drugs also possess therapeutic benefit for ADPKD treatment. For instance, it is proved that curcumin and ginkgolide B both have anti-ADPKD activities *via* inhibiting related intracellular signaling pathways (Gao et al., 2011; Zhou et al., 2012). Considering the potential anti-tumor effect of *Ganoderma* triterpenoids (GT), our group studied the effect of GT on the ADPKD using MDCK cyst model, MDCK tubulogenesis model, embryonic kidney cyst model and two ADPKD mouse models (Su et al., 2017).

Firstly, *in vitro* study showed that consecutive 7-day treatment of GT significantly inhibited FSK-stimulated MDCK cyst enlargement in a dose-dependent manner (6.25, 25, and 100 μg/mL). After washing out GT on day 8, MDCK cysts regrew to a large size. These data suggested the inhibitory effect of GT on MDCK cyst enlargement. In an embryonic kidney cyst model, 100 μM 8-bromoadenosine 3′, 5′-cyclic monophosphate (8-Br-cAMP) was used to stimulate cysts to develop rapidly in cultured embryonic kidneys. Results showed that GT significantly inhibited renal cyst development in a dose-dependent manner (6.25, 25, and 100 μg/mL) and washing out GT on day 4 led to the reformation and enlargement again of renal cysts, indicating the reversible inhibition of renal cysts by GT. In the subsequent researches, the inhibitory activity of GT on renal cysts was studied using PKD mouse models. In accordance with the results *in vitro*, in ADPKD mice, 100 mg/kg per day treatment from postnatal day 1 until day 4 significantly reduced the size of the cysts, kidney mass, fractional cyst area and kidney index without affecting other physiological index.

The studies on underlying mechanisms of GT inhibiting renal cyst development showed that GT inhibited cyst development mainly through downregulating intracellular Ras/MAPK signaling pathway *via* reducing H-ras, B-raf, p-MEK, p-ERK, Egr-1, and c-fos levels and increasing Raf-1 expression in the FSK-stimulated MDCK cell model. In the ADPKD mouse models, GT was detected to significantly downregulated the Ras/MAPK signaling pathway by reducing B-raf, p-ERK, and c-fos in ADPKD kidneys without detectable other effect on normal kidneys. Moreover, in cultured MDCK cells, 25 and 100 μg/mL GT significantly decreased cAMP levels in 10 mM FSK-treated MDCK cells.

The further study showed that GT monomer CBLZ-7 (ethyl ganoderate C2) obviously inhibited cyst enlargement and had no effect on the total numbers of colonies. Consisting with the previous results, CBLZ-7 downregulated the Ras/MAPK signaling pathway in FSK-stimulated MDCK cells in a dose-dependent manner. In conclusion, GT have potent potential to be developed as novel therapeutic agents for treating ADPKD (Fig. 1).

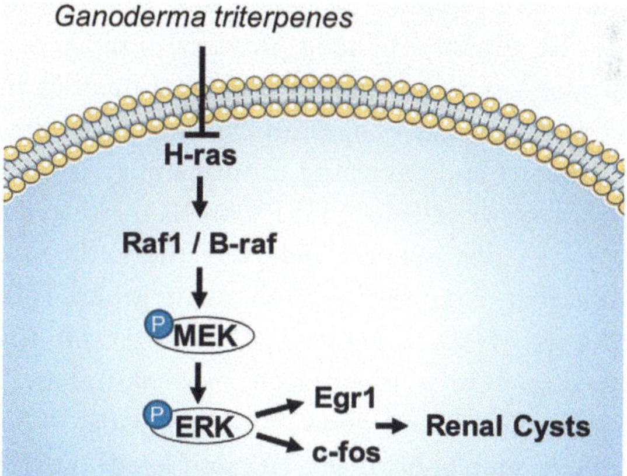

Fig. 1 Schematic diagram of the intracellular signal pathway involved in GT retarding renal cyst development in ADPKD.

3. Effect of *Ganoderma lucidum* polysaccharide peptides on renal ischemia reperfusion injury

Acute kidney injury (AKI) is a complex syndrome defined as a kidney disease with rapid loss of renal function with high morbidity and mortality. According to numerous epidemiological surveys, AKI occurs in approximately 20% of hospitalized patients especially after surgery. Specially, some AKI patients require kidney replacement therapy and have high mortality rate and increased risk of subsequent chronic kidney disease. Renal ischemia reperfusion injury (RIRI) as one type of AKI, is a common surgical complication leading to pretty high mortality, CKD and end-stage renal disease (He et al., 2017). Mechanically, both ischemia and reperfusion lead to cell injury and even death. However, there are limited effective therapies available.

G. lucidum polysaccharide peptides (GLPPs) are isolated from boiling water extract of the fruiting body of *G. lucidum*. Previous studies suggest that GLPP may exhibit protective effect in the pathophysiological mechanisms of RIRI. In 2015, it was comprehensively proved that GLPP had renoprotective activity in preventing renal ischemia reperfusion injury using *in vitro* and *in vivo* models (Zhong et al., 2015). It was identified that intraperitoneal administration of GLPP (100 mg/kg) daily for 7 days before ischemia and reperfusion significantly improved destroyed kidney function and attenuated proximal tubular damage structurally compared with vehicle control. Functionally, IR obviously increased levels of BUN and blood creatinine were significantly decreased by treatment of GLPP. Morphologically, IR directly induced proximal tubular damage including tubular brush border loss and dilatation and outer medulla injury including intertubular hemorrhage and congestion. GLPP pretreatment attenuated these structure damages and decreased tubular injury score.

To further evaluate the effect of GLPP on IR-mediated oxidative stress in the kidney. We subsequently detected the oxidative stress-related markers and found that, compared with the sham group, RIRI significantly increased the levels of myeloperoxidase (MPO) and malondialdehyde (MDA) and decreased the activities of superoxide dismutase (SOD), catalase (CAT), glutathione (GSH) and glutathione peroxidase (GSH-Px). GLPP significantly reduced such abnormally elevated levels of MPO, MDA, and increased the levels of SOD, CAT, GSH and GSH-Px in kidneys. Additionally, GLPP also inhibited the translocation of p47phox from cytosol to membrane, indicating that the renoprotective effect of GLPP could be partially attributed to alleviating the NADPH oxidase-dependent production of ROS.

All these results indicate that GLPP exerts mediating effect on renal oxidative stress and lipid peroxidation after IR. We further uncover the underlying mechanisms by detecting the apoptosis-related signaling pathways. TUNEL assay and Western blot analysis confirmed that IR obviously caused renal cell apoptosis and GLPP reduced IR-induced TUNEL-positive cells by 21.75% and the ratio of p-p53/p53 and cleaved caspase-3/caspase-3, indicating that GLPP could protect kidneys by inhibiting IR-induced apoptosis.

We measured the mitochondrial-related apoptosis level and found that GLPP significantly reduced the ratio of Bax/Bcl-2 caused by IR and inhibited the release of cytochrome C from mitochondria to the cytosol, suggesting that GLPP could inhibit the mitochondria-dependent apoptosis induced by IR. On the other hand, accumulated ROS also induced ER stress in IR model. We detected the level of ER stress-related proteins (GRP78, CHOP and caspase-12) and identified that GLPP reduced the increased expression of them and inhibited the activation of JNK, indicating that GLPP inhibit IR-induced apoptosis partially by alleviating ER stress.

Subsequently, hypoxia/reoxygenation (H/R) *in vitro* study was adopted to assess the cytotoxicity of GLPP and to confirm the GLPP renoprotective mechanisms. Results showed that at concentrations from 1.1 to 810 μg/mL, GLPP had no obvious cytotoxicity on NRK-52E cells, and improved cell viability that was decreased after hypoxia for 12 h followed by reoxygenation for 1 h. Consistent with the *in vivo* results, GLPP had the effect in anti-cellular oxidative stress induced by H/R mainly through inhibiting the activation of NADPH oxidase and increasing antioxidant activity and finally reducing the accumulation of ROS in a dose-dependent manner. Moreover, pretreatment with GLPP reversed the up-regulated ratios of p-p53/p53 and cleaved capsase-3/caspase-3, which was confirmed by TUNEL analysis. All these results proved the protective effect of GLPP in inhibiting H/R-induced apoptosis in renal tubular cells.

Further study of the protective mechanism of GLPP in H/R-induced NRK-52E cells was carried out by fluorescent, lipophilic and JC-1 (cationic probe) staining. It was proved that GLPP significantly diminished H/R-induced mitochondrial dysfunction on account of the attenuated $\Delta\Psi$m dissipation, decreased Bax and increased Bcl-2, and reduced cytochrome C in cytosol. In accordance with *in vivo* study, GLPP reversed increased expression of

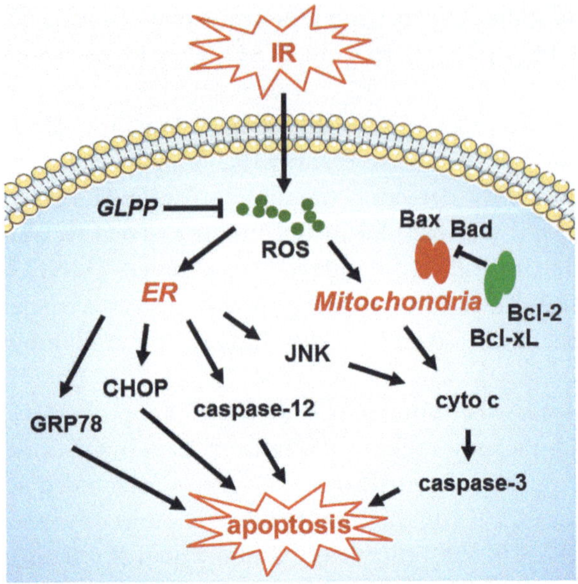

Fig. 2 Schematic diagram of the intracellular signal pathways involved in IR-induced apoptosis.

GRP78, caspase-12 and CHOP induced by H/R. Tunicamycin (TM) stimulation was adopted to create a special ER stress model and GLPP was verified to relieve ER stress-induced apoptosis partially through the JNK signaling pathway.

All these results suggest GLPP significantly rescued renal dysfunction and morphological damage in RIRI, and reversed the imbalance of redox status and reduced ROS level. Further study demonstrated that GLPP dramatically inhibited mitochondrial- and ER stress-dependent apoptosis, which identified the beneficial effects of GLPP on IR caused AKI for the first time (Fig. 2).

4. Effect of *G. lucidum* on cisplatin-induced nephrotoxicity

As the classic anti-cancer chemotherapy, cisplatin is a widely used antineoplastic agent in the treatment of many types of tumor such as bladder cancer, lung cancer, sarcomas, bone cancer, and lymphomas (Dasari & Tchounwou, 2014). However, severe side effects of cisplatin chemotherapy such as nephrotoxicity characterized as tubular dysfunction have commonly limited the effective use of this drug (Fig. 3).

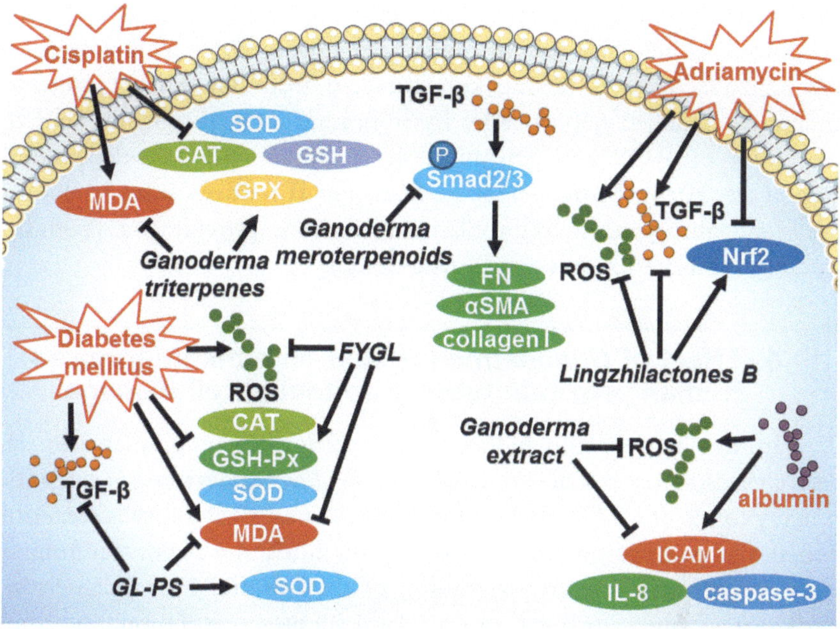

Fig. 3 Schematic diagram of the intracellular signal pathways involved in *G. lucidum* and its extractions treating cisplatin-induced nephrotoxicity, diabetic nephropathy, adriamycin-induced nephropathy, albumin-induced human proximal tubular epithelial cell damage, and fibrotic process of renal proximal tubular cells.

In 2011, Pillai et al. identified the renoprotective activity of total terpenes isolated from *G. lucidum* using cisplatin-induced nephrotoxicity mouse model. They found that treatment with *G. lucidum* terpenes (50 and 100 mg/kg) ameliorated tubular injury and significant rescued antioxidant activity by elevating GSH, SOD, CAT and GPX and by decreasing MDA that were disturbed by a single dose of cisplatin (Pillai et al., 2011). The experimental results indicate that *G. lucidum* terpenes could exert antioxidant activity and possess the renal-protection effect in cisplatin-induced nephrotoxicity and potential use in adjuvant therapy of cancer.

5. Effect of *Ganoderma lucidum* on adriamycin-induced nephropathy

As another widely acknowledged CKD mouse model, Adriamycin-induced nephropathy is characterized by initial podocyte injury and albumin urine and subsequent renal inflammation and fibrosis. In the CKD model, oxidative stress including excess ROS generation is considered associated with renal injury, and the nuclear factor erythroid 2-related factor 2 (Nrf2) is recognized as the major role in cellular defense. In 2015, Yan et al. found that lingzhilactones B (25 mg/kg) extracted from *G. lucidum* protected adriamycin-induced nephropathy by inhibiting TGF-β signaling and the generation of ROS and activating the Nrf2 *in vivo* dose-dependently (Yan et al., 2015). Moreover, lingzhilactones B reduced urinary albumin levels and abrogated myofibroblastic activation, providing a promising structure template for anti-CKD drug design.

6. Effect of *Ganoderma lucidum* on albumin-induced human proximal tubular epithelial cell damage

In the anti-chronic kidney disease drug screening, many *in vitro* researches also proposed the potential of *G. lucidum* besides those *in vivo* study. In many forms of CKD, the severity of tubulointerstitial injury is correlated with the amount of proteinuria. Such proteinuria is a major determinant of the degree and rate of progression of diseases and induces interstitial injury that is mainly attributable to concomitant presence of tubulointerstitial inflammation. In 2006, Lai et al. reported the effect of *G. lucidum* polysaccharide in anti-albumin-induced human proximal tubular epithelial cell oxidative damage and apoptosis and release of chemokines *in vitro* (Lai et al., 2006). Results showed that *G. lucidum* polysaccharide obviously inhibited the tubulointerstitial inflammation and tubular injury, suggesting that *G. lucidum* polysaccharide can be developed into a novel anti-inflammation drug targeting further downstream of proteinuria pathological processes.

7. Effect of *Ganoderma lucidum* on diabetic nephropathy

Diabetes mellitus (DM) is the most common endocrine disorder. According to the International Diabetes Federation, the prevalence of DM was almost 8.8% in 2017 and approximately 629 million people will have DM worldwide by 2045 (Jia et al., 2018). Among the complications of DM, diabetic nephropathy (DN) is the major type that is the leading cause of end-stage renal failure. DN is also the major cause of morbidity on account of the deterioration of renal function and glomerular structure (Rossing, 2006). It is valuable to develop anti-diabetic drugs with renal-protection potential. Recently, *G. lucidum* and its extractions have been studied and increasingly recognized as an alternative source for inhibiting DN.

In 2006, He et al. identified that *G. lucidum* polysaccharides (GL-PS) could prevent or delay the progression of diabetic renal complications using streptozotocin-induced type 1 diabetic mouse model (He et al., 2006). They found that GL-PS mainly decreased blood glucose and triglyceride levels in diabetic mice, suggesting the metabolic modulation of GL-PS. GL-PS decreased the level of MDA and increased the level of SOD, effectively improved the metabolic imbalance in DN. Further, GL-PS dose-dependently reduced the TGF-β expression that played a crucial role and was abnormally elevated in the development of pathologic lesions of diabetic nephropathy.

In 2014, Pan et al. investigated the effects of a novel proteoglycan (FYGL) isolated from *G. lucidum* in protecting renal function and morphology in diabetic mice (Pan et al., 2014). Their study reported that FYGL dose-dependently decreased the blood glucose and slowed the age-dependent insulin decline. 8-week administration of FYGL ameliorated the DN by three possible pathways: (1) FYGL protected oxidative stress of renal cell by directly eliminating ROS and suppressing lipid peroxidation. (2) FYGL improved oxidative injury in kidney tissues by indirectly scavenging the radicals *via* activating antioxidant enzyme systems. (3) FYGL chelated with metal ion by forming cross-bridge between carboxyl groups in galacturonic acid, decreasing ROS generation. In db/db mice, FYGL significantly rescued the reduced blood LDL-c levels and the increased HDL-c levels caused by profound alterations in lipid and lipoprotein profiles. All these results indicate that FYGL possess the anti-diabetic nephropathy advantages and can be developed novel anti-DN drugs.

8. Effect of *Ganoderma lucidum* on fibrotic process of renal proximal tubular cells

Renal fibrosis is the common pathogenesis in the progression of CKD and ESRD, The prevalence of CKD in the general population even reaches to 13% in some countries, increasingly becoming a public health problem worldwide (De Nicola & Minutolo, 2016). However, there are limited approaches to attenuate or reverse renal fibrogenesis.

In 2013, Yan et al. found that phosphorylation of Smad-3 of rat renal proximal tubular cells (NRK-52E) under the stimulation of TGF-β1 was significantly inhibited by (−)-Lingzhiol, which was isolated from *G. lucidum,* indicating the selective inhibition effect on p-Smad-3. Moreover, both (+)-Lingzhiol and (−)-Lingzhiol isolated from *G. lucidum* could significantly inhibit high-glucose-induced generation of ROS, collagen IV, fibronectin, and IL-6 and induce the transcription of Nrf2 to protect cells from oxidative damage (Yan et al., 2013). Considering the predominant role of TGF-β/Smads pathway in CKD and renal fibrosis, (−)-Lingzhiol can be developed into selective p-Smad-3 inhibitor in hindering renal fibrosis and treating chronic kidney disease.

In 2014, Dou et al. reported two meroterpenoids from *Ganoderma cochlear* with novel polycyclic skeletons and identified their renoprotective bioactivity using TGF-β1-stimulated NRK52E cells (Dou et al., 2014). Their results indicated that both racemic (+)- and (−)-cochlearols exerted renoprotection by inhibiting the expression of renal fibrosis related markers including collagen I, fibronectin, and α-SMA in a dose-dependent manner. Further study showed that these 2 compounds inhibited the phosphorylated Smad2 and Smad3, suggesting their anti-fibrotic action depended on the inhibition of TGF-β/Smads pathway. (−)-cochlearols B displayed more apparent inhibitory effect on TGF-β1 induced activation of p-Smad2 and p-Smad3 compared with cochlearols A and (+)-cochlearols B. The current results provide potential role of (−)-cochlearols B in the therapy of renal fibrosis.

9. Clinical research

Clinical researches and reports on the usefulness of *G. lucidum* in treating renal diseases are pretty limited and incomprehensive. In 2003, Xiao et al. reported their clinical observation on the effect of *G. lucidum* decoction (GLD) in treating Russula subnigricans poisoning (RSP) patients (Xiao et al., 2003). 14 patients of RSP were treated with GLD (100 g of *G. lucidum* decocted with water to 600 mL), they found that RSP induced kidney injury and GLD markedly lowered urine *N*-acetyl-D-glucosaminidase, red blood cell and protein. By comparing with 11 patients received conventional therapy, GLD exerted significant renoprotective efficacy. In 2004, Futrakul et al. conducted a clinical study in 14 nephrotic patients with focal segmental glomerulosclerosis (FSGS) (Futrakul et al., 2004). They found that treatment with *G. lucidum* successfully ameliorated injured kidney *via* inhibiting endothelial cell cytotoxicity, restoring immunocirculatory balance and suppressing proteinuria. All these researches reveal the promising prospects of the clinical value of *G. lucidum*. Further clinical researches are recommended in the future.

10. Conclusion

Until now, there have been sufficient researches and overwhelming evidences prove that *G. lucidum* contains a wide variety of bioactive components that have potent pharmacological effects. In this chapter, we mainly summarized experimental researches and clinical observations and showed abundant evidences that triterpenoids and polysaccharides isolated from *G. lucidum* possess potent activities on anti- both CKD and AKI with extreme activity and minimal toxicity (Table 1). Based on these researches, we certainly conclude that the components of *G. lucidum* exhibite renoprotective effects mainly through antioxidant, anti-apoptosis, anti-proliferation and anti-TGF-β/Smad signaling pathways.

However, the researches were mostly performed in animals or using cell models, well-designed and more reliable clinical researches are welcomed to assess and clarify the authentic biological activities of *G. lucidum* in human. Since the approaches to attenuate or reverse kidney diseases are limited, further investigations of *G. lucidum* would facilitate the development of new therapeutic strategies in treating various kidney diseases.

Table 1 Summary of the active ingredient and action mechanism of *Ganoderma lucidum*.

Active ingredient	Type of extraction	Disease	Action mechanism
Ganoderma triterpenoid	not provided	Autosomal dominant polycystic kidney disease	Downregulating Ras/MAPK signaling and promoting cell differentiation
Ganoderma lucidum polysaccharide peptides	Hydroalcoholic extraction	Renal ischemia reperfusion injury	Reducing oxidative stress, alleviating the mitochondrial and ER stress-dependent apoptosis caused by excessive ROS
Ganoderma lucidum terpenes	Chloroform extraction	Cisplatin-induced nephrotoxicity	Reducing oxidative stress
lingzhilactones B	EtOH extraction	Adriamycin-induced nephropathy	Inhibiting TGF-β signaling and the generation of ROS, activating the Nrf2

Continued

Table 1 Summary of the active ingredient and action mechanism of *Ganoderma lucidum*.—cont'd

Active ingredient	Type of extraction	Disease	Action mechanism
Ganoderma lucidum polysaccharide	Hydroalcoholic extraction	Albumin-induced human proximal tubular epithelial cell damage	Reducing oxidative damage and apoptosis
Ganoderma lucidum polysaccharides	Aqueous extraction	Diabetic nephropathy	Decreasing blood glucose and triglyceride levels, decreasing the level of MDA and increasing the level of SOD, reducing the TGF-β expression
Ganoderma lucidum proteoglycan (FYGL)	Hydroalcoholic extraction	Diabetic nephropathy	Decreasing blood glucose, reducing oxidative stress, decreasing ROS generation
Lingzhiol	EtOH extraction	Fibrotic process of renal proximal tubular cells	Inhibiting the generation of ROS, collagen IV, fibronectin, and IL-6 and inducing the transcription of Nrf2
Ganoderma cochlear meroterpenoids	Hydroalcoholic extraction	Fibrotic process of renal proximal tubular cells	Inhibiting collagen I, fibronectin, and α-SMA

Acknowledgment

Research in the author's laboratory is supported by National Natural Science Foundation of China Grants 81620108029, 81330074, 81261160507 and 81170632, Beijing Natural Science Foundation grant 7172113, Drug Discovery Program grant 2009ZX09301-010-30, the Research Fund for the Doctoral Program of Higher Education 20100001110047, the 111 project, International Science & Technology Cooperation Program of China 2012DFA11070.

Conflict of interest

The authors have no conflicts of interest to declare.

References

Chen, S., Yong, T., Zhang, Y., Su, J., Jiao, C., & Xie, Y. (2017). Anti-tumor and anti-angiogenic ergosterols from Ganoderma lucidum. *Frontiers in Chemistry*, *5*, 85. https://doi.org/10.3389/fchem.2017.00085.

Dasari, S., & Tchounwou, P. B. (2014). Cisplatin in cancer therapy: Molecular mechanisms of action. *European Journal of Pharmacology*, *740*, 364–378. https://doi.org/10.1016/j.ejphar.2014.07.025.

De Nicola, L., & Minutolo, R. (2016). Worldwide growing epidemic of CKD: Fact or fiction? *Kidney International*, *90*(3), 482–484. https://doi.org/10.1016/j.kint.2016.05.001.

Dou, M., Di, L., Zhou, L. L., Yan, Y. M., Wang, X. L., Zhou, F. J., et al. (2014). Cochlearols A and B, polycyclic meroterpenoids from the fungus Ganoderma cochlear that have renoprotective activities. *Organic Letters*, *16*(23), 6064–6067. https://doi.org/10.1021/ol502806j.

Futrakul, N., Panichakul, T., Butthep, P., Futrakul, P., Jetanalin, P., Patumraj, S., et al. (2004). Ganoderma lucidum suppresses endothelial cell cytotoxicity and proteinuria in persistent proteinuric focal segmental glomerulosclerosis (FSGS) nephrosis. *Clinical Hemorheology and Microcirculation*, *31*(4), 267–272.

Gao, J., Zhou, H., Lei, T., Zhou, L., Li, W., Li, X., et al. (2011). Curcumin inhibits renal cyst formation and enlargement in vitro by regulating intracellular signaling pathways. *European Journal of Pharmacology*, *654*(1), 92–99. https://doi.org/10.1016/j.ejphar.2010.12.008.

Harris, P. C., & Torres, V. E. (2009). Polycystic kidney disease. *Annual Review of Medicine*, *60*, 321–337. https://doi.org/10.1146/annurev.med.60.101707.125712.

He, C. Y., Li, W. D., Guo, S. X., Lin, S. Q., & Lin, Z. B. (2006). Effect of polysaccharides from Ganoderma lucidum on streptozotocin-induced diabetic nephropathy in mice. *Journal of Asian Natural Products Research*, *8*(8), 705–711. https://doi.org/10.1080/10286020500289071.

He, L., Wei, Q., Liu, J., Yi, M., Liu, Y., Liu, H., et al. (2017). AKI on CKD: Heightened injury, suppressed repair, and the underlying mechanisms. *Kidney International*, *92*(5), 1071–1083. https://doi.org/10.1016/j.kint.2017.06.030.

Jia, Y., He, J., Wang, L., Su, L., Lei, L., Huang, W., et al. (2018). Dapagliflozin aggravates renal injury via promoting gluconeogenesis in db/db mice. *Cellular Physiology and Biochemistry*, *45*(5), 1747–1758. https://doi.org/10.1159/000487783.

Lai, K. N., Chan, L. Y., Tang, S. C., & Leung, J. C. (2006). Ganoderma extract prevents albumin-induced oxidative damage and chemokines synthesis in cultured human proximal tubular epithelial cells. *Nephrology, Dialysis, Transplantation*, *21*(5), 1188–1197. https://doi.org/10.1093/ndt/gfk085.

Lin, Z. B., & Zhang, H. N. (2004). Anti-tumor and immunoregulatory activities of Ganoderma lucidum and its possible mechanisms. *Acta Pharmacologica Sinica*, *25*(11), 1387–1395.

Niu, X. M., Li, S. H., Xiao, W. L., Sun, H. D., & Che, C. T. (2007). Two new lanostanoids from Ganoderma resinaceum. *Journal of Asian Natural Products Research*, *9*(6–8), 659–664. https://doi.org/10.1080/10286020600979910.

Ong, A. C., Devuyst, O., Knebelmann, B., Walz, G., & Diseases, E.-E. W. G. f. I. K. (2015). Autosomal dominant polycystic kidney disease: The changing face of clinical management. *Lancet*, *385*(9981), 1993–2002. https://doi.org/10.1016/S0140-6736(15)60907-2.

Pan, D., Zhang, D., Wu, J., Chen, C., Xu, Z., Yang, H., et al. (2014). A novel proteoglycan from Ganoderma lucidum fruiting bodies protects kidney function and ameliorates diabetic nephropathy via its antioxidant activity in C57BL/6 db/db mice. *Food and Chemical Toxicology*, *63*, 111–118. https://doi.org/10.1016/j.fct.2013.10.046.

Pillai, T. G., John, M., & Sara Thomas, G. (2011). Prevention of cisplatin induced nephrotoxicity by terpenes isolated from Ganoderma lucidum occurring in Southern Parts of India. *Experimental and Toxicologic Pathology*, *63*(1–2), 157–160. https://doi.org/10.1016/j.etp.2009.11.003.

Qiu, J., Wang, X., & Song, C. (2016). Neuroprotective and antioxidant lanostanoid triterpenes from the fruiting bodies of Ganoderma atrum. *Fitoterapia*, *109*, 75–79. https://doi.org/10.1016/j.fitote.2015.12.008.

Rossing, P. (2006). Diabetic nephropathy: Worldwide epidemic and effects of current treatment on natural history. *Current Diabetes Reports*, *6*(6), 479–483.

Su, L., Liu, L., Jia, Y., Lei, L., Liu, J., Zhu, S., et al. (2017). Ganoderma triterpenes retard renal cyst development by downregulating Ras/MAPK signaling and promoting cell differentiation. *Kidney International*, *92*(6), 1404–1418. https://doi.org/10.1016/j.kint.2017.04.013.

Xiao, G. L., Liu, F. Y., & Chen, Z. H. (2003). Clinical observation on treatment of Russula subnigricans poisoning patients by Ganoderma lucidum decoction. *Zhongguo Zhong Xi Yi Jie He Za Zhi*, *23*(4), 278–280.

Yan, Y. M., Ai, J., Zhou, L. L., Chung, A. C., Li, R., Nie, J., et al. (2013). Lingzhiols, unprecedented rotary door-shaped meroterpenoids as potent and selective inhibitors of p-Smad3 from Ganoderma lucidum. *Organic Letters*, *15*(21), 5488–5491. https://doi.org/10.1021/ol4026364.

Yan, Y. M., Wang, X. L., Zhou, L. L., Zhou, F. J., Li, R., Tian, Y., et al. (2015). Lingzhilactones from Ganoderma lingzhi ameliorate adriamycin-induced nephropathy in mice. *Journal of Ethnopharmacology*, *176*, 385–393. https://doi.org/10.1016/j.jep.2015.11.024.

Zhang, K., Liu, Y., Zhao, X., Tang, Q., Dernedde, J., Zhang, J., et al. (2018). Anti-inflammatory properties of GLPss58, a sulfated polysaccharide from Ganoderma lucidum. *International Journal of Biological Macromolecules*, *107*(Pt. A), 486–493. https://doi.org/10.1016/j.ijbiomac.2017.09.015.

Zhong, D., Wang, H., Liu, M., Li, X., Huang, M., Zhou, H., et al. (2015). Ganoderma lucidum polysaccharide peptide prevents renal ischemia reperfusion injury via counteracting oxidative stress. *Scientific Reports*, *5*, 16910. https://doi.org/10.1038/srep16910.

Zhong, D., Xie, Z., Huang, B., Zhu, S., Wang, G., Zhou, H., et al. (2018). Ganoderma lucidum polysaccharide peptide alleviates hepatoteatosis via modulating bile acid metabolism dependent on FXR-SHP/FGF. *Cellular Physiology and Biochemistry*, *49*(3), 1163–1179. https://doi.org/10.1159/000493297.

Zhou, H., Gao, J., Zhou, L., Li, X., Li, W., Li, X., et al. (2012). Ginkgolide B inhibits renal cyst development in in vitro and in vivo cyst models. *American Journal of Physiology. Renal Physiology*, *302*(10), F1234–F1242. https://doi.org/10.1152/ajprenal.00356.2011.

Further reading

Bach, E. E., Hi, E. M. B., Martins, A. M. C., Nascimento, P. A. M., & Wadt, N. S. Y. (2018). Hypoglicemic and hypolipedimic effects of Ganoderma lucidum in streptozotocin-induced diabetic rats. *Medicines*, *5*(3). https://doi.org/10.3390/medicines5030078.

Berger, A., Rein, D., Kratky, E., Monnard, I., Hajjaj, H., Meirim, I., et al. (2004). Cholesterol-lowering properties of Ganoderma lucidum in vitro, ex vivo, and in hamsters and minipigs. *Lipids in Health and Disease*, *3*, 2. https://doi.org/10.1186/1476-511X-3-2.

Cai, Q., Li, Y., & Pei, G. (2017). Polysaccharides from Ganoderma lucidum attenuate microglia-mediated neuroinflammation and modulate microglial phagocytosis and behavioural response. *Journal of Neuroinflammation*, *14*(1), 63. https://doi.org/10.1186/s12974-017-0839-0.

Cao, L. Z., & Lin, Z. B. (2002). Regulation on maturation and function of dendritic cells by Ganoderma lucidum polysaccharides. *Immunology Letters*, *83*(3), 163–169.

Cao, L. Z., & Lin, Z. B. (2003). Regulatory effect of Ganoderma lucidum polysaccharides on cytotoxic T-lymphocytes induced by dendritic cells in vitro. *Acta Pharmacologica Sinica*, *24*(4), 321–326.

Chu, Q. P., Wang, L. E., Cui, X. Y., Fu, H. Z., Lin, Z. B., Lin, S. Q., et al. (2007). Extract of Ganoderma lucidum potentiates pentobarbital-induced sleep via a GABAergic mechanism. *Pharmacology, Biochemistry, and Behavior*, *86*(4), 693–698. https://doi.org/10.1016/j.pbb.2007.02.015.

Chung, D. J., Yang, M. Y., Li, Y. R., Chen, W. J., Hung, C. Y., & Wang, C. J. (2017). Ganoderma lucidum repress injury of ethanol-induced steatohepatitis via anti-inflammation, anti-oxidation and reducing hepatic lipid in C57BL/6J mice. *Journal of Functional Foods*, *33*, 314–322. https://doi.org/10.1016/j.jff.2017.03.059.

Cui, X. Y., Cui, S. Y., Zhang, J., Wang, Z. J., Yu, B., Sheng, Z. F., et al. (2012). Extract of Ganoderma lucidum prolongs sleep time in rats. *Journal of Ethnopharmacology*, *139*(3), 796–800. https://doi.org/10.1016/j.jep.2011.12.020.

El Zawawy, N. A., & Ali, S. S. (2016). Anti-proteolytic activity of Ganoderma lucidum methanol extract against Pseudomonas aeruginosa. *Journal of Infection in Developing Countries*, *10*(9), 1020–1024. https://doi.org/10.3855/jidc.6929.

Gokce, E. C., Kahveci, R., Atanur, O. M., Gurer, B., Aksoy, N., Gokce, A., et al. (2015). Neuroprotective effects of Ganoderma lucidum polysaccharides against traumatic spinal cord injury in rats. *Injury*, *46*(11), 2146–2155. https://doi.org/10.1016/j.injury.2015.08.017.

Hijikata, Y., & Yamada, S. (1998). Effect of Ganoderma lucidum on postherpetic neuralgia. *The American Journal of Chinese Medicine*, *26*(3–4), 375–381. https://doi.org/10.1142/S0192415X98000415.

Hijikata, Y., Yasuhara, A., & Sahashi, Y. (2005). Effect of an herbal formula containing Ganoderma lucidum on reduction of herpes zoster pain: A pilot clinical trial. *The American Journal of Chinese Medicine*, *33*(4), 517–523. https://doi.org/10.1142/S0192415X05003120.

Hsu, S. C., Ou, C. C., Chuang, T. C., Li, J. W., Lee, Y. J., Wang, V., et al. (2009). Ganoderma tsugae extract inhibits expression of epidermal growth factor receptor and angiogenesis in human epidermoid carcinoma cells: In vitro and in vivo. *Cancer Letters*, *281*(1), 108–116. https://doi.org/10.1016/j.canlet.2009.02.032.

Jang, S. H., Cho, S. W., Yoon, H. M., Jang, K. J., Song, C. H., & Kim, C. H. (2014). Hepatoprotective evaluation of Ganoderma lucidum pharmacopuncture: In vivo studies of ethanol-induced acute liver injury. *Journal of Pharmacopuncture*, *17*(3), 16–24. https://doi.org/10.3831/KPI.2014.17.022.

Koyama, K., Imaizumi, T., Akiba, M., Kinoshita, K., Takahashi, K., Suzuki, A., et al. (1997). Antinociceptive components of Ganoderma lucidum. *Planta Medica*, *63*(3), 224–227. https://doi.org/10.1055/s-2006-957658.

Lai, C. S., Yu, M. S., Yuen, W. H., So, K. F., Zee, S. Y., & Chang, R. C. (2008). Antagonizing beta-amyloid peptide neurotoxicity of the anti-aging fungus Ganoderma lucidum. *Brain Research*, *1190*, 215–224. https://doi.org/10.1016/j.brainres.2007.10.103.

Lakshmi, B., Ajith, T. A., Jose, N., & Janardhanan, K. K. (2006). Antimutagenic activity of methanolic extract of Ganoderma lucidum and its effect on hepatic damage caused by benzo[a]pyrene. *Journal of Ethnopharmacology*, *107*(2), 297–303. https://doi.org/10.1016/j.jep.2006.03.027.

Lei, L. S., & Lin, Z. B. (1993). Effects of Ganoderma polysaccharides on the activity of DNA polymerase alpha of splenocytes and immune function in aged mice. *Yao Xue Xue Bao*, *28*(8), 577–582.

Li, Y. Q., & Wang, S. F. (2006). Anti-hepatitis B activities of ganoderic acid from Ganoderma lucidum. *Biotechnology Letters*, *28*(11), 837–841. https://doi.org/10.1007/s10529-006-9007-9.

Lin, W. C., & Lin, W. L. (2006). Ameliorative effect of Ganoderma lucidum on carbon tetrachloride-induced liver fibrosis in rats. *World Journal of Gastroenterology*, *12*(2), 265–270. https://doi.org/10.3748/wjg.v12.i2.265.

Matsuzaki, H., Shimizu, Y., Iwata, N., Kamiuchi, S., Suzuki, F., Iizuka, H., et al. (2013). Antidepressant-like effects of a water-soluble extract from the culture medium of Ganoderma lucidum mycelia in rats. *BMC Complementary and Alternative Medicine*, *13*, 370. https://doi.org/10.1186/1472-6882-13-370.

Meng, G. L., Zhu, H. Y., Yang, S. J., Wu, F., Zheng, H. H., Chen, E., et al. (2011). Attenuating effects of Ganoderma lucidum polysaccharides on myocardial collagen cross-linking relates to advanced glycation end product and antioxidant enzymes in high-fat-diet and streptozotocin-induced diabetic rats. *Carbohydrate Polymers*, *84*(1), 180–185. https://doi.org/10.1016/j.carbpol.2010.11.016.

Miyamoto, I., Liu, J., Shimizu, K., Sato, M., Kukita, A., Kukita, T., et al. (2009). Regulation of osteoclastogenesis by ganoderic acid DM isolated from Ganoderma lucidum. *European Journal of Pharmacology*, *602*(1), 1–7. https://doi.org/10.1016/j.ejphar.2008.11.005.

Pan, D., Zhang, D., Wu, J., Chen, C., Xu, Z., Yang, H., et al. (2013). Antidiabetic, antihyperlipidemic and antioxidant activities of a novel proteoglycan from Ganoderma lucidum fruiting bodies on db/db mice and the possible mechanism. *PLoS One*, *8*(7). e68332https://doi.org/10.1371/journal.pone.0068332.

Ren, H., Meng, X., Yin, J., Sun, J., Huang, Q., & Yin, Z. (2018). Ganoderma lucidum polysaccharide peptide attenuates skin flap ischemia-reperfusion injury in a thioredoxin-dependent manner. *Plastic and Reconstructive Surgery*, *142*(1), 23e–33e. https://doi.org/10.1097/PRS.0000000000004503.

Ren, Z. L., Wang, C. D., Wang, T., Ding, H., Zhou, M., Yang, N., et al. (2019). Ganoderma lucidum extract ameliorates MPTP-induced parkinsonism and protects dopaminergic neurons from oxidative stress via regulating mitochondrial function, autophagy, and apoptosis. *Acta Pharmacologica Sinica*, *40*(4), 441–450. https://doi.org/10.1038/s41401-018-0077-8.

Shen, J., Park, H. S., Xia, Y. M., Kim, G. S., & Cui, S. W. (2014). The polysaccharides from fermented Ganoderma lucidum mycelia induced miRNAs regulation in suppressed HepG2 cells. *Carbohydrate Polymers*, *103*, 319–324. https://doi.org/10.1016/j.carbpol.2013.12.044.

Socala, K., Nieoczym, D., Grzywnowicz, K., Stefaniuk, D., & Wlaz, P. (2015). Evaluation of anticonvulsant, antidepressant-, and anxiolytic-like effects of an aqueous extract from cultured mycelia of the Lingzhi or Reishi medicinal mushroom Ganoderma lucidum (higher basidiomycetes) in mice. *International Journal of Medicinal Mushrooms*, *17*(3), 209–218.

Su, J., Su, L., Li, D., Shuai, O., Zhang, Y., Liang, H., et al. (2018). Antitumor activity of extract from the sporoderm-breaking spore of Ganoderma lucidum: Restoration on exhausted cytotoxic T cell with gut microbiota remodeling. *Frontiers in Immunology*, *9*, 1765. https://doi.org/10.3389/fimmu.2018.01765.

Sudheesh, N. P., Ajith, T. A., Ramnath, V., & Janardhanan, K. K. (2010). Therapeutic potential of Ganoderma lucidum (Fr.) P. Karst. Against the declined antioxidant status in the mitochondria of post-mitotic tissues of aged mice. *Clinical Nutrition*, *29*(3), 406–412. https://doi.org/10.1016/j.clnu.2009.12.003.

Sun, X. Z., Liao, Y., Li, W., & Guo, L. M. (2017). Neuroprotective effects of Ganoderma lucidum polysaccharides against oxidative stress-induced neuronal apoptosis. *Neural Regeneration Research*, *12*(6), 953–958. https://doi.org/10.4103/1673-5374.208590.

Tie, L., Yang, H. Q., An, Y., Liu, S. Q., Han, J., Xu, Y., et al. (2012). Ganoderma lucidum polysaccharide accelerates refractory wound healing by inhibition of mitochondrial oxidative stress in type 1 diabetes. *Cellular Physiology and Biochemistry*, *29*(3–4), 583–594. https://doi.org/10.1159/000338512.

Tran, P. T., Dat, N. T., Dang, N. H., Van Cuong, P., Lee, S., Hwangbo, C., et al. (2019). Ganomycin I from Ganoderma lucidum attenuates RANKL-mediated osteoclastogenesis by inhibiting MAPKs and NFATc1. *Phytomedicine*, *55*, 1–8. https://doi.org/10.1016/j.phymed.2018.10.029.

Wan, F., & Huang, D. (1992). Anti-inflammatory and analgesic actions of artificial and fermentative Ganoderma sinense (AFGS). *Zhongguo Zhong Yao Za Zhi*, *17*(10), 619–622. 640.

Wang, S. Y., Hsu, M. L., Hsu, H. C., Tzeng, C. H., Lee, S. S., Shiao, M. S., et al. (1997). The anti-tumor effect of Ganoderma lucidum is mediated by cytokines released from activated macrophages and T lymphocytes. *International Journal of Cancer*, *70*(6), 699–705.

Wang, G. J., Huang, Y. J., Chen, D. H., & Lin, Y. L. (2009). Ganoderma lucidum extract attenuates the proliferation of hepatic stellate cells by blocking the PDGF receptor. *Phytotherapy Research*, *23*(6), 833–839. https://doi.org/10.1002/ptr.2687.

Wang, G. H., Li, X., Cao, W. H., Li, J., & Wang, L. H. (2018). A retrospective study of Ganoderma Lucidum spore powder for patients with epilepsy. *Medicine (Baltimore)*, *97*(23). e10941https://doi.org/10.1097/MD.0000000000010941.

Wang, S. Q., Li, X. J., Qiu, H. B., Jiang, Z. M., Simon, M., Ma, X. R., et al. (2014). Anti-epileptic effect of Ganoderma lucidum polysaccharides by inhibition of intracellular calcium accumulation and stimulation of expression of CaMKII alpha in epileptic hippocampal neurons. *PLoS One*, *9*(7). e102161https://doi.org/10.1371/journal.pone.0102161.

Wang, S. Q., Li, X. J., Zhou, S., Sun, D. X., Wang, H., Cheng, P. F., et al. (2013). Intervention effects of Ganoderma lucidum spores on epileptiform discharge hippocampal neurons and expression of neurotrophin-4 and N-cadherin. *PLoS One*, *8*(4). e61687https://doi.org/10.1371/journal.pone.0061687.

Wang, X., Zhao, X., Li, D., Lou, Y. Q., Lin, Z. B., & Zhang, G. L. (2007). Effects of Ganoderma lucidum polysaccharide on CYP2E1, CYP1A2 and CYP3A activities in BCG-immune hepatic injury in rats. *Biological & Pharmaceutical Bulletin*, *30*(9), 1702–1706.

Weng, C. J., Fang, P. S., Chen, D. H., Chen, K. D., & Yen, G. C. (2010). Anti-invasive effect of a rare mushroom, Ganoderma colossum , on human hepatoma cells. *Journal of Agricultural and Food Chemistry*, *58*(13), 7657–7663. https://doi.org/10.1021/jf101464h.

Wu, Y. W., Fang, H. L., & Lin, W. C. (2010). Post-treatment of Ganoderma lucidum reduced liver fibrosis induced by thioacetamide in mice. *Phytotherapy Research*, *24*(4), 494–499. https://doi.org/10.1002/ptr.2949.

Wu, J. G., Kan, Y. J., Wu, Y. B., Yi, J., Chen, T. Q., & Wu, J. Z. (2016). Hepatoprotective effect of Ganoderma triterpenoids against oxidative damage induced by tert-butyl hydroperoxide in human hepatic HepG2 cells. *Pharmaceutical Biology*, *54*(5), 919–929. https://doi.org/10.3109/13880209.2015.1091481.

Wu, X., Zeng, J., Hu, J., Liao, Q., Zhou, R., Zhang, P., et al. (2013). Hepatoprotective effects of aqueous extract from Lingzhi or Reishi medicinal mushroom Ganoderma lucidum (higher basidiomycetes) on alpha-amanitin-induced liver injury in mice. *International Journal of Medicinal Mushrooms*, *15*(4), 383–391.

Xie, Y. Z., Yang, F., Tan, W., Li, X., Jiao, C., Huang, R., et al. (2016). The anti-cancer components of Ganoderma lucidum possesses cardiovascular protective effect by regulating circular RNA expression. *Oncoscience*, *3*(7–8), 203–207. https://doi.org/10.18632/oncoscience.316.

Yang, Z., Chen, C., Zhao, J., Xu, W., He, Y., Yang, H., et al. (2018). Hypoglycemic mechanism of a novel proteoglycan, extracted from Ganoderma lucidum, in hepatocytes. *European Journal of Pharmacology*, *820*, 77–85. https://doi.org/10.1016/j.ejphar.2017.12.020.

Yang, X. J., Liu, J., Ye, L. B., Yang, F., Ye, L., Gao, J. R., et al. (2006). In vitro and in vivo protective effects of proteoglycan isolated from mycelia of Ganoderma lucidum on carbon tetrachloride-induced liver injury. *World Journal of Gastroenterology*, *12*(9), 1379–1385. https://doi.org/10.3748/wjg.v12.i9.1379.

Yang, Z. W., Wu, F., & Zhang, S. L. (2016). Effects of ganoderic acids on epileptiform discharge hippocampal neurons: Insights from alterations of BDNF, TRPC3 and apoptosis. *Pharmazie*, *71*(6), 340–344.

Zeng, Q., Zhou, F., Lei, L., Chen, J., Lu, J., Zhou, J., et al. (2017). Ganoderma lucidum polysaccharides protect fibroblasts against UVB-induced photoaging. *Molecular Medicine Reports*, *15*(1), 111–116. https://doi.org/10.3892/mmr.2016.6026.

Zhang, Q., & Lin, Z. (1999). Study on antitumor activity and mechanism of Ganoderma polysaccharides B. *Zhongguo Zhong Xi Yi Jie He Za Zhi*, *19*(9), 544–547.

Zhang, J., Tang, Q., Zhou, C., Jia, W., Da Silva, L., Nguyen, L. D., et al. (2010). GLIS, a bioactive proteoglycan fraction from Ganoderma lucidum, displays anti-tumour activity by increasing both humoral and cellular immune response. *Life Sciences*, *87*(19–22), 628–637. https://doi.org/10.1016/j.lfs.2010.09.026.

Zhao, H. B., Wang, S. Z., He, Q. H., Yuan, L., Chen, A. F., & Lin, Z. B. (2005). Ganoderma total sterol (GS) and GS1 protect rat cerebral cortical neurons from hypoxia/reoxygenation injury. *Life Sciences*, *76*(9), 1027–1037. https://doi.org/10.1016/j.lfs.2004.08.013.

Zhou, Z. Y., Tang, Y. P., Xiang, J., Wua, P., Jin, H. M., Wang, Z., et al. (2010). Neuroprotective effects of water-soluble Ganoderma lucidum polysaccharides on cerebral ischemic injury in rats. *Journal of Ethnopharmacology*, *131*(1), 154–164. https://doi.org/10.1016/j.jep.2010.06.023.

CHAPTER TEN

Fungal polysaccharides

Zhiyong Xiao[a,b], Wenxia Zhou[a,b], Yongxiang Zhang[a,b,*]
[a]Beijing Institute of Pharmacology and Toxicology, Beijing, China
[b]State Key Laboratory of Toxicology and Medical Countermeasures, Beijing, China
*Corresponding author: e-mail address: zhangyx@bmi.ac.cn

Contents

Abstract

Fungal bioactive polysaccharides are well known and have been widely used in Asia as a part of the traditional diet and medicine. In fact, some biopolymers (mainly β-glucans or glycoconjugate) have already made their way to the market as antitumor or immunostimulating drugs. In the last decades, the relationship between structure and activity of polysaccharides and their detailed mode of action have been the core of intense research to understand and utilize their medicinal properties. Most of the antitumor polysaccharides belong to conserved β-glucans, with a linear β-(1 → 3)-glucan backbone and attached β-(1 → 6) branch. Structurally different β-glucans appear to have different affinities toward their receptors and thus generate markedly different host responses. However, their antitumor activities are mainly influenced by molecular mass, degree of branching, conformation, and structure modification of the polysaccharides. β-Glucans act on several immune receptors including Dectin-1, complement receptor (CR3) and TLR-2/6, then trigger both innate and adaptive response and enhance opsonic and nonopsonic phagocytosis. Various receptor interactions explain the possible mode of actions of polysaccharides.

Advances in Pharmacology, Volume 87
ISSN 1054-3589
https://doi.org/10.1016/bs.apha.2019.08.003

Abbreviations

ADCC	antibody-dependent cell-mediated cytotoxicity
CLR	C-type lectin receptor
CR3	complement receptor 3
CR3-DCC	CR3-dependent cellular cytotoxicity
DB	degree of branching
FAE	follicle-associated epithelium
iC3b	inactivated complement 3b
IL	interleukin
ITAM	immunoreceptor tyrosine-based activation motif
LPS	lipopolysaccharide
MAMPs	microbe-associated molecular patterns
M cells	microfold cells
MW	molecular weight
MyD88	myeloid differentiation factor 88
NF-κB	nuclear factor-κB
PAMPs	pathogen-associated molecular patterns
PRRs	pattern recognition receptors
Syk	spleen tyrosine kinase
TLRs	toll-like receptors
TNF-α	tumor necrosis factor-α

1. Introduction

Fungi are widely used in medicine, food and health care products and have been used for a long time. Fossil records prove the existence of fungi as far back in time as the Paleozoic era (408–438 million years ago) in the Silurian period (Alexopoulos, Mims, & Blackwell, 1996; Ren, Perera, & Hemar, 2012). As early as 6000–7000 years ago in the Yangshao culture period, eating mushrooms and other edible fungi was very common in China. Many books, such as *The Annals of Lu Buwei* (Lüshi Chunqiu, 吕氏春秋) and *Book of Rites* (Li Ji, 礼记), written ~2000 years ago offer detailed descriptions of human dietary intake of edible mushrooms. Based on this long-term consumption, the nutritional and therapeutic benefits of fungi gradually gained attention. For example, in the most ancient Chinese pharmaceutical work, *Shen Nong's Herbal Classic* (Shennong Bencaojing, 神农本草经), documents about 10 varieties of fungi, such as *Poria cocos Wolf* (*P. cocos Wolf*), *Tremella fuciformis* (*T. fuciformis*), *Polypori umbellatus* (*P. umbellatus*), *Omphalia lapidescens* (*O. lapidescens*) and *Phellinus*

Quél (*P. Quél*), etc. The medicinal properties of the aforementioned fungi range from delaying aging, clearing dampness and promoting diuresis, invigorating the spirit, relieving cough and asthma to improving learning and memory. Mushrooms have also played an important role in the treatment of ailments in eastern European countries. The most important species in these countries are *Inonotus obliquus*, Pilát (Chaga), *Fomitopsis officinalis*, *Piptoporus betulinus* and *Fomes fomentarius* (Chang & Wasser, 2012; Wasser, 2014), which have been widely used for treating gastrointestinal disorders, various forms of cancers, bronchial asthma, night sweats, etc. There is also a long history of traditional use of mushrooms as cultivating objects in Mesoamerica (especially for species of the genus *Psilocybe*), Africa (Yoruba populations in Nigeria and Benin), Algeria, and Egypt (Wasser, 2014).

Most fungi with immunomodulation and anti-cancer activities belong to the class of Basidiomycetes and, to a lesser extent, Ascomycetes. Traditionally used fungi possessing immunomodulation and anti-cancer activities are *Ganoderma lucidum* (*G. lucidum*), *Lentinus edodes* (*Shiitake, L. edodes*), *Tremella fuciformis* (*T. fuciformis*), *Griflola frondosa* (*common name: Maitake, G. frondosa*), *Hericium erinaceus* (*H. erinaceus*), *Agaricus blazei Murrill* (*A. blazei Murrill*), *Coriolus versicolor* (*C. versicolor*), *Inonotus obliquus* (*I. bliquus*) *and Poria cocos Wolf* (*P. cocos Wolf*), etc. All of these species belong to the class Basidiomycetes, whereas *Cordyceps militaris* (*C. militaris*) is in the class of Ascomycetes. In recent decades, the bioactivities of fungus have been confirmed by extensive studies. The antitumor activity of the Basidiomycetes was first demonstrated by Byerrum and co-workers (1957). They discovered that an extract from Basidiomycetes mushrooms exerted a significant inhibitory effect against Sarcoma S-180 tumor cells (Byerrum et al., 1957). Since then the substances in Basidiomycetes mushrooms that possess antitumor and immunomodulation activity have been widely studied. Through various separation and purification methods, compounds such as proteins, peptides, terpenoids, phenolic and polyphenolics, ergosterols, lectins and polysaccharides or glycans from different types of fungus have been isolated, identified and explored (El Enshasy & Hatti-Kaul, 2013; Kalac, 2013). Among these, polysaccharides or glycans have been considered one of the most important components that are responsible for the immunostimulating and anti-cancer functions of fungus (Chen et al., 2004; Giavasis, 2014; Ivanova, Krupodorova, Barshteyn, Artamonova, & Shlyakhovenko, 2014; Wasser, 2014).

Recently, several fungal polysaccharides or glycans have been subjected to Phase I, II, and III clinical trials. Commercial polysaccharides are used extensively in Asia to treat various cancers and other diseases. This chapter will focus on the fungal polysaccharides with antitumor and immunomodulation activities, especially those have already been marketed and used in clinic, such as lentinan from *L. edodes*, grifolan from *G. frondosa*, schizophyllan from *S. commune*, PSP (polysaccharide peptide) and krestin (polysaccharide protein) from *T. versicolor*, etc. Among the polysaccharides drugs on the market, lentinan, schizophyllan and krestin were first developed by Japan, while most of the others are marketed in China as polysaccharides extracted from fungus.

2. Structure-activity relationship of polysaccharides with antitumor activity

Most studies show that fungal polysaccharides perform their antitumor actions not through a direct tumor-killing activity, but through their effects of immunopotentiation or immunomodulation as systemic reactions. Fungal polysaccharides can be classified into different groups according to structure (linear and branched), sugar composition (homo- and heteropolysaccharides), and the type of bonds between the monomers (β-(1 → 3), β-(1 → 6), or α-(1 → 3), etc.). To gain full activity, some polysaccharides need to form more complex conformation (Liu et al., 2011; Wang, Xu, & Zhang, 2008; Xin, Wang, Luo, & Meng, 2018). Antitumor polysaccharides differ greatly in their chemical structure and physical properties, but most of them belong to conserved β-glucans with a backbone of glucose residues linked by β-(1 → 3)-glycosidic bonds and attached β-(1 → 6) branch, although other side branches such as (1 → 2) and (1 → 4) branching also occur (Devi & Maiti, 2016; Snarr, Qureshi, & Sheppard, 2017). Structurally different β-glucans appear to have different affinities toward their receptors and thus generate markedly different host responses (Chen & Seviour, 2007). However, their antitumor activities are mainly influenced by molecular mass, degree of branching, conformation, and structure modification of the polysaccharides (Devi et al., 2016; El Enshasy & Hatti-Kaul, 2013; Meng, Liang, & Luo, 2016; Ren et al., 2012).

2.1 Effect of molecular mass

The molecular weight (MW) of fungal polysaccharides is usually required to be within a certain range to facilitate its biological activity. It used to be widely believed that higher molecular weight usually exhibited higher antitumor activity (Fadok et al., 2000; Goodridge et al., 2011).

For example, a (1→3)-β-glucan, the fraction isolated from *G. frondosa* with the highest molecular mass (800 kDa) shows the most potent antitumor and immunomodulatory activities, including activation of alternative complement pathway, glucose consumption by macrophages, macrophage-mediated lysosomal enzyme activity in culture supernatant and cell lysate, and interleukin (IL)-1 activity, etc. Medium molecular mass fraction (250 and 21 kDa) exhibited low levels of activities such as activation of alternative complement pathway and lysosomal enzyme secretion. Low molecular mass fraction (6.4 kDa) only activated glucose consumption and synthesis of lysosomal enzyme. These results suggest that a large molecular weight is required to augment multiple immunological activities (Adachi, Ohno, Ohsawa, Oikawa, & Yadomae, 1990). Another study about (1→3)-β-glucans from *G. frondosa* also showed that the tumoricidal cytokine tumor necrosis factor-α (TNF-α) release was correlated with the molecular weight, since the highest molecular weight fraction (≥45 kDa) exhibited the strongest activity (Okazaki, Adachi, Ohno, & Yadomae, 1995).

The superior activity of polysaccharides with high molecular weight may be attributed to more active unit and the better binding affinity to the carbohydrate receptors of the immune cells (El Enshasy & Hatti-Kaul, 2013). In addition, small β-glucans compete with large β-glucans for binding sites and interfere with the activities of large β-glucans (Hayashi, Shoubayashi, Kondo, & Fukudome, 2019). The Kururu no β-glu® (KBG) is a commercial hydrothermal-treated *Aureobasidium pullulans* β-glucan that can suppress lipopolysaccharide (LPS) induced nitrogen oxide (NO) synthesis and TNF-α production in RAW264.7 cells. Reprocessed KBG has more low molecular weight fractions (approx. MW of 10 kDa), and simultaneously markedly enhanced suppressive activities (Hayashi et al., 2019).

2.2 Effect of degree of branching (DB)

Fungal (1→3)-β-glucans differ with respect to their degree of branching (DB) and branch distribution. Lentinan and schizophyllan are both (1→3)-β-D-glucans consisting of a main chain of (1→3)-linked β-D-glucopyranosyl units with β-D-glucopyranosyl branch units linked 1→6 at an interval of two/one branches for every five β-D-glucopyranosyl (DB = 2/5 or 40%) or three β-D-glucopyranosyl (DB = 1/3 or 33%) residue, respectively (Tabata, Ito, Kojima, Kawabata, & Misaki, 1981) (Fig. 1). The polysaccharide moiety of PSK is composed of (1→3)-β−/(1→4)-β-D-glucan with one branch for every five β-D-glucopyranosyl residue

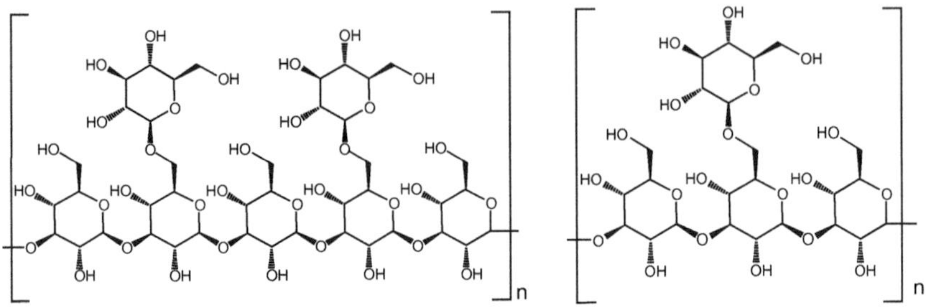

Fig. 1 Structure units of polysaccharides showing antitumor activity: lentinan (CAS No. 37339-90-5) and schizophyllan (CAS No. 9050-67-3).

(DB = 1/5 or 20%) (Tsukagoshi et al., 1984). Actually, other β-D-glucans with both higher (0.75) and lower DB (0.04) also exist. The highly branched glucans of *Auricularia auricular-judae* (Kikurage) (DB = 0.75) and of *Pestalotia* Sp. 815 (DB = 0.67) have limited activity against tumors. The much less branched glucan from *G. lucidum* (DB = 0.06) also possesses only marginal activity (Misaki et al., 1984; Misaki, Kakuta, Sasaki, Tanaka, & Miyaji, 1981). The most active polymers generally have a degree of branching between 20% and 33% (Bohn & BeMiller, 1995).

Debranching polysaccharides sometimes increases their bioactivity. For example, a highly branched (1 → 3)-β-D-glucan from fungus *Sclerotinia sclerotiorum* IFO 9395 could not activate macrophages and release TNF-α in vitro. After debranching modification removed 50%, 75% and 100% of the branching glucose residues of native glucan, the derivatives gain the activity of inducing TNF-α release (Okazaki et al., 1995). Debranching lentinan also increases its biological activity. Modified lentinan with 32% DB exhibits the most impressive antitumor activity (Bae et al., 2013).

The distribution of the branch units along the backbone chain is also responsible for the biological activities of fungal polysaccharides. The phytopathogenic fungus *Phytophthora parasitica* produces several (1 → 3)-β-glucans, which have occasional disaccharides βGlcp(1 → 3) βGlcp as branch units. Trisaccharide side chains are present in their highest molecular weight fraction, which also has the highest antitumor activity when tested against the allogeneic sarcoma 180 in CD-1 mice (Bruneteau et al., 1988).

2.3 Effect of conformation

The conformation of polysaccharides means the shape and size of polysaccharides in solution, including monosaccharide conformation, flexibility, spatial structure, etc. (Wang et al., 2017). The conformations of polysaccharides in solution are categorized as random coil, single helix, double helix, triple helix, worm-like shape, rod-like shape, and aggregate. Because of relatively small space steric hindrance and higher spin degree of freedom, linear α- or β-(1→3)-glucans show the random thread chain conformation. However, β-(1→3)-glucans with branches tend to form helix conformations because of the numerous hydrogen bonds on their side chains. The most bioactive fungal polysaccharides known, lentinan, schizophyllan, PSK and scleroglucan, all form triple helix structure under most experimental conditions (Misaki et al., 1981; Palleschi, Bocchinfuso, Coviello, & Alhaique, 2005). The anti-tumor activity of lentinan is accompanied by its β-helix structures. If lentinan were to be dissolved in DMSO, the bioactivity would be dismissed because the conformation is destroyed (Zhang, Li, Xu, & Zeng, 2005). Under most experimental conditions, the structure of schizophyllan is that of a very stiff triple helix with a persistent length between 150 to 200 nm, as illustrated in Fig. 2 (Kony et al., 2007). The core of the helix is formed by three (1→3)-β-D-glucan chains, held together by hydrogen bonds. The (1→6)-β-D-glucan lateral residues, branched from every third glucose unit along each chain, are directed toward the exterior of the helix (Fig. 2). In contrast to most polysaccharides, which usually dissolve poorly in water, schizophyllan exhibits a fairly high solubility due to the presence of its lateral residues (Kony et al., 2007). Schizophyllan-OH derived from the alkaline-treated schizophyllan has a single helix structure because hydrogen bonds fail to form. It results in a reduced ability to inhibit tumor growth as

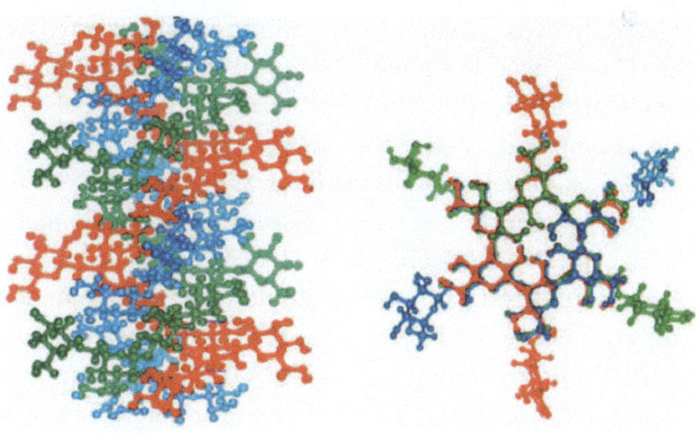

Fig. 2 Hypothetical type of hydrogen bond in schizophyllan triple helix (Kony, Damm, Stoll, van Gunsteren, & Hunenberger, 2007).

compared with native schizophyllan (Ooi & Liu, 2000). These data suggest that the configuration of polysaccharide is fundamental for the biological system to recognize it.

2.4 Effect of structure modification

In recent years, a lot of biological, physical, and chemical methods have been developed to modify polysaccharides for desired bioactivities (Wang et al., 2017). Among biological modifications, β-Glucanase is commonly used to decrease the MW and increase the water solubility and bioactivity of β-glucans. Ultrasonic, irradiation, microwave, and heating are traditional and feasible modification methods that cause structural changes in polysaccharides by breaking glucosidic bonds, enhancing the stretching of the molecular chain, initiating oxidation-reduction reaction of free radicals, etc. High pressure microfluidization is a new physical method used to modify polysaccharides. This technology is implemented by pumping and splitting a solution into two microstreams, which then collide against each other in the interaction chamber, where shear, turbulent, and cavitation forces are generated (Kasaai, Charlet, Paquin, & Arul, 2003). High pressure microfluidization could decrease the MW, change the microstructure, promote hydroscopicity, and enhance the solubility of polysaccharides (Wang et al., 2017). Dynamic high pressure microfluidization was used to prepare water-soluble yeast β-glucan. According to the conformational parameters calculated from the worm-like cylinder model, the β-glucan obtained exists as a semi-stiff chain in aqueous solution (Liu et al., 2016).

To improve the biological activity of polysaccharides, various carboxymethylated, hydroxylated, formylmethylated, aminoethylated and sulfated products have been designed. A (1 → 3)-α-D-glucan from *L. edodes*, exhibits higher immunomodulatory and anti-cancer activity after sulfated modification compared with the native polysaccharide (Zhang & Cheung, 2002). A hydroxylated form of schizophyllan, sulfonation of TAPA1 (a polysaccharide extracted from *Tremella aurantialba* fruiting bodies), carboxymethylated-sulfated β-(1 → 3)-D-glucan from *P. Cocos* and formylmethylated and aminoethylated derivatives of schizophyllan also show greater anti-cancer activity compared to their native polysaccharides (Du et al., 2010; Ohno, Miura, Chiba, Adachi, & Yadomae, 1995; Usui, Tomono, Sakai, Kiho, & Ukai, 1995). The introduction of carboxymethyl and sulfate groups enhance the backbone flexibility (Carlucci, Ciancia, Matulewicz, Cerezo, & Damonte, 1999), thus increases the possible contact between the modified polysaccharides with the immune cell receptor through hydrogen binding and electrostatic attraction (Chen, Zhang, & Cheung, 2010). In addition, carboxymethylation helps to transform β-glucans into a water-soluble form, which also contributes to its activity.

From the above research findings, it appears that molecular weight, branching, structure configuration, and modification have strong influences on the bioactivity of polysaccharides. Thus, all these polysaccharide features should be considered in an inter-related context for better understanding of the immunomodulatory potency of the compounds.

3. Immune recognition of fungal polysaccharides

The biological activities of polysaccharides mainly depend on their recognition and binding by specific receptors. Fungal β-glucans are absent in vertebrate tissue. Acting as microbe-associated molecular patterns (MAMPs), formerly called pathogen-associated molecular patterns (PAMPs), β-glucans mediate their stimulation mechanism by binding to cell surface pattern recognition receptors (PRRs), mainly Dectin-1, complement receptor 3 (CR3), Toll-like receptors (TLRs), and scavenger receptors (Devi et al., 2016). Generally, β-glucans initiate innate immunity by binding to the specific β-glucan receptor Dectin-1 on macrophages (Batbayar, Kim, & Kim, 2011) and DCs (Kim et al., 2010) or to CR3 on granulocytes and natural killer (NK) cells (Thornton, Vetvicka, Pitman, Goldman, & Ross, 1996). β-Glucans also directly activate other immune cells such as B cells (Dong et al., 2007), T cells (Tian et al., 2011), eosinophils (Mahauthaman et al., 1988), and neutrophils (van Bruggen et al., 2009). In addition, the above receptors express on intestinal epithelial cells. As humans cannot metabolize the β-glycosidic bonds in β-glucans, it has long been believed that the bacterial fermentation process taking place within the intestinal system is involved in the disposal of β-glucans (Brown et al., 2003; Chan, Chan, & Sze, 2009; Rice et al., 2005). Solubility, molecular mass, tertiary structure, degree of branching, polymer charge and solution conformation (triple or single helix or random coil) are characteristics of polysaccharides that also influence the interactions with their receptors (Brown & Gordon, 2005). Therefore, it is worthwhile to explore the receptors recognizing β-glucans.

3.1 Dectin-1

Dectin-1 is a primary and well-studied C-type lectin receptor (CLR) that is primarily responsible for β-glucan recognition and control of fungal infection (Ferwerda et al., 2010; Taylor et al., 2007). It is a type II (asialoglycoprotein and DC receptors, Ca^{2+} binding) membrane receptor with an extracellular C-type lectin-like carbohydrate recognition domain, separated from the cell membrane by a short stalk region, and an intracellular domain containing an immunoreceptor tyrosine-based activation motif (ITAM) (Brown & Gordon, 2001; Brown et al., 2003, 2002; Taylor et al., 2002; Willment, Gordon, & Brown, 2001). Dectin-1 is expressed by various myeloid cells (DCs, monocytes, macrophages) and subsets of B- and T cells (Seo et al., 2013; Taylor et al., 2002; Willment et al., 2001). It only recognizes (1→3)-β linked glucans, so does not interact with a mixed-linkage (1→3)/(1→4)-β-glucan backbone structure derived from barley, nor a glucan exclusively composed of a (1→6)-β-linked glucose backbone. The recognition of dectin-1 differs according to the structure of glucans, including polymer length and side-chain branching. The minimal binding subunit for recombinant Dectin-1 is a (1→3)-β-D-glucan oligosaccharide containing a backbone with seven glucose subunits and a single (1→6)-β-linked side-chain branch at the nonreducing terminus (Adams et al., 2008). Greater molecular size increases the affinity of Dectin-1 for glucans (Adams et al., 2008; Mueller et al., 2000). Dectin-1 interacts with (1→3)-β-D-glucans over a very wide range of binding affinities ranging from 2.6 mM to 2.2 pM (Adams et al., 2008; Sahasrabudhe et al., 2016). Glucan phosphate, a derivative from saprophytic yeast, has an extremely high affinity (2.2 pM) when binding to Dectin-1, indicating that the (1→6) side-chain branches located on the surface of glucan phosphate modulate this recognition (Kanagawa et al., 2011; Nakashima et al., 2018). In addition, within the crystal structure of Dectin-1, there is a shallow groove running between Trp221 and His223 (Brown et al., 2007). The (1→3)-β-D-glucans with a polymer backbone composed of seven or more glucose repeat subunits can interact with the Trp221/His223 groove in Dectin-1. Mutations of one or both residues significantly affected the ability of various glucans when binding to Dectin-1. Helical conformation of glucan polymers may facilitate the interaction of glucans with the Trp221/His223 groove in Dectin-1 (Adams et al., 2008).

β-Glucans binding to Dectin-1 induces Dectin-1 oligomerization (Brown et al., 2007). Engaging Dectin-1 results in tyrosine phosphorylation of the ITAMs/hemITAMs motif. Then spleen tyrosine kinase (Syk) is recruited and canonical NF-κB signaling is activated via a Card9/Bcl10/Malt1 complex (Geijtenbeek & Gringhuis, 2009; Patin, Thompson, & Orr, 2019; Rogers et al., 2005). Immune activation, including phagocytosis, oxidative burst, neutrophil degranulation, and the production of cytokines and chemokines occurs consequently (Murphy, Davis, & Carmichael, 2010; Schnaar, 2016). Independent of Syk, Dectin-1 activates Raf-1, resulting in the phosphorylation and acetylation of p65 (Ifrim et al., 2013). Engaging Dectin-1 also involves phospholipase Cγ2–induced activation of MAPK, activator protein-1, and NF-κB, resulting in cytokine production and Th1 and Th17 differentiation (Bryant et al., 2015). Recent research focusing on pathogen sensor and handling aspects of Dectin-1 has found that Dectin-1 activates the noncanonical caspase-8 inflammasome and canonical NLRP3/caspase-1 inflammasome, causing IL-1β transcription and processing (Gringhuis et al., 2012; Li et al., 2011). Dectin-1 induces activation of macrophage-1 antigen (Mac-1) that is coordinated by guanine nucleotide exchange factors Vav1 and Vav3, a pathway that may localize cytotoxic responses of circulating neutrophils to infected tissue (Li et al., 2011). In macrophages, Dectin-1 also interacts with Bruton's tyrosine kinase (BTK) and Vav1 to elicit phagocytosis (Strijbis et al., 2013). Moreover, Dectin-1 collaborates with several other receptors, such as TLR2, Galactin-3, tetraspanins CD37 and CD63, etc. (Dennehy et al., 2008; Esteban et al., 2011; Meyer-Wentrup et al., 2007).

Dectin-1 binds both soluble and particulate β-glucans, however, it is only activated by particulate β-glucans. When particulate β-glucans bind to Dectin-1, the CD45 and CD148 tyrosine phosphatases are excluded from the clustered sites of dectin-1, enabling downstream signal transduction through hemITAM (Goodridge et al., 2011). Soluble β-glucans are unable to exclude CD45 and CD148 around Dectin-1, and thus signal propagation fails. As a negative feedback mechanism, phagocytosis of particulate β-glucans following Dectin-1 binding results in reduced Dectin-1 signaling and cytokine responses (Brown et al., 2003; Patin et al., 2019; Rosas et al., 2008).

3.2 CR3

CR3 (CD11b/CD18, αMβ2-integrin, Mac-1) is the first receptor identified in innate immune cells that involves in β-glucan recognition and serves as the major receptor on human neutrophils recognizing β-glucan-bearing particles (Albeituni & Yan, 2013; van Bruggen et al., 2009). Orally administered β-glucans can be absorbed at intestinal Peyer's patches through microfold cells (M cells) or follicle-associated epithelium (FAE), subsequently bound to dectin-1 and TLR2. The macrophages or DCs internalize and fragment β-glucans into smaller sized ones (~25 kDa), then release them to the lymph nodes. The small β-glucan fragments, like the soluble β-glucans mentioned above, bind to Dectin-1, but are unable to activate macrophages or DCs, due to their inability to cluster Dectin-1 on the membrane (Goodridge et al., 2011). Instead, the small β-glucan fragments released from the cells activate NK cells and granulocytes by binding to CR3 on them (Chan et al., 2009). As far as intravenously administered soluble β-glucans is concerned, they can be delivered directly to the CR3 on circulating granulocytes (Chan et al., 2009).

CR3 is a dimeric integrin consisting of two transmembrane proteins (CD11b/CD18) and two functional domains. The inserted domain (I-domain) contains opsonic inactivated complement 3b (iC3b)-binding site, while the cation-independent lectin domain at the C-terminal to the I-domain binds to β-glucan (Thornton et al., 1996; Xia & Ross, 1999). Currently, the lectin domain of CR3 contains no known lectin-like sequence and the exact binding mechanism is unclear as well (Jin, Li, & Wang, 2018; Vorup-Jensen & Jensen, 2018). β-Glucans bind to the lectin domain and prime it for binding to iC3b on the surface of reactor cells, including cancer cells tagged with monoclonal antibody and coated with iC3b. Then the activated CR3 containing cells, such as the neutrophils, are recruited into tumor milieu. Meanwhile, tumor specific antigens recruit antibodies bound to the tumor cell surface and mediate opsonization to tumor cells through iC3b (Chan et al., 2009; Hong et al., 2004; Salvador et al., 2008). Eventually, neutrophils recognize iC3b-opsonized tumor cells and lead to the antibody-dependent cell-mediated cytotoxicity (ADCC) and CR3-mediated cytotoxicity (CR3-DCC) to kill tumor cells (Jin et al., 2018). β-Glucan-mediated CR3-DCC response is Syk and PI3K-dependent. It might be ineffective if these signaling molecules were blocked (Li et al., 2006).

The cytotoxic effect produced by β-glucans-primed CR3-dependent neutrophils is extremely important in tumor immunotherapy because it causes neutrophils to produce double ligands dependent cytotoxic responses. This feature has been applied in tumor immunotherapy. For example, barley β-(1 → 3), (1 → 4)-glucan given orally can potentiate the activity of an antitumor monoclonal antibody (anti-ganglioside-2 or "3F8"), leading to enhanced tumor regression and survival in a human neuroblastoma xenografts mouse model (Cheung, Modak, Vickers, & Knuckles, 2002). On the basis of that characteristic, the joint use of β-glucan and 3F8 antibody was tested in a recent phase I study. It was found that the combination exhibited good tolerance and showed antitumor activity in patients with either recurrent or refractory neuroblastoma (Modak et al., 2013).

3.3 TLRs

TLRs are the best described PRR family for pathogen recognition. There are 13 functional TLRs in mice, of which 10 have been identified in humans.

TLRs 1, 2, 4, 5, 10, 11, and 12 are all expressed in the plasma membrane, whereas TLRs 3, 7, 8, and 9 are expressed in the endosome. Ligand binding to either the extracellular or endosomal ectodomain of TLRs leads to dimerization of the cytoplasmic Toll/IL-1R (TIR) domain. All TLRs members form homodimer, except TLR2, which forms a heterodimer with TLR1 or TLR6 (Jin et al., 2007; Kang et al., 2009; Ozinsky et al., 2000). Adaptor proteins are subsequently recruited and downstream signaling is induced dependent on myeloid differentiation factor 88 (MyD88) (engaged by all TLRs except TLR3) and/or TIR domain-containing adaptor (TRIF, engaged by TLR3 and TLR4). MyD88-dependent activation of NF-κB induces transcription of proinflammatory cytokines, while IFN regulatory factors-3 (IRF-3) nuclear translocation and transcription of type I IFN genes are central events downstream of TRIF (Patin et al., 2019; Takeuchi & Akira, 2010). Actually, the TLR and dectin-1 signaling pathways share the IKK/IκB/NF-κB complex to initiate NF-kB transcription, thus synergistic effects might be implicated between these two signaling pathways.

Transmembrane TLRs recognize PAMPs, including β-glucans present in fungal cell walls (Batbayar, Lee, & Kim, 2012; Zhang, Zhang, Zhang, & Tian, 2019). Upon binding to β-glucans, such as zymosan, TLR2 cooperates with Dectin-1 in producing interleukins, TNF-α and ROS to induce a proinflammatory response in murine macrophages and DCs (Batbayar et al., 2012; Gantner, Simmons, Canavera, Akira, & Underhill, 2003; Taghavi et al., 2018). Similar results can also be obtained from TLR2, TLR3, TLR4, TLR5, TLR7, or TLR9 stimulated with particulate β-glucans (Dennehy et al., 2008; Dragicevic et al., 2012). Enhanced NF-κB translocation resulted in increased production of not only proinflammatory cytokines TNF, IL-23, IL-6, and IL-10, but also anti-inflammatory cytokine IL-10 (Dennehy et al., 2008; Ostrop & Lang, 2017). Some of these cytokines may play important roles in cancer therapy, such as TNF-α enhances leukocyte recruitment to inflammatory sites and promotes infiltration of cytotoxic T cells into the tumor vicinity (Taghavi et al., 2018). Furthermore, blocking TLR-4 inhibits the production of IL-12 p40 and IL-10 induced by purified Ganoderma glucan via the augmentation of the IκB kinase, NF-κB activity and MAPK phosphorylation, suggesting that TLR-4 signaling involves glucan induced DCs maturation (Lin, Liang, Lee, & Chiang, 2005). TLR2 is also highly expressed on DC. Polysaccharide krestin (PSK), a selective TLR-2 agonist, inhibits breast cancer in mice by inducing type I immunity characterized by IL-12 production via TLR2 activation (Lu et al., 2011).

Summarily, the recognition of β-glucans on immunocytes and subsequent actions of β-glucans on tumor cells are presented in Fig. 3.

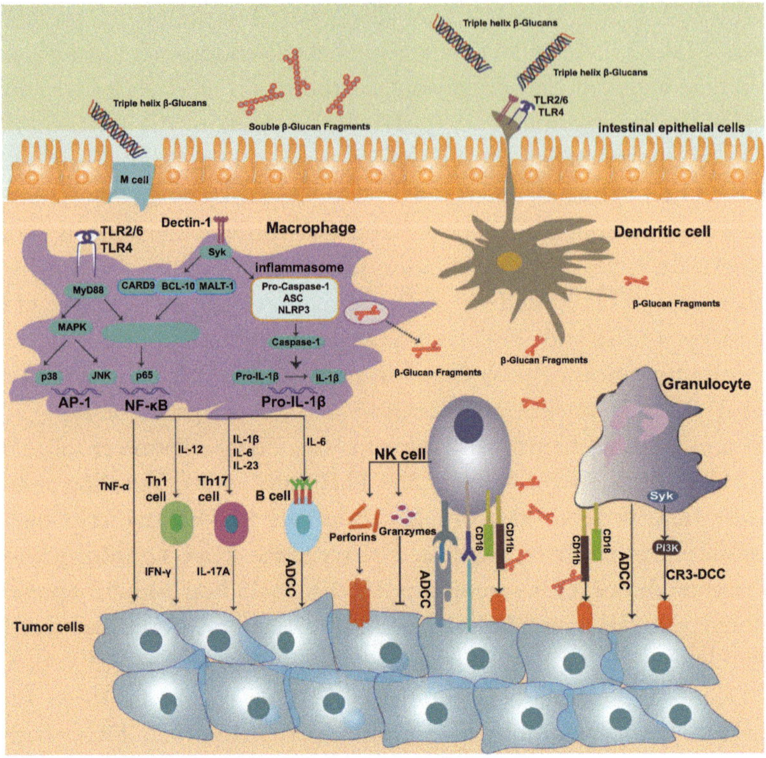

Fig. 3 Schematic representation of the recognition of β-glucans on immunocytes and subsequent actions of β-glucans on tumor cells. Orally administered β-glucans pass through the epithelial lumen by active transport mediated by M cells and subsequently captured by macrophages or bind to the projected tips of dendritic cells (DCs) in the follicle-associated epithelium (FAE) of Peyer's patches via dectin-1 receptor with or without TLR-2/6/4. Dectin-1 activation will recruit Syk and then trigger NF-κB mainly through CARD9 to produce multiple cytokines, such as IL-2, IL-23, IL-6, TNF-α, and IL-10, resulting in T and B cells proliferation/differentiation, DCs maturation and respiratory burst, and subsequently cytolysis of the tumor cells. NLRP3 inflammasome is simultaneously activated via a dectin-Syk pathway. TLRs activation is mainly MyD88-dependent manner here and also triggers NF-κB, in addition MAPK pathways (p38 and JNK) are also activated to induce subsequent AP-1 activation. In addition, the large β-glucan molecules can be internalized and fragmented into smaller sized β-glucan fragments within the macrophages and released in the lymph nodes. These small β-glucan fragments, like soluble β-glucans, bind to dectin-1, but are unable to activate macrophages and DCs. However, they are taken up by the circulating granulocytes and natural killer (NK) cells via the complement receptor (CR)-3. The NK cells secrete perforins and granzymes, which make pores and fragmenting the DNA in tumor cells, respectively. The granulocytes kill tumor cells through antibody-dependent cell-mediated cytotoxicity (ADCC), mAb-CR3-dependent cellular cytotoxicity (DCC) and initiating opsonization to coat tumor with iC3b.

4. Conclusion

Fungal polysaccharides are the subject of research in many bioscience fields. Research on fungal polysaccharides focuses mainly on identifying the factors responsible for their biological activity, optimization of production (connected with the cost and productivity), and elucidation of their role and application in interactions between various chemical medicine. Although the anti-cancer and immunomodulatory activities of fungal polysaccharides have been studied for many years, the modes of their immune regulation, structure-function relationship and receptor interactions are still poorly understood.

Structure identification of polysaccharides and the investigation of their mechanisms depends on the availability of isolation, purification and chemical structure confirmation methods. Fungal polysaccharides isolation methods are mostly based on fractionation. However, due to the inherent difficulties in completely deciphering the fine structure of a polysaccharide isolated from a natural source, the results of different studies tend to be incomparable, or even contradictory. Improving the techniques of isolation, purification, and exploration of properties is required to better understand the role of polysaccharides in a variety of processes and the possible applications in the food or pharmaceutical industries (Osinska-Jaroszuk et al., 2015).

Nowadays, homopolysaccharides from fungus characterized by β-D-glucans are thought to be the major class of polysaccharides with therapeutic properties. Actually, studies have shown that the heteropolysaccharides also present pronounced biological activities, such as antitumor, anti-oxidative, immunomodulatory, anti-nociceptive and anti-inflammatory effects. For example, heteropolysaccharide with a heterogeneous main chain (Glcp, Galp and Rhap) from *Boletus edulis* demonstrates antitumor activity on mouse renal cancer cell line Renca and tumor-bearing BALB/c mice (Wang, Sun, Wu, Yang, & Tan, 2014). Heteropolysaccharides are also one of the major components in traditional herbal medicines in China, which are more complex than D-glucans, because there is more variability in their monosaccharide composition, anomeric configuration, linkage and branching type (Ruthes, Smiderle, & Iacomini, 2016). The advanced tools available to determine carbohydrate structures should be applied and a careful analysis will be required to determine their medical application potential in the future.

In any case, as our knowledge of the structure of fungal polysaccharides becomes increasingly clearer, details about the mechanisms of action of polysaccharides in various systems are being revealed. Wider applications of polysaccharides in both biotechnology and medicine can be expected in the future.

Acknowledgments

This work was supported by the National Science and Technology Major Projects (2016ZX09J16104-001) and the National Natural Science Foundation of China (81001652).

Conflict of interest

No conflict of interest.

References

Adachi, Y., Ohno, N., Ohsawa, M., Oikawa, S., & Yadomae, T. (1990). Change of biological activities of (1——3)-beta-D-glucan from *Grifola frondosa* upon molecular weight reduction by heat treatment. *Chemical & Pharmaceutical Bulletin, 38*(2), 477–481.

Adams, E. L., Rice, P. J., Graves, B., Ensley, H. E., Yu, H., Brown, G. D., et al. (2008). Differential high-affinity interaction of dectin-1 with natural or synthetic glucans is dependent upon primary structure and is influenced by polymer chain length and side-chain branching. *The Journal of Pharmacology and Experimental Therapeutics, 325*(1), 115–123. https://doi.org/10.1124/jpet.107.133124.

Albeituni, S. H., & Yan, J. (2013). The effects of beta-glucans on dendritic cells and implications for cancer therapy. *Anti-Cancer Agents in Medicinal Chemistry, 13*(5), 689–698.

Alexopoulos, C. J., Mims, C. W., & Blackwell, M. (1996). *Introductory mycology* (4th ed.). New York: Wiley.

Bae, I. Y., Kim, H. W., Yoo, H. J., Kim, E. S., Lee, S., Park, D. Y., et al. (2013). Correlation of branching structure of mushroom β-glucan with its physiological activities. *Food Research International, 51*(1), 195–200.

Batbayar, S., Kim, M. J., & Kim, H. W. (2011). Medicinal mushroom Lingzhi or Reishi, *Ganoderma lucidum* (W.Curt.:Fr.) P. Karst., beta-glucan induces Toll-like receptors and fails to induce inflammatory cytokines in NF-kappaB inhibitor-treated macrophages. *International Journal of Medicinal Mushrooms, 13*(3), 213–225.

Batbayar, S., Lee, D. H., & Kim, H. W. (2012). Immunomodulation of fungal beta-glucan in host defense signaling by Dectin-1. *Biomolecules & Therapeutics, 20*(5), 433–445. https://doi.org/10.4062/biomolther.2012.20.5.433.

Bohn, J. A., & BeMiller, J. N. (1995). (1→3)-β-D-glucans as biological response modifiers: A review of structure-functional activity relationships. *Carbohydrate Polymers, 28*(1), 3–14.

Brown, G. D., & Gordon, S. (2001). Immune recognition. A new receptor for beta-glucans. *Nature, 413*(6851), 36–37. https://doi.org/10.1038/35092620.

Brown, G. D., & Gordon, S. (2005). Immune recognition of fungal beta-glucans. *Cellular Microbiology, 7*(4), 471–479. https://doi.org/10.1111/j.1462-5822.2005.00505.x.

Brown, G. D., Herre, J., Williams, D. L., Willment, J. A., Marshall, A. S., & Gordon, S. (2003). Dectin-1 mediates the biological effects of beta-glucans. *The Journal of Experimental Medicine, 197*(9), 1119–1124. https://doi.org/10.1084/jem.20021890.

Brown, J., O'Callaghan, C. A., Marshall, A. S., Gilbert, R. J., Siebold, C., Gordon, S., et al. (2007). Structure of the fungal beta-glucan-binding immune receptor dectin-1: Implications for function. *Protein Science, 16*(6), 1042–1052. https://doi.org/10.1110/ps.072791207.

Brown, G. D., Taylor, P. R., Reid, D. M., Willment, J. A., Williams, D. L., Martinez-Pomares, L., et al. (2002). Dectin-1 is a major beta-glucan receptor on macrophages. *The Journal of Experimental Medicine, 196*(3), 407–412. https://doi.org/10.1084/jem.20020470.

Bruneteau, M., Fabre, I., Perret, J., Michel, G., Ricci, P., Joseleau, J. P., et al. (1988). Antitumor active beta-D-glucans from *Phytophthora parasitica. Carbohydrate Research, 175*(1), 137–143.

Bryant, C. E., Orr, S., Ferguson, B., Symmons, M. F., Boyle, J. P., & Monie, T. P. (2015). International union of basic and clinical pharmacology. XCVI. Pattern recognition receptors in health and disease. *Pharmacological Reviews, 67*(2), 462–504. https://doi.org/10.1124/pr.114.009928.

Byerrum, R. U., Clarke, D. A., Lucas, E. H., Ringler, R. L., Stevens, J. A., & Stock, C. C. (1957). Tumor inhibitors in *Boletus edulis* and other Holobasidiomycetes. *Antibiotics & Chemotherapy*, 7(1), 1–4.

Carlucci, M. J., Ciancia, M., Matulewicz, M. C., Cerezo, A. S., & Damonte, E. B. (1999). Antiherpetic activity and mode of action of natural carrageenans of diverse structural types. *Antiviral Research, 43*(2), 93–102.

Chan, G. C., Chan, W. K., & Sze, D. M. (2009). The effects of beta-glucan on human immune and cancer cells. *Journal of Hematology & Oncology, 2*, 25. https://doi.org/10.1186/1756-8722-2-25.

Chang, S. T., & Wasser, S. P. (2012). The role of culinary-medicinal mushrooms on human welfare with a pyramid model for human health. *International Journal of Medicinal Mushrooms, 14*(2), 95–134.

Chen, J., & Seviour, R. (2007). Medicinal importance of fungal beta-(1–>3), (1–>6)-glucans. *Mycological Research, 111*(Pt. 6), 635–652. https://doi.org/10.1016/j.mycres.2007.02.011.

Chen, H. S., Tsai, Y. F., Lin, S., Lin, C. C., Khoo, K. H., Lin, C. H., et al. (2004). Studies on the immuno-modulating and anti-tumor activities of *Ganoderma lucidum* (Reishi) polysaccharides. *Bioorganic & Medicinal Chemistry, 12*(21), 5595–5601. https://doi.org/10.1016/j.bmc.2004.08.003.

Chen, X., Zhang, L., & Cheung, P. C. (2010). Immunopotentiation and anti-tumor activity of carboxymethylated-sulfated beta-(1–>3)-d-glucan from *Poria cocos. International Immunopharmacology, 10*(4), 398–405. https://doi.org/10.1016/j.intimp.2010.01.002.

Cheung, N. K., Modak, S., Vickers, A., & Knuckles, B. (2002). Orally administered beta-glucans enhance anti-tumor effects of monoclonal antibodies. *Cancer Immunology, Immunotherapy, 51*(10), 557–564. https://doi.org/10.1007/s00262-002-0321-3.

Dennehy, K. M., Ferwerda, G., Faro-Trindade, I., Pyz, E., Willment, J. A., Taylor, P. R., et al. (2008). Syk kinase is required for collaborative cytokine production induced through Dectin-1 and toll-like receptors. *European Journal of Immunology, 38*(2), 500–506. https://doi.org/10.1002/eji.200737741.

Devi, K. S., Krishna, D., Das, J., Agarwal, T., Kumari, K., Maji, S., et al. (2016). Molecular mechanisms associated with particulate and soluble heteroglycan mediated immune response. *Journal of Cellular Biochemistry, 117*(7), 1580–1593. https://doi.org/10.1002/jcb.25449.

Devi, K. S., & Maiti, T. K. (2016). Immunomodulatory and anti-cancer properties of pharmacologically relevant mushroom glycans. *Recent Patents on Biotechnology, 10*(1), 72–78.

Dong, S. F., Chen, J. M., Zhang, W., Sun, S. H., Wang, J., Gu, J. X., et al. (2007). Specific immune response to HBsAg is enhanced by beta-glucan oligosaccharide containing an alpha-(1–>3)-linked bond and biased towards M2/Th2. *International Immunopharmacology*, 7(6), 725–733. https://doi.org/10.1016/j.intimp.2007.01.004.

Dragicevic, A., Dzopalic, T., Vasilijic, S., Vucevic, D., Tomic, S., Bozic, B., et al. (2012). Signaling through Toll-like receptor 3 and Dectin-1 potentiates the capability of human monocyte-derived dendritic cells to promote T-helper 1 and T-helper 17 immune responses. *Cytotherapy*, *14*(5), 598–607. https://doi.org/10.3109/14653249.2012.667873.

Du, X. J., Zhang, J. S., Yang, Y., Tang, Q. J., Jia, W., & Pan, Y. J. (2010). Purification, chemical modification and immunostimulating activity of polysaccharides from *Tremella aurantialba* fruit bodies. *Journal of Zhejiang University Science B*, *11*(6), 437–442. https://doi.org/10.1631/jzus.B0900402.

El Enshasy, H. A., & Hatti-Kaul, R. (2013). Mushroom immunomodulators: Unique molecules with unlimited applications. *Trends in Biotechnology*, *31*(12), 668–677. https://doi.org/10.1016/j.tibtech.2013.09.003.

Esteban, A., Popp, M. W., Vyas, V. K., Strijbis, K., Ploegh, H. L., & Fink, G. R. (2011). Fungal recognition is mediated by the association of dectin-1 and galectin-3 in macrophages. *Proceedings of the National Academy of Sciences of the United States of America*, *108*(34), 14270–14275. https://doi.org/10.1073/pnas.1111415108.

Fadok, V. A., Bratton, D. L., Rose, D. M., Pearson, A., Ezekewitz, R. A., & Henson, P. M. (2000). A receptor for phosphatidylserine-specific clearance of apoptotic cells. *Nature*, *405*(6782), 85–90. https://doi.org/10.1038/35011084.

Ferwerda, G., Netea, M. G., Joosten, L. A., van der Meer, J. W., Romani, L., & Kullberg, B. J. (2010). The role of Toll-like receptors and C-type lectins for vaccination against *Candida albicans*. *Vaccine*, *28*(3), 614–622. https://doi.org/10.1016/j.vaccine.2009.10.082.

Gantner, B. N., Simmons, R. M., Canavera, S. J., Akira, S., & Underhill, D. M. (2003). Collaborative induction of inflammatory responses by dectin-1 and Toll-like receptor 2. *The Journal of Experimental Medicine*, *197*(9), 1107–1117. https://doi.org/10.1084/jem.20021787.

Geijtenbeek, T. B., & Gringhuis, S. I. (2009). Signalling through C-type lectin receptors: Shaping immune responses. *Nature Reviews. Immunology*, *9*(7), 465–479. https://doi.org/10.1038/nri2569.

Giavasis, I. (2014). Bioactive fungal polysaccharides as potential functional ingredients in food and nutraceuticals. *Current Opinion in Biotechnology*, *26*, 162–173. https://doi.org/10.1016/j.copbio.2014.01.010.

Goodridge, H. S., Reyes, C. N., Becker, C. A., Katsumoto, T. R., Ma, J., Wolf, A. J., et al. (2011). Activation of the innate immune receptor Dectin-1 upon formation of a 'phagocytic synapse'. *Nature*, *472*(7344), 471–475. https://doi.org/10.1038/nature10071.

Gringhuis, S. I., Kaptein, T. M., Wevers, B. A., Theelen, B., van der Vlist, M., Boekhout, T., et al. (2012). Dectin-1 is an extracellular pathogen sensor for the induction and processing of IL-1beta via a noncanonical caspase-8 inflammasome. *Nature Immunology*, *13*(3), 246–254. https://doi.org/10.1038/ni.2222.

Hayashi, N., Shoubayashi, Y., Kondo, N., & Fukudome, K. (2019). Hydrothermal processing of beta-glucan from *Aureobasidium pullulans* produces a low molecular weight reagent that regulates inflammatory responses induced by TLR ligands. *Biochemical and Biophysical Research Communications*, *511*(2), 318–322. https://doi.org/10.1016/j.bbrc.2019.02.042.

Hong, F., Yan, J., Baran, J. T., Allendorf, D. J., Hansen, R. D., Ostroff, G. R., et al. (2004). Mechanism by which orally administered beta-1,3-glucans enhance the tumoricidal activity of antitumor monoclonal antibodies in murine tumor models. *Journal of Immunology*, *173*(2), 797–806. https://doi.org/10.4049/jimmunol.173.2.797.

Ifrim, D. C., Joosten, L. A., Kullberg, B. J., Jacobs, L., Jansen, T., Williams, D. L., et al. (2013). *Candida albicans* primes TLR cytokine responses through a Dectin-1/Raf-1-mediated pathway. *Journal of Immunology*, *190*(8), 4129–4135. https://doi.org/10.4049/jimmunol.1202611.

Ivanova, T. S., Krupodorova, T. A., Barshteyn, V. Y., Artamonova, A. B., & Shlyakhovenko, V. A. (2014). Anticancer substances of mushroom origin. *Experimental Oncology*, *36*(2), 58–66.

Jin, M. S., Kim, S. E., Heo, J. Y., Lee, M. E., Kim, H. M., Paik, S. G., et al. (2007). Crystal structure of the TLR1-TLR2 heterodimer induced by binding of a tri-acylated lipopeptide. *Cell*, *130*(6), 1071–1082. https://doi.org/10.1016/j.cell.2007.09.008.

Jin, Y., Li, P., & Wang, F. (2018). Beta-glucans as potential immunoadjuvants: A review on the adjuvanticity, structure-activity relationship and receptor recognition properties. *Vaccine*, *36*(35), 5235–5244. https://doi.org/10.1016/j.vaccine.2018.07.038.

Kalac, P. (2013). A review of chemical composition and nutritional value of wild-growing and cultivated mushrooms. *Journal of the Science of Food and Agriculture*, *93*(2), 209–218. https://doi.org/10.1002/jsfa.5960.

Kanagawa, M., Satoh, T., Ikeda, A., Adachi, Y., Ohno, N., & Yamaguchi, Y. (2011). Structural insights into recognition of triple-helical beta-glucans by an insect fungal receptor. *The Journal of Biological Chemistry*, *286*(33), 29158–29165. https://doi.org/10.1074/jbc.M111.256701.

Kang, J. Y., Nan, X., Jin, M. S., Youn, S. J., Ryu, Y. H., Mah, S., et al. (2009). Recognition of lipopeptide patterns by Toll-like receptor 2-Toll-like receptor 6 heterodimer. *Immunity*, *31*(6), 873–884. https://doi.org/10.1016/j.immuni.2009.09.018.

Kasaai, M. R., Charlet, G., Paquin, P., & Arul, J. (2003). Fragmentation of chitosan by microfluidization process. *Innovative Food Science & Emerging Technologies*, *4*(4), 403–413.

Kim, H. S., Kim, J. Y., Lee, H. K., Kim, M. S., Lee, S. R., Kang, J. S., et al. (2010). Dendritic cell activation by glucan isolated from *umbilicaria esculenta*. *Immune Network*, *10*(6), 188–197. https://doi.org/10.4110/in.2010.10.6.188.

Kony, D. B., Damm, W., Stoll, S., van Gunsteren, W. F., & Hunenberger, P. H. (2007). Explicit-solvent molecular dynamics simulations of the polysaccharide schizophyllan in water. *Biophysical Journal*, *93*(2), 442–455. https://doi.org/10.1529/biophysj.106.086116.

Li, B., Allendorf, D. J., Hansen, R., Marroquin, J., Ding, C., Cramer, D. E., et al. (2006). Yeast beta-glucan amplifies phagocyte killing of iC3b-opsonized tumor cells via complement receptor 3-Syk-phosphatidylinositol 3-kinase pathway. *Journal of Immunology*, *177*(3), 1661–1669. https://doi.org/10.4049/jimmunol.177.3.1661.

Li, X., Utomo, A., Cullere, X., Choi, M. M., Milner, D. A., Jr., Venkatesh, D., et al. (2011). The beta-glucan receptor Dectin-1 activates the integrin Mac-1 in neutrophils via Vav protein signaling to promote *Candida albicans* clearance. *Cell Host & Microbe*, *10*(6), 603–615. https://doi.org/10.1016/j.chom.2011.10.009.

Lin, Y. L., Liang, Y. C., Lee, S. S., & Chiang, B. L. (2005). Polysaccharide purified from *Ganoderma lucidum* induced activation and maturation of human monocyte-derived dendritic cells by the NF-kappaB and p38 mitogen-activated protein kinase pathways. *Journal of Leukocyte Biology*, *78*(2), 533–543. https://doi.org/10.1189/jlb.0804481.

Liu, H., Li, Y., Gao, J., Shi, A., Liu, L., Hu, H., et al. (2016). Effects of microfluidization with ionic liquids on the solubilization and structure of beta-D-glucan. *International Journal of Biological Macromolecules*, *84*, 394–401. https://doi.org/10.1016/j.ijbiomac.2015.12.014.

Liu, J., Zhang, C., Wang, Y., Yu, H., Liu, H., Wang, L., et al. (2011). Structural elucidation of a heteroglycan from the fruiting bodies of Agaricus blazei Murill. *International Journal of Biological Macromolecules*, *49*(4), 716–720. https://doi.org/10.1016/j.ijbiomac.2011.07.003.

Lu, H., Yang, Y., Gad, E., Wenner, C. A., Chang, A., Larson, E. R., et al. (2011). Polysaccharide krestin is a novel TLR2 agonist that mediates inhibition of tumor growth via stimulation of CD8 T cells and NK cells. *Clinical Cancer Research*, *17*(1), 67–76. https://doi.org/10.1158/1078-0432.CCR-10-1763.

Mahauthaman, R., Howell, C. J., Spur, B. W., Youlten, L. J., Clark, T. J., Lessof, M. H., et al. (1988). The generation and cellular distribution of leukotriene C4 in human eosinophils stimulated by unopsonized zymosan and glucan particles. *The Journal of Allergy and Clinical Immunology*, *81*(4), 696–705.

Meng, X., Liang, H., & Luo, L. (2016). Antitumor polysaccharides from mushrooms: A review on the structural characteristics, antitumor mechanisms and immunomodulating activities. *Carbohydrate Research*, *424*, 30–41. https://doi.org/10.1016/j.carres.2016.02.008.

Meyer-Wentrup, F., Figdor, C. G., Ansems, M., Brossart, P., Wright, M. D., Adema, G. J., et al. (2007). Dectin-1 interaction with tetraspanin CD37 inhibits IL-6 production. *Journal of Immunology*, *178*(1), 154–162. https://doi.org/10.4049/jimmunol.178.1.154.

Misaki, A., Kakuta, M., Sasaki, T., Tanaka, M., & Miyaji, H. (1981). Studies on interrelation of structure and antitumor effects of polysaccharides: Antitumor action of periodate-modified, branched (1 goes to 3)-beta-D-glucan of *Auricularia auricula-judae*, and other polysaccharides containing (1 goes to 3)-glycosidic linkages. *Carbohydrate Research*, *92*(1), 115–129.

Misaki, A., Kawaguchi, K., Miyaji, H., Nagae, H., Hokkoku, S., Kakuta, M., et al. (1984). Structure of pestalotan, a highly branched (1——3)-beta-D-glucan elaborated by Pestalotia sp. 815, and the enhancement of its antitumor activity by polyol modification of the side chains. *Carbohydrate Research*, *129*, 209–227.

Modak, S., Kushner, B. H., Kramer, K., Vickers, A., Cheung, I. Y., & Cheung, N. K. (2013). Anti-GD2 antibody 3F8 and barley-derived (1-> 3),(1-> 4)-beta-D-glucan: A phase I study in patients with chemoresistant neuroblastoma. *Oncoimmunology*, *2*(3). e23402https://doi.org/10.4161/onci.23402.

Mueller, A., Raptis, J., Rice, P. J., Kalbfleisch, J. H., Stout, R. D., Ensley, H. E., et al. (2000). The influence of glucan polymer structure and solution conformation on binding to (1->3)-beta-D-glucan receptors in a human monocyte-like cell line. *Glycobiology*, *10*(4), 339–346. https://doi.org/10.1093/glycob/10.4.339.

Murphy, E. A., Davis, J. M., & Carmichael, M. D. (2010). Immune modulating effects of beta-glucan. *Current Opinion in Clinical Nutrition and Metabolic Care*, *13*(6), 656–661. https://doi.org/10.1097/MCO.0b013e32833f1afb.

Nakashima, A., Yamada, K., Iwata, O., Sugimoto, R., Atsuji, K., Ogawa, T., et al. (2018). Beta-glucan in foods and its physiological functions. *Journal of Nutritional Science and Vitaminology (Tokyo)*, *64*(1), 8–17. https://doi.org/10.3177/jnsv.64.8.

Ohno, N., Miura, N. N., Chiba, N., Adachi, Y., & Yadomae, T. (1995). Comparison of the immunopharmacological activities of triple and single-helical schizophyllan in mice. *Biological & Pharmaceutical Bulletin*, *18*(9), 1242–1247.

Okazaki, M., Adachi, Y., Ohno, N., & Yadomae, T. (1995). Structure-activity relationship of (1->3)-beta-D-glucans in the induction of cytokine production from macrophages, in vitro. *Biological & Pharmaceutical Bulletin*, *18*(10), 1320–1327.

Ooi, V. E., & Liu, F. (2000). Immunomodulation and anti-cancer activity of polysaccharide-protein complexes. *Current Medicinal Chemistry*, 7(7), 715–729.

Osinska-Jaroszuk, M., Jarosz-Wilkolazka, A., Jaroszuk-Scisel, J., Szalapata, K., Nowak, A., Jaszek, M., et al. (2015). Extracellular polysaccharides from Ascomycota and Basidiomycota: Production conditions, biochemical characteristics, and biological properties. *World Journal of Microbiology and Biotechnology*, *31*(12), 1823–1844. https://doi.org/10.1007/s11274-015-1937-8.

Ostrop, J., & Lang, R. (2017). Contact, collaboration, and conflict: Signal integration of Syk-coupled C-type lectin receptors. *Journal of Immunology*, *198*(4), 1403–1414. https://doi.org/10.4049/jimmunol.1601665.

Ozinsky, A., Underhill, D. M., Fontenot, J. D., Hajjar, A. M., Smith, K. D., Wilson, C. B., et al. (2000). The repertoire for pattern recognition of pathogens by the innate immune system is defined by cooperation between toll-like receptors. *Proceedings of the National Academy of Sciences of the United States of America*, *97*(25), 13766–13771. https://doi.org/10.1073/pnas.250476497.

Palleschi, A., Bocchinfuso, G., Coviello, T., & Alhaique, F. (2005). Molecular dynamics investigations of the polysaccharide scleroglucan: First study on the triple helix structure. *Carbohydrate Research*, *340*(13), 2154–2162. https://doi.org/10.1016/j.carres.2005.06.026.

Patin, E. C., Thompson, A., & Orr, S. J. (2019). Pattern recognition receptors in fungal immunity. *Seminars in Cell & Developmental Biology*, *89*, 24–33. https://doi.org/10.1016/j.semcdb.2018.03.003.

Ren, L., Perera, C., & Hemar, Y. (2012). Antitumor activity of mushroom polysaccharides: A review. *Food & Function*, *3*(11), 1118–1130. https://doi.org/10.1039/c2fo10279j.

Rice, P. J., Adams, E. L., Ozment-Skelton, T., Gonzalez, A. J., Goldman, M. P., Lockhart, B. E., et al. (2005). Oral delivery and gastrointestinal absorption of soluble glucans stimulate increased resistance to infectious challenge. *The Journal of Pharmacology and Experimental Therapeutics*, *314*(3), 1079–1086. https://doi.org/10.1124/jpet.105.085415.

Rogers, N. C., Slack, E. C., Edwards, A. D., Nolte, M. A., Schulz, O., Schweighoffer, E., et al. (2005). Syk-dependent cytokine induction by Dectin-1 reveals a novel pattern recognition pathway for C type lectins. *Immunity*, *22*(4), 507–517. https://doi.org/10.1016/j.immuni.2005.03.004.

Rosas, M., Liddiard, K., Kimberg, M., Faro-Trindade, I., McDonald, J. U., Williams, D. L., et al. (2008). The induction of inflammation by dectin-1 in vivo is dependent on myeloid cell programming and the progression of phagocytosis. *Journal of Immunology*, *181*(5), 3549–3557. https://doi.org/10.4049/jimmunol.181.5.3549.

Ruthes, A. C., Smiderle, F. R., & Iacomini, M. (2016). Mushroom heteropolysaccharides: A review on their sources, structure and biological effects. *Carbohydrate Polymers*, *136*, 358–375. https://doi.org/10.1016/j.carbpol.2015.08.061.

Sahasrabudhe, N. M., Tian, L., Berg, M. v. d., Bruggeman, G., Bruininx, E., Schols, H. A., et al. (2016). Endo-glucanase digestion of oat β-glucan enhances Dectin-1 activation in human dendritic cells. *Journal of Functional Foods*, *21*, 104–112.

Salvador, C., Li, B., Hansen, R., Cramer, D. E., Kong, M., & Yan, J. (2008). Yeast-derived beta-glucan augments the therapeutic efficacy mediated by anti-vascular endothelial growth factor monoclonal antibody in human carcinoma xenograft models. *Clinical Cancer Research*, *14*(4), 1239–1247. https://doi.org/10.1158/1078-0432.CCR-07-1669.

Schnaar, R. L. (2016). Glycobiology simplified: Diverse roles of glycan recognition in inflammation. *Journal of Leukocyte Biology*, *99*(6), 825–838. https://doi.org/10.1189/jlb.3RI0116-021R.

Seo, B. S., Lee, S. H., Lee, J. E., Yoo, Y. C., Lee, J., & Park, S. R. (2013). Dectin-1 stimulation selectively reinforces LPS-driven IgG1 production by mouse B cells. *Immune Network*, *13*(5), 205–212. https://doi.org/10.4110/in.2013.13.5.205.

Snarr, B. D., Qureshi, S. T., & Sheppard, D. C. (2017). Immune recognition of fungal polysaccharides. *Journal of Fungi*, *3*(3), 47. https://doi.org/10.3390/jof3030047.

Strijbis, K., Tafesse, F. G., Fairn, G. D., Witte, M. D., Dougan, S. K., Watson, N., et al. (2013). Bruton's tyrosine kinase (BTK) and Vav1 contribute to Dectin1-dependent phagocytosis of *Candida albicans* in macrophages. *PLoS Pathogens*, *9*(6). e1003446. https://doi.org/10.1371/journal.ppat.1003446.

Tabata, K., Ito, W., Kojima, T., Kawabata, S., & Misaki, A. (1981). Ultrasonic degradation of schizophyllan, an antitumor polysaccharide produced by *Schizophyllum commune* fries. *Carbohydrate Research*, *89*(1), 121–135.

Taghavi, M., Mortaz, E., Khosravi, A., Vahedi, G., Folkerts, G., Varahram, M., et al. (2018). Zymosan attenuates melanoma growth progression, increases splenocyte proliferation and induces TLR-2/4 and TNF-alpha expression in mice. *Journal of Inflammation*, *15*, 5. https://doi.org/10.1186/s12950-018-0182-y.

Takeuchi, O., & Akira, S. (2010). Pattern recognition receptors and inflammation. *Cell*, *140*(6), 805–820. https://doi.org/10.1016/j.cell.2010.01.022.

Taylor, P. R., Brown, G. D., Reid, D. M., Willment, J. A., Martinez-Pomares, L., Gordon, S., et al. (2002). The beta-glucan receptor, dectin-1, is predominantly expressed on the surface of cells of the monocyte/macrophage and neutrophil lineages. *Journal of Immunology*, *169*(7), 3876–3882. https://doi.org/10.4049/jimmunol.169.7.3876.

Taylor, P. R., Tsoni, S. V., Willment, J. A., Dennehy, K. M., Rosas, M., Findon, H., et al. (2007). Dectin-1 is required for beta-glucan recognition and control of fungal infection. *Nature Immunology*, *8*(1), 31–38. https://doi.org/10.1038/ni1408.

Thornton, B. P., Vetvicka, V., Pitman, M., Goldman, R. C., & Ross, G. D. (1996). Analysis of the sugar specificity and molecular location of the beta-glucan-binding lectin site of complement receptor type 3 (CD11b/CD18). *Journal of Immunology*, *156*(3), 1235–1246.

Tian, J., Ma, J., Wang, S., Yan, J., Chen, J., Tong, J., et al. (2011). Increased expression of mGITRL on D2SC/1 cells by particulate beta-glucan impairs the suppressive effect of CD4+CD25+ regulatory T cells and enhances the effector T cell proliferation. *Cellular Immunology*, *270*(2), 183–187. https://doi.org/10.1016/j.cellimm.2011.05.003.

Tsukagoshi, S., Hashimoto, Y., Fujii, G., Kobayashi, H., Nomoto, K., & Orita, K. (1984). Krestin (PSK). *Cancer Treatment Reviews*, *11*(2), 131–155.

Usui, S., Tomono, Y., Sakai, M., Kiho, T., & Ukai, S. (1995). Preparation and antitumor activities of beta-(1–>6) branched (1–>3)-beta-D-glucan derivatives. *Biological & Pharmaceutical Bulletin*, *18*(12), 1630–1636.

van Bruggen, R., Drewniak, A., Jansen, M., van Houdt, M., Roos, D., Chapel, H., et al. (2009). Complement receptor 3, not Dectin-1, is the major receptor on human neutrophils for beta-glucan-bearing particles. *Molecular Immunology*, *47*(2–3), 575–581. https://doi.org/10.1016/j.molimm.2009.09.018.

Vorup-Jensen, T., & Jensen, R. K. (2018). Structural immunology of complement receptors 3 and 4. *Frontiers in Immunology*, *9*, 2716. https://doi.org/10.3389/fimmu.2018.02716.

Wang, Q., Sheng, X., Shi, A., Hu, H., Yang, Y., Liu, L., et al. (2017). Beta-glucans: Relationships between modification, conformation and functional activities. *Molecules*, *22*(2). https://doi.org/10.3390/molecules22020257.

Wang, D., Sun, S. Q., Wu, W. Z., Yang, S. L., & Tan, J. M. (2014). Characterization of a water-soluble polysaccharide from Boletus edulis and its antitumor and immunomodulatory activities on renal cancer in mice. *Carbohydrate Polymers*, *105*, 127–134. https://doi.org/10.1016/j.carbpol.2013.12.085.

Wang, X., Xu, X., & Zhang, L. (2008). Thermally induced conformation transition of triple-helical lentinan in NaCl aqueous solution. *The Journal of Physical Chemistry B*, *112*(33), 10343–10351. https://doi.org/10.1021/jp802174v.

Wasser, S. P. (2014). Medicinal mushroom science: Current perspectives, advances, evidences, and challenges. *Biomedical Journal*, *37*(6), 345–356. https://doi.org/10.4103/2319-4170.138318.

Willment, J. A., Gordon, S., & Brown, G. D. (2001). Characterization of the human beta-glucan receptor and its alternatively spliced isoforms. *The Journal of Biological Chemistry*, *276*(47), 43818–43823. https://doi.org/10.1074/jbc.M107715200.

Xia, Y., & Ross, G. D. (1999). Generation of recombinant fragments of CD11b expressing the functional beta-glucan-binding lectin site of CR3 (CD11b/CD18). *Journal of Immunology*, *162*(12), 7285–7293.

Xin, Y., Wang, X., Luo, L., & Meng, F. (2018). Conformation-dependent manipulation of human islet amyloid polypeptide fibrillation by shiitake-derived Lentinan. *ACS Applied Materials & Interfaces*, *10*(37), 31069–31079. https://doi.org/10.1021/acsami.8b11078.

Zhang, P., & Cheung, P. C. (2002). Evaluation of sulfated *Lentinus edodes* alpha-(1−>3)-D-glucan as a potential antitumor agent. *Bioscience, Biotechnology, and Biochemistry*, *66*(5), 1052–1056. https://doi.org/10.1271/bbb.66.1052.

Zhang, L., Li, X., Xu, X., & Zeng, F. (2005). Correlation between antitumor activity, molecular weight, and conformation of lentinan. *Carbohydrate Research*, *340*(8), 1515–1521. https://doi.org/10.1016/j.carres.2005.02.032.

Zhang, M., Zhang, Y., Zhang, L., & Tian, Q. (2019). Mushroom polysaccharide lentinan for treating different types of cancers: A review of 12 years clinical studies in China. *Progress in Molecular Biology and Translational Science*, *163*, 297–328. https://doi.org/10.1016/bs.pmbts.2019.02.013.

CHAPTER ELEVEN

Toxicity of traditional Chinese medicine herbal and mineral products

Runping Liu[a], Xiaojiaoyang Li[a], Nana Huang[b], Mengyue Fan[c], Rong Sun[b,c,d,*]

[a]Beijing University of Chinese Medicine, Beijing, China
[b]The Second Hospital of Shandong University, Shandong University, Jinan, China
[c]Tianjin University of Traditional Chinese Medicine, Tianjin, China
[d]Advanced Medical Research Institute, Shandong University, Jinan, China
*Corresponding author: e-mail address: sunrong@sdu.edu.cn

Contents

Abstract

Traditional Chinese medicine (TCM) has been used to treat numerous kinds of diseases for more than 2000 years in eastern Asian countries. A portion of the TCM herbal and mineral products are believed to be toxic according to modern standards, and are still widely prescribed in the clinic. However, some TCM products considered to be non-toxic or low-toxic have been reported to possess significant toxicological effects on different organs in both animal and human models. In this review, we define the term "toxic" in TCM, and then we summarize the advances in pharmacology and toxicology

Advances in Pharmacology, Volume 87
ISSN 1054-3589
https://doi.org/10.1016/bs.apha.2019.08.001

research of Toxic Traditional Chinese Medicine (TTCM), including Chinese aconite (Fu Zi), Arsenic Trioxide, *Tripterygium wilfordii* Hook f. (Thunder God Vine), herbal drugs derived from plants in the Aristolochiaceae Juss. family (Ma Dou Ling), and other TCM products. Finally, the compatibility art of TCM and modern pharmaceutical approaches to manage undesired toxicity of TTCM is discussed. Promoting pharmacology and toxicology studies of TTCM and non-toxic TCM is critical for the further development and safety of TCM in clinical practice.

Abbreviation

AA	aristolochic acid
AAN	AA-related nephropathy
AL	aristolactam
AMPK	AMP-activated protein kinase
APL	acute promyelocytic leukemia
ATF4	activating transcription factor 4
ATO	Arsenic trioxide
ATRA	all-trans retinoic acid
CHOP	C/EBP-homologous protein
CNS	central nervous system
DDAs	diester-diterpenoid alkaloids
DNMT	DNA methyltransferase
ER	endoplasmic reticulum
GABAα	gamma-aminobutyric acid
HIF-1α	hypoxia-inducible factor 1α
HLA-B	human leukocyte antigen-B
HO-1	oxygenase
HSP	heat shock protein
HVOD	hepatic veno-occlusive disease
IRE1	inositol-requiring ER-to-nucleus signal kinase 1
JNK	c-Jun N-terminal kinases
MAO	monoamine oxidase enzymes
MDAs	monoester-diterpenoid alkaloids
NMDA	*N*-methyl-D-aspartic acid receptor
Nrf2	nuclear factor (erythroid-derived 2)-like 2
PERK	PKR-like ER kinase
PAs	pyrrolizidine alkaloids
PM	*Polygonum multiflorum*
PML-RARα	promyelocytic leukemia protein-retinoic acid receptor α
RA	rheumatoid arthritis
RB	*Radix Bupleuri*
ROS	reactive oxygen species
SAM	S-adenosyl methionine
SIRT1/3	sirtuin 1/3
STAT3	signal transducing activator of transcription 3
TCM	traditional Chinese medicine

TFIIH	the basal transcription factor IIH
TP	triptolide
Th17	T helper cell 17
Treg	regulatory T cell
TTCM	toxic traditional Chinese medicine
TW	*Tripterygium wilfordii* Hook f., Thunder God Vine
UDAs	unesterified-diterpenoid alkaloids

1. Introduction

Traditional Chinese medicine (TCM) is an evidence- and clinic-based medical system which has been used to treat various diseases, from physical to psychological, in eastern Asia for over 2000 years. Treating patients with TCM helped China having 100 million people by the end of 1000 AD and having 400 million people by the end of 1900. Long history has proved TCM to be benefit over risk to people's health. According to the annual pharmacovigilance report from China FDA (2013–2017), TCM products-related adverse effects contributed to about 16% of all 1.5 million cases/year reported cases, which is 240,000 cases/year, whereas, synthetic chemical drugs-induced adverse effects contributed to more than 80% of all reports. Based on the estimated TCM consuming population in China, which is more than 140 million people or cases/year, the risk of TCM-induced adverse effects is pretty low (0.17%). The lack of systemic evaluation of pharmacology and toxicology using modern approaches and the not-well-identified material base of TCM products are the major reasons why TCM is not accepted as drugs by the western world. Nowadays, many doctors and scientists around the world are dedicated to investigating the pharmacology and toxicology of TCM products and to discovering the scientific principles of TCM theory.

Approximately 6000 TCM herbals and mineral products were historically documented in *Material Medica* books. Among the vast number of drugs, several are considered to be toxic based on both TCM and western medicine theory. Some of these toxic TCM (TTCM) agents are still widely used in clinics, either alone or in complex TCM formulations. With the development of modern pharmacology and toxicology, verification of toxicity of TCM products and evaluation of therapeutic effects of TTCM have attracted growing attention of researchers globally. Several potential toxic chemicals in TCM products have been identified and are restricted by newly designed administrative regulations to improve the safety of TCM during clinical practice in China. On the other hand, with the extensive preclinical studies and promising evidence from clinical studies, some of the classic TTCM drugs achieved success in the treatment of various fetal or previous untreatable diseases. Here, we first discuss the definition of "Toxic," or "Du" in Chinese, in the TCM theory system and provide a general introduction of documented TTCM cases in China Pharmacopeia. Specific products and formulations discussed include Chinese aconite (Fu Zi), Arsenic Trioxide, *Tripterygium wilfordii* Hook f. (Thunder God Vine) and herbal drugs derived from Aristolochiaceae Juss. plants (Ma Dou Ling). Toxicity induced by non-toxic TCM drugs and their management are also discussed. We aim to provide insights into the understanding of potential pharmacological effects of TTCM and the tight connection between therapeutic effects and toxicity in TCM theory.

2. Definition of "Du" or "Toxic" in traditional Chinese medicine (TCM)

In the theory system of TCM, the definition of "Toxic," or "Du" in Chinese, is different from the definition of toxicity that in modern medicine and toxicology. General defined "Du" in TCM indicates the integrative effects of a TCM product, including both pharmacological and toxicological effects. From this perspective, all drugs have toxicity and all toxins are potential medicines. This is the ancient philosophy of TCM. As recorded in *Zhou Li-Tian Guan Zhong Zai* (*The Rites of Zhou*), a constitutional file formed at Han Dynasty (200 AD), "Doctors follow the rules of medicine, and manipulate toxic to treat diseases." In addition, "Du" represents any special effect of an individual TCM product against human, which is also called "Pian Xing." *Shen Nong Ben Cao Jing (Shen Nong's Materia Medica)*, written during the Han dynasty more than 1700 years ago, first mentioned several basal concepts describing "Pian Xing," as one of the five flavors ("Wei" in Chinese) (sour, salty, sweet, bitter and spicy), four properties ("Qi" in Chinese) (cold, cool, warm and hot), and "Du" of TCM products. In TCM theory, pharmacological effects of any herbal or TCM drugs depend on "Du" or "Pian Xing." Generally speaking, the biological effects of the herbal or other TCM products that have greater "Du" or "Pian Xing" are usually rapid onset and intense. On the other hand, narrowly defined "Du" in TCM is similar to the definition of toxicity in western medicine and the narrowly defined toxic TCM (TTCM) is the focus of this review. The safe pharmacological dose range of TTCM is limited in clinical practice. Misuse or drug overdose of TTCM will usually lead to severe organ injury or even death.

The concept of "Du" grade has been known in TCM for more than two millenia. The term, "Du," in this context is usually is the combination of both "Pianxing" and narrowly defined "Du." In Shen Nong Ben Cao Jing, 365 documented TCM products were first archived into three categories, including "top grade," "average grade" and "lowest grade," based on the "Du" grade. For this categorization, the term of "Du" usually reflects "Pian Xing" rather than toxicity of a TCM product. For instance, "Zhu Sha," which is HgO with significant toxicity, was listed in "top grade," simply because it has no "Flavor." Whereas, the authors have also noticed the potential toxicity of TCM products. As paraphrased, it states the "lowest grade" TCM products were "only used to treat diseases in specific regions that lack sufficient herbal resources, and were usually toxic during long-term use". Later on, the definition of "Du" evolved to include both the concept of "Pian Xing" and toxicity, since the ancient TCM practices had become aware of the "Pian Xing"-related toxicity of TCM products. Famous TCM experts, Jingyue Zhang and Zihe Zhang, further emphasized the concept of "great Du," "average Du," "mild Du," and "no Du" and the relationship between "Du" of a TCM product and their pharmacological effects. As recorded in *Huang Di Nei Jing- Su Wen*, the first medical book of TCM theory, "To avoid harm to the body from TCM products, stop the treatment when 60% of the disease is removed when using TCM product of 'great Du'; stop the treatment when 70% of the disease is removed when using TCM product of 'average Du'; stop the treatment when 80% of the disease is removed when using TCM product of 'mild Du'; stop the treatment when 90% of the disease is removed when using TCM product of 'no Du'; and then using proper foods to improve the homeostasis of the body and cure the disease completely." This record represents the ancient philosophy of TCM for managing toxicity during the therapy. Systemic "Du" records for individual TCM products were first found in *Wu Pu's Materia Medica* written at the era of Three Kingdoms. Since then, most of the *Materia Medica* books, including *Xin Xiu Ben Cao* at Tang Dynasty, *Zheng Lei Ben Cao* at Song Dynasty and *Ben Cao Gang Mu* at Ming Dynasty by Shizhen Li, recorded "Du" grade of a TCM product as essential information.

3. Documented TTCM in China pharmacopeia

With the development of modern pharmacology and toxicology, studies regarding the toxicity of TTCM and other TCM drugs have drawn great attention. However, systemic toxicity evaluation and clinical pharmacovigilance of TCM drugs or formulas are still lacking, leading to incomparable experimental evidence and vague national regulatory standards. The China Pharmacopeia has clear records regarding the collection, processing, regular dose of clinical use, however, the description of the "Du" grade of TCM drugs is mainly based on the summary of ancient TCM articles or *Materia Medica* books and is more similar to the concept of toxicity in modern medicine. The current China Pharmacopeia (2015) recorded 618 TCM products, in which 83 products (13.43%) are documented as TTCM and are further divided into three grades, including "great toxic," "average toxic," and "mild toxic," according to the severity of toxicity or toxic dose threshold.

General information of TTCM documented in the China Pharmacopeia and widely used TCM drugs with potential toxicity which are not recorded as toxic in the China Pharmacopeia are shown in Table 1.

4. Advances in pharmacology studies and application of classic TTCM

According to the established TCM theory, the connection between "toxic" and pharmacological effects is dialectic but not antagonistic. In TCM clinical practice, syndrome differentiation ("Bian Zheng" in Chinese) is critical for determining the treatment, requiring the identification of the age, gender, constitution (physical fitness) and the specific condition of disease progression of the individual patient. Under successful syndrome differentiation, even TTCM with relatively high toxicity will be well tolerated by patients and will usually achieve better therapeutic effects when compared to TCM drugs with mild or no toxicity. On the other hand, failed syndrome differentiation will lead to adverse or toxic effects induced by non-toxic or mild toxic TCM drugs. Although the TCM theory is substantially different from modern medicine, numerous efforts have been dedicated in the past decades to elucidating the underlying mechanism of TTCM clinical practice by using modern pharmacology and toxicology approaches.

Table 1 General information for toxic TCM.

Name	Chinese Name	Bioactive compounds	Toxic chemicals	Target organs clinical (symptoms)	Target organs experimental	Daily dose[a]	"Toxic" grade	Recorded as toxic in CP?
Aconiti Radix	Chuan wu	Aconitine, Hypaconitine, Neoaconitine, Deoxyaconitine, Neoaconine	Aconitine, Mesaconitine, Hypaconitine, Higenamine	Heart, nervous system (nausea, vomiting, abdominal pain and diarrhea, muscle tremor, arrhythmias, central paralysis when severe) (Li et al., 2019)	Uterus, ovary (Ren, 2009), testes (Zhang, Wang, Wang, Wang, & Li, 2007)	Processing needed. Usually no direct use	Highly toxic	Yes
Aconiti Kusnezoffii Folium	Cao wu ye	Aconitum alkaloids	Aconitum alkaloids	Heart, nervous system (similar to Chuan wu) (Wang, Gong, Duan, Lv, & Du, 2019; Zan et al., 2018)		1–1.2 g	Mild toxic	Yes
Aconiti Kusnezoffii Radix	Cao wu	Aconitine, Hypaconitine, Neoaconitine	Aconitine, Hypaconitine, Neoaconitine	Heart, brain, kidney (similar to Chuan wu, shock or death when severe) (Wang et al., 2018)	Genotoxicity (Wei, Yan, Liu, & Zhao, 2011), embryo, testes, ovary (Miao et al., 2018)	Processing needed. Usually no direct use	Highly toxic	Yes
Aconiti Kusnezoffii Radix Cocta	Zhi cao wu (processed Cao wu)	Isaconatine, Benzoylhypacoitine, Benzoylmesaconine, Aconitine, Hypaconitine, Neoaconitine	–	–	Heart (Ye et al., 2019), nervous system (Wang, Wang, & Zhu, 2018)	1.5–3 g	Average toxic	Yes
Aconiti Radix Cocta	Zhi chuan wu (processed Chuan wu)	Isaconatine, Benzoylhypacoitine, Benzoylmesaconine	–	–	–	1.5–3 g	Average toxic	Yes
Aconm Lateralis Radix Praeparaia	Fu zi	Aconitine, Hypaconitine, Neoaconitine	Aconitine, Hypaconitine, Neoaconitine	Nervous system, heart, digestive system (numb limbs, numb tongue and mouth, nausea, vomiting, abdominal pain and diarrhea, palpitation, arrhythmias) (Yang, Xia, Tian, Li, & Sun, 2017)	–	3–15 g	Average toxic	Yes

Continued

Table 1 General information for toxic TCM.—cont'd

Name	Chinese Name	Bioactive compounds	Toxic chemicals	Target organs clinical (symptoms)	Target organs experimental	Daily dose[a]	"Toxic" grade	Recorded as toxic in CP?
Agkistrodon	Qi she	Proteins and amino acids, Phospholipids, Nucleosides	Hemolytic toxin	Blood system (bleeding, local tissue swelling and necrosis) (Liu, Liu, Feng, Guo, & Liu, 2018)	–	3–9 g, 1–3 g per time and 3 times/day	Average toxic	Yes
Anemones Raddeanae Rhizoma	Liang tou jian	Raddeanin A	Anemonin, Ranunculin, Protoanemonin, Raddeanin A	–	Heart (Zhou, Sun, Li, Wang, & Liu, 2007)	1–3 g	Average toxic	Yes
Arisaematis Rhizoma	Tian nan xing	Apigenin	CaC_2O_4	Oral, pharynx, larynx and skin mucosa (burning throat, numb tongue and mouth, mucosa edema and erosion, difficult in opening mouth, asphyxia when severe) (Fan, Li, Xiao, & Lin, 2003)	Kidney (Dong et al., 2015)	External use. Processing needed for internal use	Average toxic	Yes
Arisaematis Rhizoma Preparatum	Zhi tian nan xing (processed Tian nan xing)	Apigenin	–	–	–	3–9 g	Average toxic	Yes
Armeniacae Semen Amarum	Ku xing ren	Amygdalin	Amygdalin (decomposed to prussic acid by acid or enzyme)	Lung, colon, nervous system (at first: nausea, vomiting, abdominal pain and diarrhea, headache, palpitation, hypertension; severe intoxication: hypotension, loss of consciousness, tachypnea, mydriasis, death due to respiratory paralysis) (Du, Zhang, & Zhao, 2013)	–	5–10 g	Mild toxic	Yes
Artemisiae Argyi Folium	Ai ye	Eucalyptol, Thujone, 6-Methoxyflavone, Luteolin, B-Amyrin, Acidic Polysaccharides, Catecholamine, Trace Element	Moxa volatile oil	Liver, digestive system (nausea, vomiting, abdominal pain and diarrhea, acute gastroenteritis; abnormal liver function) (Sun, Wang, Huang, Chi, & Miao, 2010)	Kidney, genotoxicity, embryo (Zhang, Kang, Guo, & Zhou, 2017)	3–9 g	Mild toxic	Yes

Berberidis Radix	San ke zhen	Berberine hydrochloride	–	–		9–15 g	Average toxic	Yes
Bruceae Fructus	Ya dan zi	Fatty acids: Oleic acid, Nigakilactone	Nigakilactone	–	Stomach, intestine, liver, kidney (Sun & Yang, 2010)	0.5–2 g	Mild toxic	Yes
Bufonis Venenum	Chan su	Cifogenin, Resibufogenin	Bufadienolides	Heart, nervous system, digestive system (palpitation, paroxysmal atrial arrhythmia, sinus arrhythmia, atrioventricular block, atrial fibrillation; dizziness and headache, numb limbs and mouth, convulsion) (Li, Li, Wang, & Ma, 2016)	–	Internal use: 0.015–0.03 g	Average toxic	Yes
Bungarus Parvus	Jin qian bai hua she	Phosphatidic constituents	Cadmium	–	–	2–5 g	Average toxic	Yes
Calomelas	Qing fen	Mercurous chloride	Mercurous chloride	Liver, kidney, cardiovascular system, nervous system (elevation of serum ALT and AST, kidney failure, hypertension, allergy, skin irritation) (Qiu & Wang, 2015)	–	Internal use: 0.1–0.4 g	Average toxic	Yes
Carotae Fructus	Nan he shi	Asarone, Bisabolene, Crotonic acid, Asarylaldehyde	–	–	–	3–9 g	Mild toxic	Yes
Carpesii Fructus	He shi	Valerianic acid, N-hexanoic acid, Oleic acid, Stigmasterol	–	–	–	3–9 g	Mild toxic	Yes
Chelidonii Herba	Bai qu cai	Chelerythrine, Chelidonine	Macleyine, Coptisine, Chelerythrine	–	Multi-organ (Luo, Ma, & Lin, 2014)	9–18 g	Average toxic	Yes
Cinnabaris	Zhu sha	Mercury sulfide	Mercury sulfide	Nervous system, liver, kidney (nausea, vomiting, abdominal pain and diarrhea; difficult in opening mouth, body tremor; oliguria, anuria, kidney failure; arrhythmia; coma and even death) (Ding et al., 2016)	Lung (Yen et al., 2008), reproductive system (Gu et al., 2011), genotoxicity (Zhang, Wu, & Tang, 2011)	0.1–0.5 g	Average toxic	Yes

Continued

Table 1 General information for toxic TCM.—cont'd

Name	Chinese Name	Bioactive compounds	Toxic chemicals	Target organs clinical (symptoms)	Target organs experimental	Daily dose[a]	"Toxic" grade	Recorded as toxic in CP?
Cnidii Fructus	She chuang zi	Osthole	–	–	–	Internal use: 3–10 g	Mild toxic	Yes
Crotonis Fructus	Ba dou	Crotonoside, Croton oil, Magnoflorine, Croton total protein	Croton oil, Crotin	Intestine (abdominal pain) (Shan et al., 2018)	–	0.1–0.3 g	Highly toxic	Yes
Crotonis Semen Pulveratum	Ba dou shuang	Crotonoside, Croton oil, Magnoflorine, Croton total protein	Croton oil, Crotin	–	Intestine (Shan et al., 2018)	0.1–0.3 g	Highly toxic	Yes
Curculiginis Rhizoma	Xian mao	Curculigoside	–	Nervous system, heart (hyperhydrosis, numb limbs; palpitation, irritability, arrhythmia) (Wang, Zhang, Kong, & Du, 2018)	Liver, kidney, ovary, testis (Bao, Zhao, Song, & Li, 2011)	3–10 g	Average toxic	Yes
Daturae Flos	Yang jin hua	Scopolamine, Scopolamine, Atropine	–	Lung, heart, nervous system, digestive system (tachypnea, dyspnea; arrhythmia; irritability, dizziness; nausea, vomiting, constipation) (Jiang, Gao, Tian, Peng, & Xia, 2016)		0.3–0.6 g	Average toxic	Yes
Dichroae Radix	Chang shan	Dichroine A, B and C	Dichroine A, B and C	–	Digestive system, nervous system (Li et al., 2018)	5–9 g	Average toxic	Yes
Dryopteridis Crassirhizomatis Rhizoma	Mian ma guan zhong	Phloroglucinol derivatives	–	–	–	4.5–9 g	Mild toxic	Yes
Dryopteridis Crassirhizomatis Rhizoma Carbonisatum	Mian ma guan zhong tan (processed Mian ma guan zhong)	Filicic acid, Flavaspidic acid, Albaspidin	–	–	–	5–10 g	Mild toxic	Yes
Entadae Semen	Ke teng zi	–	–	–	–	10–15 g	Mild toxic	Yes

Erycibes Caulis	Ding gong teng	Erycib alkaloid, Scopolamine, Scopoletin	–	Liver, spleen, stomach (hyperhidrosis, numb limbs, nausea, vomiting, hypertension; allergy: allergic shock and death) (Fan & Mei, 2012)		3–6 g	Mild toxic	Yes
Euodiae Fructus	Wu zhu yu	Evodiamine, Rutaecarpine, Limonin, Evodin	Evodiamine, Rutaecarpine, Evodin	Nervous system (blurred vision, illusion, chest distress) (Cai, Meng, & Yang, 2006)	Liver, kidney, genotoxicity (Chen, Dong, Li, & Yuan, 2017)	2–5 g	Mild toxic	Yes
Euphorbiae Ebracteolatae Radix	Lang du	Diterpenoids, Acetophenones, Flavones	Euphorbia Ebiacteolata Hayata Water Extract	Stomach, intestine, heart (nausea, vomiting, abdominal pain, diarrhea, dizziness, irritability, palpitation) (Han, Qu, Ma, Cao, & Wang, 2013)	Spleen, kidney, liver (Liwei et al., 2018)	External use	Average toxic	Yes
Euphorbiae Hirtae Herba	Fei yang cao	Flavonoids, Tannins, Triterpenes	Diterpenoids	Intestine (abdominal pain, diarrhea) (Xin, Sun, Long, Wang, & Cheng, 2014)	–	6–9 g	Mild toxic	Yes
Euphorbiae Semen	Qian jin zi	Euphorbia sterol	–	–	–	1–2 g	Average toxic	Yes
Euphorbiae Semen Pulveratum	Qian jin zi Shuang (processed Qian jin zi)	Fatty oil	–	–	–	0.5–1 g	Average toxic	Yes
Eupolyphaga Steleophaga	Tu bie chong	Amino acid, Naphthalene, Aliphatic aldehyde, Aromatic aldehydes	–	–	Liver, brain, cardiovascular system (Yang, 2002)	3–10 g	Mild toxic	Yes
Genkwa Flos	Yuan hua	Daphnetin, Genkwanin	–	–	Liver, kidney (Zhou, Sun, Xiao, Liu, & Zhang, 2019)	1.5–3 g	Average toxic	Yes
Ginkgo Semen	Bai guo	Kaempferin, Quercetin, Rutin, Bilobetin, Ginkgetin	Ginkgol, Hydrocyanic acid	Central nervous system, respiratory system, liver, kidney (fatigue, sleepiness, convulsion; vomiting, abdominal pain; kidney injury: proteinuria, erythrocyturia) (Zhao & Wei, 2016)	–	5–10 g	Average toxic	Yes

Continued

Table 1 General information for toxic TCM.—cont'd

Name	Chinese Name	Bioactive compounds	Toxic chemicals	Target organs clinical (symptoms)	Target organs experimental	Daily dose[a]	"Toxic" grade	Recorded as toxic in CP?
Gleditsiae Fructus Abnormalis	Zhu ya zao	Triterpenoid saponins	–	Digestive system (vomiting and diarrhea)	–	1–1.5 g	Mild toxic	Yes
Gleditsiae Sinensis Fructus	Da zao jiao	Total saponins, Echinocystic acid	–	Lung, colon (abdominal pain, diarrhea) (Lu & Zhang, 2013)	–	1–1.5 g	Mild toxic	Yes
Hirudo	Shui zhi	Hirudin, Heparin, Histamine	–	–	–	1–3 g	Average toxic	Yes
Hydrargyri Oxydum Rubrum	Hong fen	HgO	HgO	Nervous system (abnormal of motor and sensory nervous system, tremor, ataxia) (Fields, Borak, & Louis, 2017)	Kidney, liver (Wang et al., 2017)	External use only	Highly toxic	Yes
Hyoscyami Semen	Tian xian zi	Scopolamine, Atropine	Scopolamine, Atropine	Heart, brain (xerostomia, difficult to swallow, dry mucosa and skin, headache, tachycardia, blurred vision, dysuria; when severe: dizziness, mania, or mental deterioration, sleepiness; death due to hypotension and respiratory failure) (Wang, Qiao, Li, & Xu, 2018)	–	0.06–0.6 g	Highly toxic	Yes
Illicii Cortex	Di feng pi	Difengpin, Magnolol, B-Sitosterol, Linalool	Safrole	–	Liver (Chien et al., 2018; Yang et al., 2018)	6–9 g	Mild toxic	Yes
Impatientis Semen	Ji xing zi	Hosenkosidek, A	Sterols	(Dry throat, nausea, inappetence) (Kong, Li, & Du, 2018)	–	3–5 g	Mild toxic	Yes
Kansui Radix	Gan sui	Euphol	–	Heart, liver, kidney (abdominal pain, diarrhea, dehydration, respiratory failure and central paralysis when severe) (Zhang, 2014)	–	0.5–1.5 g	Average toxic	Yes
Knoxiae Radix	Hong da ji	Lucidin, 3-Hydroxy Morinda Quinone	Lucidin	–	Kidney, genotoxicity (Wu, Wang, Cheng, Zhao, & Li, 2017)	Internal use 1.5–3 g	Mild toxic	Yes
Laggerae Herba	Chou ling dan cao	Sbsinthin	–	–	–	9–15 g	Average toxic	Yes

Meliae Cortex	Ku lian pi	Mersosin, Toosendanin, Isotoosendanin, Kulinone, Kulactone, Kulolactone	Toosendanin	–	Liver, kidney (Luo, Lu, Chen, & Wang, 2016)	3–6 g	Average toxic	Yes
Menispermi Rhizoma	Bei dou gen	Daurisoline, Dauricine, Sinomenine	Dauricine, Sinomenine	Stomach, intestine (diarrhea, inappetence) (Sun & Wang, 2009)	Liver, kidney (Zhou, Jin, & Yao, 2012)	3–9 g	Mild toxic	Yes
Momordicae Semen	Mu bie zi	Gypsogenin	–	–	–	Internal use 0.9–1.2 g	Average toxic	Yes
Murrayae Folium Et Cacumen	Jiu li xiang	Murrayone, Murpanidin, Isomexoticin	–	–	Liver, stomach (Huang, Yang, Huang, & Yang, 2017)	6–12 g	Mild toxic	Yes
Mylabris	Ban mao	Cantharidin	Cantharidin	Multi-organ, internal use: digestive system, urinary system External use: skin (nausea, vomiting, abdominal pain, diarrhea, alimentary tract hemorrhage; acute kidney injury, hematuresis, frequent urination, oliguria; dizziness, headache, fever, shock) (Yu & Yu, 2019)	–	0.03–0.06 g, internal use after processed	Highly toxic	Yes
Osmundae Rhizoma	Zi qi guan zhong	Ponasteronea, Ecdysterone, Ecdysone	–	–	–	5–9 g	Mild toxic	Yes
Papaveris Pericarpium	Ying su qiao	Morphine	Morphine, Codeine, Narcotine, Papaverine	Nervous system, digestive system (addiction, withdrawal symptom) (Tan, Yang, Zhang, & Du, 2019)	–	3–6 g	Average toxic	Yes
Paridis Rhizoma	Chong lou	Polyphyllini, Ii,Vi, Vii	–	–	Digestive system, nervous system , reproductive system (Chen & Yan, 2012)	3–9 g	Mild toxic	Yes

Continued

Table 1 General information for toxic TCM.—cont'd

Name	Chinese Name	Bioactive compounds	Toxic chemicals	Target organs clinical (symptoms)	Target organs experimental	Daily dose[a]	"Toxic" grade	Recorded as toxic in CP?
Periplocae Cortex	Xiang jia pi	4-Methoxysalicylaldehyde, Periplocin, Isovanillin	Periplocin	–	Heart, liver, kidney (Wang, Yang, Li, & Li, 2016)	3–6 g	Average toxic	Yes
Pharbitidis Semen	Qian niu zi	Pharbitisin, Chanoclavine, Ergoklinine, Cinnamic acid	Ergot alkaloids, Pharbitisin	–	Intestine, kidney, nervous system (He, Yu, Yang, & Du, 2018)	3–6 g	Average toxic	Yes
Physochlainae Radix	Hua shan shen	Hyoscyamine, Scopoletin, Anisodamine, Scopolamine, Atropine	Tropane alkaloids	–	Central nervous system, cardiovascular system, respiratory system, liver, kidney (Li, Lei, Yan, & Luo, 2008)	0.1–0.2 g	Average toxic	Yes
Phytolaccae Radix	Shang lu	Esculentoside A	Esculentoside	Digestive system, cardiovascular system, respiratory system, nervous system (nausea, vomiting, dizziness, headache, blurred vision, fatigue, trance, sinus tachycardia; When severe: convulsion, coma, shock and even death) (Li & Yao, 2011)		3–9 g	Average toxic	Yes
Picrasmae Ramulus Et Folium	Ku mu	4-Methoxy-5-Hydroxycanthin-6-One, Nigakihemiacetal A, B, C, D, E, F	Quassinoids, Alkaloids	Colon, lung (vomiting, diarrhea, dizziness, convulsion, cough, tachypnea) (Fu, Wang, Li, Wang, & Du, 2019)		1–4.5 g	Mild toxic	Yes
Pinelliae Rhizoma	Ban xia	Succinic acid, Amino acid, Pinellin, Alkaloids	Lectin protein	Nervous system (at first: numb mouth, dry throat, throat hyperemia, dysphagia, intensive vomiting, diarrhea, fever, hyperhidrosis, palpitation; when severe: laryngeal spasm, death due to respiratory paralysis) (Hu, Wang, Zhang, & Sun, 2016)	Kidney, liver, embryotoxicity (Hu et al., 2016; Zhang et al., 2011)	Internal use, 3–9 g after processed	Average toxic	Yes

Psammosilenes Radix	Jin tie suo	Triterpenoid Saponin, Cyclic Peptides, Lactam Alkaloids, Alkaloids, Maltophenols, Lignans	Saponins	Mucosa irritation (throat discomfort) (Wang, Zhang, et al., 2018)	–	0.1–0.3 g	Mild toxic	Yes
Pseudolaricis Cortex	Tu jing pi	Pseudolaric acid B	–	–	–	External use	Average toxic	Yes
Pterocephali Herba	Yi shou cao	Oleanolic acid	–	–	–	1–3 g	Mild toxic	Yes
Realgar	Xiong huang	As_2S_2	Arsenic	Nervous system, digestive system, urinary system, cardiovascular system, hemopoietic system, skin (nausea, vomiting, headache, dizziness, fatigue, pain of limbs; when severe: convulsion, acute kidney failure, coma and death) (Li, Wang, & Du, 2018)	–	0.05–0.1 g	Average toxic	Yes
Rhododendri Mollis Flos	Nao yang hua	Farrerol, Grayanotoxini, Rhodojaponiniii, Rhodomolleinii, Ericolin, Kalmitoxin	Grayanotoxini, Rhodojaponiniii, Rhodomolleinii, Ericolin, Kalmitoxin	Heart, lung, brain (nausea, vomiting, abdominal pain, diarrhea, slow heartbeat, hypotension, dyspnea, respiratory failure and death) (Li, Li, Huang, Liu, & Sun, 2018)	–	0.6–1.5 g	Highly toxic	Yes
Ricini Semen	Bi ma zi	Ricinine	Ricin	Liver, kidney, stomach, intestine, central nervous system, respiratory system (throat irritation, nausea, abdominal pain, diarrhea; liver injury; kidney injury; hemorrhagic gastritis, hemorrhagic enteritis; when severe: reparatory and vasomotor central paralysis, death) (Yan et al., 2017)	–	2–5 g	Average toxic	Yes

Continued

Table 1 General information for toxic TCM.—cont'd

Name	Chinese Name	Bioactive compounds	Toxic chemicals	Target organs clinical (symptoms)	Target organs experimental	Daily dose[a]	"Toxic" grade	Recorded as toxic in CP?
Scolopendra	Wu gong	Aflatoxin	Substances, Hemolytic protein	Digestive system, nervous system, respiratory system (nausea, vomiting, abdominal pain, diarrhea, fatigue, unconsciousness, slow heartbeat, hypotension and low body temperature) (Qiang, Fang, & Du, 2019)	–	3–5 g	Average toxic	Yes
Scorpio	Quan xie	Scorpion Venom, Trimethylamine, Betaine, Nucleosides	Insect toxins, Mammalian toxins	–	Nervous system, respiratory system (Liang, Zhao, B5ao, Yang, & Liu, 2017)	3–6 g	Average toxic	Yes
Sinopodophylli Fructus	Xiao ye lian	8,2′-Diisoprenyl Quercetin-3-Methyl Ether, 8-Isoprenyl Kaempferol, Podophyllotoxin, Deoxypodophyllotoxin, 4′-Nordeoxypodophyllotoxin	–	–	–	3–9 g	Mild toxic	Yes
Sophorae Tonkinensis Radix Et Rhizoma	Shan dou gen	Matrine, Oxymatrine	–	Digestive system, nervous system (dizziness, headache, nausea, vomiting, chest distress, palpitation, fatigue; when severe: pale face, body tremor, alalia, hobble) (Nie et al., 2018)	Kidney (Zhang & Shen, 2018)	3–6 g	Average toxic	Yes
Strychni Semen	Ma qian zi	Strychnine, Brucine	Strychnine, Brucine	Nervous system, heart (early stage: nausea, dizziness, vomiting, anxiety; middle stage: convulsion, hypersensitive to environment, entasia, opisthotonos, tonic convulsion; late stage: dyspnea, death from suffocation due to intensive spasm of respiratory muscles) (Zhang, Li, & Du, 2018)	Kidney, liver (Fan et al., 2018)	0.3–0.6 g, processing needed for internal use	Highly toxic	Yes

Strychni Semen Pulveratum	Ma qian zi Fen (processed Ma qian zi)	Strychnine, Brucine	Strychnine, Brucine	Nervous system, heart (similar to Ma qian zi) (Bao & Tu, 2000)	Kidney (Wu et al., 2016)	0.3–0.6 g	Highly toxic	Yes
Sulfur	Liu huang	S, As, Se, Te	S, As, Se, Te	Multi-organ (mild intoxication: photophobia, watering, foreign body sensation, keratitis, conjunctivitis; burning throat; moderate intoxication: central nervous system symptoms, vomiting, dizziness, headache, palpitation, tachypnea, fatigue, large liver; severe intoxication: dyspnea, low levels of consciousness, corestenoma, convulsion, coma, respiratory central paralysis, death) (Liu, 2012)	–	External use	Average toxic	Yes
Toosendan Fructus	Chuan lian zi	Toosendanin, Melianone, Melianol	Toosendanin	–	Liver, kidney, central nervous system (Chen, Wang, & Du, 2018)	5–10 g	Mild toxic	Yes
Toxicodendri Resina	Gan qi	Urushiol	–	Multi-organ (dizziness, headache, liver and kidney injury, convulsion when severe) (Wang, Lu, Meng, & Ji, 2014)	–	2–5 g	Average toxic	Yes
Tribuli Fructus	Ji li	Total saponins of tribulus	–	–	–	6–10 g	Mild toxic	Yes
Typhonii Rhizoma	Bai fu zi (processed Fu zi)	Hypaaconitine	–	Stomach, intestine, oropharynx (numb mouth, burning throat, stiff tongue, followed by numb limbs and muscle tremor; vomiting, salivation) (Huang, Dai, & Ma, 2015; Ni, Qi, Ma, & Wang, 2014)	–	3–6 g, processing needed for internal use	Average toxic	Yes

Continued

Table 1 General information for toxic TCM.—cont'd

Name	Chinese Name	Bioactive compounds	Toxic chemicals	Target organs clinical (symptoms)	Target organs experimental	Daily dose[a]	"Toxic" grade	Recorded as toxic in CP?
Xanthii Fructus	Cang er zi	Chlorogenic acid, 1,5-Dicaffeoylquinic acid, Carboxyatractyloside	Atractyloside, Dicaffeoylquinic acid	Liver, heart, kidney, skin, nervous system (nausea, vomiting, abdominal pain; liver injury/necrotic liver damage; chest distress, hyperhidrosis, cough, sinus tachycardia; oliguria, tea-colored urine, face edema; rash; convulsion and abnormal electroencephalogram) (Nie et al., 2019)	–	3–10 g	Average toxic	Yes
Zanthoxyl Radix	Liang mian zhen	Nitidine, Oxynitidine, Nitidine chloride	Oxynitidine, Nitidine chloride	Nervous system (dizziness, vomiting, dumb whole body, dyspnea, disturbance of consciousness) (Li & Liu, 2018)	Liver, kidney (Wei, Liu, Li, & Liu, 2009)	5–10 g	Mild toxic	Yes
Radix Et Rhizoma Tripterygii Wilfordii	Lei gong teng	Triptolide, Tripterygium Glycosides, Celastrol	Triptolide, Tripterygium glycosides, Celastrol	Heart, kidney, liver, testes, ovary (chest distress, palpitation, arrhythmia; oliguria, hematuresis, acute kidney injury, inappetence, fatigue, large liver; reproductive organs atrophy, sexual hypoactivity) (Li, Jiang, & Zhang, 2014)	Liver, kidney, reproductive system, multi-organs (Li et al., 2014)	Internal use: 15–25 g (*Chinese Material Medica*, not recorded in CP)	Highly toxic	Not recorded in CP
Acori Tatarinowii Rhizoma	Shi chang pu	Volatile oil (Asaryl ether)	Volatile oil (Asaryl ether)	–	Brain, kidney, liver, genotoxicity (Li et al., 2014)	3–10 g	Mild toxic	No
Angelicae Sinensis Radix	Dang gui	Volatile Oils, Polysaccharides, Flavonoids, Ferulic acid	Arsenic	–	Liver, kidney (Wang, Jia, & Li, 2012)	6–12 g	Mild toxic	No

Asari Radix Et Rhizoma	Xi xin	Heterotropan, Asarone, Aristolochic acid	Asarone, Aristolochic acid	–	Lung (Li, Han, et al., 2018; Li, Du, et al., 2018; Li, Wang, & Du, 2018), kidney (Michl, Bello, Kite, Simmonds, & Heinrich, 2017), testes (Cui et al., 2019), ovary (Tan et al., 2019), genotoxicity (Stegmuller, Schrenk, & Cartus, 2018)	1–3 g	Average toxic	No
Bupleuri Radix	Chai hu	Bupleurum Saikosaponins, Volatile oil of Radix Bupleuri, Flavonoids from Radix Bupleuri, Bupleurum Polysaccharide	Bupleurum Saikosaponins, Volatile oil of Radix Bupleuri	Liver (liver injury, allergic shock) (Li, Du, et al., 2018; Li, Wang, & Du, 2018)	Liver (Li, Du, et al., 2018; Li, Wang, & Du, 2018)	3–10 g	Mild toxic	No
Chuanxiong Rhizoma	Chuan xiong	Ferulic acid, Ligustilide, Senkyunolide A, Senkyunolide I, Tetramethylpyrazine	Tetramethylpyrazine	–	Embryotoxicity (Wang, Bao, Yi, & Xia, 2019)	3–10 g	Mild toxic	No
Coptidis Rhizoma	Huang lian	Berberine Hydrochloride, Berberine, Coptisine, Palmatine	Berberine, Alkaloids	Allergy (rash) (Li, 2006)	Liver (Wang et al., 2019)	2–5 g	Mild toxic	No
Dipsaci Radix	Xu duan	Dipsacus Total Saponins: Dipsacus Saponins Vi	Radix Dipsaci Water Extract	–	Genotoxicity (Liu et al., 2016)	9–15 g	Mild toxic	No
Epimedii Folium	Yin yang huo	Epimediun flavonoids, Icariin, Epimedium polysaccharide	Herba Epimedii Alcohol Extract	–	Liver (Zhang et al., 2018; Zhang, Li, & Du, 2018)	6–10 g	Mild toxic	No
Leonuri Herba	Yi mu cao	Stachydrine Hydrochloride, Leonurine Hydrochloride	Stachydrine Hydrochloride, Leonurine Hydrochloride	Liver, kidney (fatigue, hyperhidrosis, kidney failure) (Luo, Liu, Zhou, & Song, 2018)	–	9–30 g, dried; 12–40 g, fresh	Mild toxic	No
Paeoniae Radix Alba	Bai shao	Total Glycosides of Paeony	Total Glycosides of Paeony	–	Embryotoxicity (Han & He, 2008)	6–15 g	Mild toxic	No

Continued

Table 1 General information for toxic TCM.—cont'd

Name	Chinese Name	Bioactive compounds	Toxic chemicals	Target organs clinical (symptoms)	Target organs experimental	Daily dose[a]	"Toxic" grade	Recorded as toxic in CP?
Polygoni Multiflori Radix	He shou wu	Stilbene Glycosides, Anthraquinones, Flavonoids	Stilbene Glycosides, Anthraquinones	Liver (acute liver injury) (Lin et al., 2019)	Liver (Li et al., 2019)	3–6 g	Mild toxic	No
Psoraleae Fructus	Bu gu zhi	Psoralen, Isopsoralen, Bavachin	Psoralen, Isopsoralen, Bavachinin	–	Liver, reproductive system (Alam, Khan, & Asad, 2018), kidney (Zhao & Sun, 2014)	6–10 g	Highly toxic	No
Stephaniae Tetrandrae Radix	Fang ji	Tetrandrine Fangchinoline	Tetrandrine	–	Liver, kidney (Liang et al., 2010)	5–10 g	Mild toxic	No
Aristolochia Fructus	Ma dou ling	Aristolochic acid, Alkaloids, Lignans	Aristolochic acid	Kidney (kidney dysfunction, (proximal) renal tubular injury, elevated urine NAG and RBP, proteinuria, amino-aciduria, hypouricemia, renal tubular acidosis) (Zhang et al., 2019)	Kidney, liver (Liang et al., 2010)	3–9 g	Mild toxic	No
Aristolochia fangchi	Guang fang ji	Aristolochic acid, Tetrandrine	Aristolochic acid	Kidney (similar to Ma dou ling) (Zhang, Zhao, et al., 2019)	Kidney, liver (Liang et al., 2010)	4.5–9 g, (Chinese Material Medica)	Mild toxic	Removed from CP
Caulis aristolochiae manshuriensis	Guan mu tong	Aristolochic acid, Oleanolic acid, Akebosides	Aristolochic acid	Kidney (Similar to Ma dou ling) (Zhang, Zhao, et al., 2019)	Kidney, liver (Liang et al., 2010)	3–6 g (Chinese Material Medica)	Highly toxic	Removed form CP

[a]Daily dose recommended in China Pharmacopeia, based on 70 kg body weight.
CP, China Pharmacopeia.

4.1 Chinese aconite (Fu Zi), "resurrection" drug or poison?

4.1.1 Definition

"Fu Zi" refers to the processed root of *Aconitum carmichaelii* Debeaux, which is also known as Chinese Aconite. "Fu Zi" was first recorded in *Shen Nong Ben Cao Jing*, and was categorized in "lowest grade" due to its severe toxicity when misused, overdose, improper processing or wrong compatibility with herbs. Zhenshi Li also provided comments on "Fu Zi" as quoted here "frizzle up the juice from Fuzi to be poison, then shoot preys."

4.1.2 Use

However, as summarized by Zhang et al., "Fu Zi" is broadly used in all kinds of TCM preparations and presents in 13.20% among 500 well-known and historically successful prescriptions (Zhou et al., 2015). There are two famous TCM decoctions named "Si Ni Tang" and "Fu Shen Tang," in which the composition of "Fu Zi" is more than 50% and 60%, respectively. For centuries these preparations were used to treat heart failure and collapse, myocardial infarction, and shock. In the past decades, a group of TCM doctors became famous for their bold, but successful clinical practice of prescribing extremely high doses of "Fu Zi." Based on promising and powerful therapeutic effects against heart failure and shock, "Fu Zi" earned a reputation as a "resurrection" drug and "the first key herb to recuperate the depleted 'Yang' and rescue the patient from danger" despite its potential toxicity (Zhou et al., 2015).

4.1.3 Mechanism

Modern phytochemistry studies identified 122 chemical constituents, most of which are alkaloids, in *Aconitum carmichaelii* Debeaux. Alkaloids have been suggested as the most bioactive, as well as toxic, compounds among all isolated chemicals, and can be further categorized into diester-diterpenoid alkaloids (DDAs), monoester-diterpenoid alkaloids (MDAs) and unesterified-diterpenoid alkaloids (UDAs) (Wu et al., 2018). Emerging animal studies have demonstrated that various types of compounds, including fuzinoside, mesaconine, higenamine and benzoylmesaconine contributed to the significant cardiotonic activity (Jian et al., 2012; Zhou et al., 2015). Adrenergic β-receptor and release of catecholamine may serve as the predominant mechanisms. In addition to cardiotonic action, bidirectional regulation of arrhythmia by "Fu Zi" has been demonstrated by several studies. DDAs, especially aconitine, contributed to arrhythmia, however, alcoholic and aqueous extracts of "Fu Zi," along with several alkaloids, such as

Lappaconitine, exert anti-arrhythmia activities through unidentified mechanisms (Bryzgalov, Romanov, Tolstikova, & Shults, 2013; Lou et al., 2018). It has also been reported that "Fu Zi" polysaccharide protects cardiomyocytes from ischemia-reperfusion injury by targeting calcium homeostasis and mitochondrial function (Deng, Liu, Sun, Dong, & Huang, 2019; Liu et al., 2012; Wang, He, et al., 2016; Wang, Yang, et al., 2016; Wang et al., 2019). Activation of cell survival signaling, such as Signal Transducing Activator of Transcription 3 (STAT3) and AMP-activated protein kinase (AMPK), was also plausibly involved (Liao et al., 2013; Zhou et al., 2015). Furthermore, pharmacological effects targeting other organs or systems have also been demonstrated, including anti-inflammation, immunoregulation, analgesic, and activities on energy metabolism (Zhou et al., 2015).

4.1.4 Toxicity

In China Pharmacopeia, daily safety dose of "Fu Zi" is 3–15 g, however, the actual "Fu Zi" consumption during clinical salvage of heart failure or shock patients is usually much higher (from 30 g to even 300 g), which leads to increased risk of intoxication. Nausea, vomiting, dizziness, palpitations, hypotension, arrhythmia, shock and coma were identified as typical symptoms of "Fu Zi" poisoning. Lethal dose studies revealed that DDAs plays a critical role in "Fu Zi" related toxicity, and the toxicity of MDAs and UDAs was about 1000-fold weaker (Singhuber, Zhu, Prinz, & Kopp, 2009). Pharmacokinetic and toxicokinetic studies revealed the distribution of DDAs mainly in liver, kidney and heart and its elimination through liver and kidney after oral administration. Consistently, cardiac, hepatic and renal toxicity of "Fu Zi" preparations were widely reported. However, direct experimental evidence regarding DDAs-induced liver and kidney damage is still lacking. Recent studies suggested that DDAs, such as acotinine, mesaconitine, and hypaconitine, modulated Na^+ channel function and Na^+/Ca^{2+} homeostasis, which are the possible arrhythmogenic mechanisms (Chen, Guo, et al., 2018; Chen, Wang, & Du, 2018; Zhang, Cai, Zhang, Qi, & Lu, 2018; Zong et al., 2019). Whether regulation of ion channels functions also contributes to the pharmacological effects of "Fu Zi" is still elusive. Additionally, several studies suggested that DDAs-induced dysregulation of cell signaling, mitochondrial dysfunction and apoptosis were also responsible for "Fu Zi"-induced cardiomyocytes death and cardiac toxicity (Huang et al., 2018; Liu, Han, Li, Liu, & Kang, 2019; Zhuang et al., 2016).

Unfortunately, despite wide clinical use and extensive pharmacology and toxicology studies, no specific dose-toxicity relationship has been discovered in clinical studies, and there is no specific detoxification therapy other than regular cardiovascular supportive treatment when "Fu Zi" intoxication occurrs (Yang, Ji, & Zuo, 2018). Hence, further pharmacokinetic, toxicokinetic, mechanistic studies are urgently required, and use of "Fu Zi" as personalized medicine is strongly recommended (Wu, Guo, et al., 2018).

4.2 Arsenic compounds, from poison to drug

4.2.1 Definition and toxicity

Arsenic trioxide (As_2O_3: ATO), one of the most famous poisons, has been documented in almost all TCM *Material Medica* books as a compound with "great Toxic" for over a century. In TCM, ATO was only used as an emetic drug. Arsenicals were also applied in the treatment of syphilis in the early 20th century in Europe. However, human exposure to environmental arsenic, especially in drinking water, has become a severe worldwide health issue. Chronic exposure to arsenic is related to broad-targeting toxicity against almost all vital organs and systems, including cardiotoxicity, nephrotoxicity, hepatotoxicity, and reproductive toxicity. Acute arsenic poisoning usually leads to nausea, vomiting, severe diarrhea, and even death.

4.2.2 Use

From the early 1970s to 1990s, inspired by local TCM pharmacists, Tingdong Zhang and colleagues at Harbin Medical University investigated the therapeutic effects of ATO against different types of leukemia, including acute leukemia. These pioneer findings clearly demonstrated that ATO is effective for the treatment of acute promyelocytic leukemia (APL) (Rao, Li, & Zhang, 2013). In the late 1990s, several systemic clinical and experimental studies further confirmed the previous studies, attracting the attention of the western world. Recently published recommendations by an expert panel of the European LeukemiaNet on the management of acute promyelocytic leukemia supported ATO in combination with all-trans retinoic acid (ATRA) as the new standard for non-high-risk patients (WBC count $<10 \times 10^9$/L) (Sanz et al., 2019). In the past decade, oral arsenic plus ATRA has been commercially available as Realgar-Indigo Naturalis formula (RIF) (Zhu, Hu, Lo Coco, & Jin, 2019). Oral arsenic promotes a safe profile, improved quality of life, lowered medical costs, and achieved comparable clinical efficacy to that of normal intravenous formulations

(Zhu et al., 2019, 2018). These recent therapy developments made acute promyelocytic leukemia, once the most health-threatening type of leukemia, the most treatable leukemia.

4.2.3 Mechanism

Previous studies demonstrated that the metabolism of ATO and other arsenic compounds required multiple methylations by using S-adenosyl methionine (SAM), which is also an essential co-factor of DNA methyltransferases (DNMTs). Depletion of SAM after arsenic metabolism leads to global DNA hypomethylation and increased expression of tumor suppressors in leukemia cells (Yi et al., 2000). However, other studies suggested that the DNA hypomethylation induced upregulation of several oncogenes and promoted carcinogenesis in various organs (Cohen, Arnold, Eldan, Lewis, & Beck, 2006). As described in a previous review, methylated arsenic metabolites interrupted mitochondrial electron transport chain (ETC), which contributed to reactive oxygen species (ROS) generation and, subsequently, oxidative stress-induced apoptosis (Khairul, Wang, Jiang, Wang, & Naranmandura, 2017). It has also been reported that some metabolites mainly targeted the endoplasmic reticulum (ER) and induced ER stress-related apoptosis through activation of PKR-like ER kinase-activating transcription factor 4-C/EBP-homologous protein (PERK-ATF4-CHOP) axis or inositol-requiring ER-to-nucleus signal kinase 1(IRE1)-related c-Jun N-terminal kinases (JNKs) apoptotic signaling activation (Naranmandura et al., 2012; Szegezdi, Logue, Gorman, & Samali, 2006). Promyelocytic leukemia protein (PML)-retinoic acid receptor alpha (RARα) is the most common fusion protein found specifically in APL patients, which drives the disease development and progression by arresting leukemia cells differentiation and maturation. Both ATRA and ATO exert their anti-leukemia activities by promoting the degradation of this protein and further differentiation of leukemia cells. As previously reported, ATO directly bound to a cysteine residue of PML and PML-RARα fusion protein and resulted in SUMOylation and following degradation of these proteins (Zhang et al., 2010).

In combining increased risk of experimental exposure with wide clinical practice for the treatment of APL, the severe and broad targeting toxicity of arsenic has attracted significant attention from researchers. A growing number of studies revealed that ROS production-induced oxidative stress, ER stress, and apoptosis are major mechanisms underlying ATO-induced various organ toxicity (Khairul et al., 2017). In addition, due to arsenic-induced global DNA hypomethylation and ROS production in normal cells, ATO exposure significantly increased risk of cancer initiation in skin, bladder, and lung (Cohen et al., 2006; Kitchin, 2001). The International Agency for Research on Cancer (IARC) and the US Environmental Protection Agency (EPA) also categorized arsenic as a carcinogen based on epidemiological studies, making arsenic both an anti-cancer drug and a carcinogen at the same time. Although several studies suggested that ATO also exhibited inhibitory effects against various solid tumor growth, severe adverse effects and potential carcinogenicity obstructed further development of arsenic compounds as treatment of cancers other than APL (Miller Jr., 2002). A better understanding of the mechanisms of action of ATO and better management of undesired side effects may be beneficial. Overall, most of the toxicological activities of arsenic are essential for its pharmacological effects as an anti-cancer drug, highlighting the connection between "toxic" and therapeutic effects of TCM drugs.

4.3 *Tripterygium wilfordii* Hook f. and its bioactive compounds

4.3.1 Definition and clinical use

Tripterygium wilfordii Hook f. (TW, Thunder God Vine or Lei Gong Teng) is one of the most representative TTCM herb with great therapeutic potential that has been broadly studied by scientists, not only from China, but also in western laboratories due to its significant immunosuppressive effects and anti-cancer activity. Currently, several patented TCM, made only from TW (a single component TCM prescription), are approved by China FDA and are clinically available, including Tripterygium wilfordii tablets, Tripterygium wilfordii glycosides tablets, and Tripterygium hypoglaucum hutch tablets. These drugs are widely used in clinical settings with a daily dose of 1–1.5 mg tripterygium glycosides (including triptolide and celastrol)/kg/day for immunosuppression following organ transplantation and the treatment of autoimmune and inflammation-related diseases, such as rheumatoid arthritis (RA), multiple sclerosis, diabetic nephritic syndrome, Lupus, Behcet's disease, and central nervous system (CNS) diseases. Although occasional, but severe, adverse effects were found during clinical practice, these drugs are still not replaceable due to their significantly stronger efficacy against diseases when compared to other drugs. Thus, emerging clinical evidence regarding pharmacology and toxicology properties of these drugs has accumulated, and continuous efforts are dedicated to investigating the underlying mechanisms of TW and its bioactive compounds.

4.3.2 Pharmacological effects and mechanisms

According to biochemical and pharmacokinetic studies, triptolide (TP) and celastrol are two of the most bioactive, yet toxic, constituents identified in TW as well as in those FDA approved medicines in China (Du et al., 2018; Wang, Huang, et al., 2018). Triptolide is considered as the most potent systematic anti-inflammatory and immunoregulating natural products (Graziose, Lila, & Raskin, 2010). As summarized in previous reviews by Li et al. and Chen et al., the mechanisms associated with the significant therapeutic effects of TP and celastrol against T helper cell-mediated immunity, including RA and inflammatory bowel diseases, have been extensively studied. Emerging evidence suggests that TP suppresses inflammatory responses by attenuating MAPK/NF-κB activation and inhibiting downstream responses (Chen et al., 2018; Li et al., 2014). Triptolide also abrogated the activation of innate immune responses through decreasing the leukocyte numbers and myeloid cells trafficking, suppression of Toll-like receptors (TLRs) signaling and NLRP3 inflammasome activation, and reduced expression of pro-inflammatory cytokines, thus protected other systems, including the lung, the kidney, and the central nervous system (CNS), from inflammation-related injury.

Both TP and celastrol have drawn substantial attention for their potential bioactivity targeting cancer. A growing number of studies suggests that TP arrested cancer cell proliferation and induced apoptosis in various cancer cells and xenograft mouse models. Reported plausible mechanisms include accumulation of tumor suppressor p53, oxidative stress and mitochondrial damage, XPB subunit-dependent disruption of RNA polymerase II (RNAPII) function, and cell cycle arrest (Hou, Tong, Peng, Zhang, & Yan, 2018). In addition, the anti-inflammatory effects of TP also contribute to its anti-cancer activity. Furthermore, it has been suggested that TP reversed multidrug-resistance and sensitized cancer cells to chemotherapy through modulation of drug efflux transporters, specifically, ATP-binding cassette (ABC) transporters (Joshi, Vishwakarma, & Bharate, 2017). Celastrol has been well established as a heat shock protein (HSP) 90 inhibitor by inducing degradation of HSP90 and its client proteins. By inhibiting HSP90 activity, celastrol promotes degradation of various oncogenic proteins, interrupts several proliferating signaling pathways, including AKT, MEK, EGFR and further inhibits cancer cell growth (Fan et al., 2014; Wei et al., 2014). Several HSP90 independent mechanisms were also identified, including ROS accumulation-induced oxidative stress, attenuated cancer surviving signalings, including inflammation, AKT, hypoxia-inducible factor 1α(HIF-1α) and Wnt/β-catenine pathways, and ER stress (Kashyap et al., 2018).

4.3.3 Toxicity and mechanisms

During the past decades, an accumulation of clinical studies report severe adverse effects of TW containing preparations targeting almost all main organs, including alimentary tracts, liver, kidney, reproductive system, cardiovascular system and immune system, however, without a clear dose-toxicity correlation (Xi, Peng, Wu, Zhou, & Zhou, 2017). Most of these adverse effects were also observed in animal models or found in *in vitro* studies. However, contrary to several animal studies using $IL10^{-/-}$ colitis mice where TP protects against severe intestinal inflammation and epithelium damage, several clinical observations suggest TP-induced ulcerative colitis is a common adverse effect of TW preparations for the digestive system. Although both experimental evidence and clinical practice suggested TW preparation and TP as a therapeutic option for diabetic nephropathy, occasional clinical cases have been reported that TP and TW preparations showed significant nephrotoxicity by inducing cell apoptosis. Mechanisms explaining these contradictory results are still elusive.

Oxidative stress is well recognized as one of the most critical mechanisms of TW- and TP-induced liver, kidney, heart, and reproductive system toxicity. TP leads to ROS accumulation and mitochondrial damage through increased ROS production and suppressed anti-oxidant mechanisms, including NF-E2-related factor 2 (Nrf2), heme oxygenase 1 (HO-1), and Sirtuin 3 (SIRT3) (Cao et al., 2016; Fu, Jiang, & Zhang, 2013; Yang et al., 2016). Oxidative stress will further contribute to apoptosis, autophagy, inflammation, and thus induce toxicity in different organs. Interestingly, these mechanisms are essential for the anti-cancer activities of TP and TW. In addition, it has been reported that TP-mediated immunomodulation of T helper cell 17 (Th17) and regulatory T cell (Treg) balance and the resulting inflammatory response is not only important for the immunotherapeutic effect of TP but is also critical for its liver toxicity (Xi et al., 2017). Recent studies demonstrated the common mechanism underlying both immunosuppressive effects and broad targeting toxicity of TP. A human-based gene expression study demonstrated that more than 90% of the genes moderated by TP were downregulated, suggesting TP as a global transcription inhibitor (Vispe et al., 2009). Further molecular mechanic studies confirmed that TP primarily targeted XPB, a critical subunit of the basal transcription factor IIH (TFIIH), by covalent modification, and thus reduced RNAPII-induced transcription (Chen, Gao, & Shilatifard, 2015; He et al., 2015). Taken together, these findings reflect the connection between the toxicity and pharmacological effects of the same drug and support TCM theory.

4.4 Herbal drugs derived from Aristolochiaceae Juss. family of plants

4.4.1 Definition

Several common TCM herbal drugs, including *Asari Radix Et Rhizoma* (Xi Xin), *Caulis aristolochiae manshuriensis* (Guan Mu Tong), and *Aristolochia Fructus* (Ma Dou Ling), are derived from plants belonging the Aristolochiaceae Juss. family. These herbal products were all identified as "mild Toxic" or "average Toxic" in ancient TCM books. The major toxic substances in these herbals have been identified as aristolochic acids (AAs). Other bonaticals known to contain AAs were well-documented in a previous review (Debelle, Vanherweghem, & Nortier, 2008). Used alone or in combination with other TCM products, these herbals were widely prescribed for the treatment of various neurological disorders and epilepsy.

4.4.2 Pharmacological effects and mechanisms

Alpha (α)- and beta (β)-asarone are the most bioactive compounds identified in the essential oil components of these herbal compounds during isolation (Rajput, Tonge, & Karuppayil, 2014). As reviewed previously, both α- and β-asarone have significant neuroprotective, antipyretic, analgesic, and anticonvulsant activities, as well as offering therapeutic effects against depression, anxiety, epilepsy and anxiety (Chellian, Pandy, & Mohamed, 2017). The anti-epilepsy effects of α-asarone are dependent on gamma-aminobutyric acid (GABAα) receptor activation, *N*-methyl-D-aspartic acid receptor (NMDA) receptor antagonism, and NaV channel inhibition. The anti-anxiety effects of α-asarone are also dependent on the activation of the GABAα receptor. However, the anti-epilepsy and anti-anxiety effects of β-asarone are still considered controversial. The significant inhibition of monoamine oxidase enzymes (MAO), both MAO-A and B, is critical for the anti-depressive, anti-Alzheimer's and anti-Parkinson activities of α- and β-asarone (Tao, Irie, Li, & Keung, 2005; Tian et al., 2017). Direct neuroprotective effects of α- and β-asarone through modulation of ER stress, Beclin-1 dependent autophagy and inflammation are also important for the treatment of neurodegeneration diseases (Deng et al., 2016; Ning, Zhang, Wang, Deng, & Fang, 2019). Although other pharmacological effects, such as anti-cancer and anti-inflammation activities were reported, pre-clinical and clinical evidence is still limited (Chellian et al., 2017). The toxicity of α- and β-asarone is not well studied. Some preclinical evidence suggested that α- and β-asarone had potential genotoxicity in cell line studies or animal models (Chellian et al., 2017). Further verification and investigation of underlying mechanisms are still required.

4.4.3 Toxicity and mechanisms

The most extensively studied toxic compounds in these herbal concoctions are AAs. In the early 1990s, a severe safety incidence of AA-containing Chinese herbals erupted, causing renal fibrosis and kidney failure in over a hundred women in a Belgium weight loss clinic (Vanherweghem et al., 1993). Subsequent clinical reports regarding AA-related nephropathy (AAN) and urothelial cancers have continued to emerge. A previous clinical study including 300 AAN patients further demonstrated that the intake of AA-I was correlated with features of AAN. Specifically, highest daily intake (0.0063–0.314 g/day, median 0.0366 g/day) and highest cumulative AA-I (0.02–3.96 g, median 1.04 g) within 1–120 days (median 14 days) was found in acute AAN patients; an AA-I daily dose at 0.0037–0.078 g/day (median 0.0187 g/day) for a relatively short medication period (8–365 days, median 105 days) was associated with tubular dysfunction AAN; the lowest daily dose (0.00001–0.237 g/day, median 0.00005 g/day) but highest cumulative AA-I (0.025–16.3 g, median 1.01 g) in the longest period (6–14,965 days, median 1825 days) contributed to chronic AAN (Yang et al., 2012). Numerous experiments suggest that kidney proximal tubule epithelial cells were primary targets of metabolic-activated AAs (Jelakovic et al., 2019). Covalent aristolactam (AL)-DNA adducts formation, mitochondrial damage, autophagy related epithelial to myofibroblast transversion, NF-kB related cytokine secretion and inflammation-promoted fibrosis have been demonstrated as predominant molecular mechanisms under the pathogenesis of AAN (Man et al., 2017; Michl et al., 2017; Wang, Liu, Xue, & Zhou, 2019). It has been further elucidated that excessive AL-DNA-adducts triggered loss-of-function mutation of tumor suppressor p53, a A:T-to-T:A mutation, and further contributed to the upper urinary tract and kidney cancers (Ng et al., 2017; Rosenquist & Grollman, 2016; Zhang, Zhao, et al., 2019). This mutational signature has been used as a biomarker for the detection of environmental and herals-related AA exposure. Previous studies indicated that ingestion of more than 60 g of herbals containing AAs and cumulative intake of 250 mg AAs significantly increased the risk of urinary tract cancer and renak cell carcinoma, respectively (Chen et al., 2013; Hoang et al., 2016). In addition, using the signature genetic mutation, it was suggested that AA and their derivatives were widely implicated in hepatocellular carcinoma (HCC) throughout Asian countries (Ng et al., 2017). Most recently, a clinical study based on a larger population further indicated that cumulative comsumption of AAs containing herbals less than 200 g was not associated with HCC (Chen, Tsai, & Lai, 2019). Taken together, these clinical and experimental findings resulted in several AA-containing TCM herbal products being withdrawn from the China Pharmacopeia, including *Caulis aristolochiae manshuriensis* (Guan Mu Tong) and *Aristolochia fangchi* (Guang Fang Ji). Although *Asari Radix Et Rhizoma* (Xi Xin) are still recorded in the China Pharmacopeia, the presence of AAs is limited to 0.001% of raw material. China Food and Drug Administration provided a list of 43 approved AAs-containing TCM remedies in 2017 (Zhou et al., 2019). The International Agency for Research on Cancer, the World Health Organization's cancer agency, also categorized AA-I, AA-II, and aristolactam as a proven group-1 human carcinogens in 2012 (Zhou, Pei, et al., 2019).

It is interesting that herbal drugs from the Aristolochiaceae Juss. family have been used medicinally for centuries, however, are well defined as carcinogens and toxins targeting kidney at the same time. Based on previous findings, the material basis of therapeutic effects and toxicity of these herbals are separated, specifically, α- and β-asarone are responsible for major pharmacological effects, and the toxicity is mainly dependent on the existence of AA. Separating these compounds and adjusting the herbal composition of previous TCM remedies may be helpful to improve the efficiency of these drugs and to diminish toxicity. As mentioned in a previous review, further studies focusing on pharmacokinetic studies, the relationship between AA exposure-related mutation signature and various cancers, immune responses after AA exposure, and potential anti-tumor activities of AA will benefit the rediscovery of AA-containing TCM herbal drugs as valuable and safe medicines (Zhou, Pei, et al., 2019).

5. Potential toxicity of non-toxic TCM

In addition to documented TTCM, clinical reports regarding undesired toxicity-induced by non-toxic TCM drugs are still emerging. In some cases, it is hard to exclude the involvement of non-TCM risks, since the combined use of TCM drugs with western medicine, including drugs with a known risk of toxicity, such as acetaminophen, are very common in clinical practice. In other cases, the potential risks of non-toxic TCM-induced toxicity have been verified by both clinical and experimental evidence. The liver, kidney, and intestine are the most commonly targeted organs, indicating the important role of drug metabolism and elimination in TCM-induced toxicity. Among these adverse effects, herb-induced liver injury (HILI) is usually the leading concern with the safety of TCM products. Although limited in its reliability, the Roussel Uclaf Causality Assessment Method (RUCAM) is a well established and widely used tool to quantitatively assess causality in suspected cases of drug-induced liver injury (DILI) and HILI, especially idiosyncratic DILI and HILI. The use and update of RUCAM were well summarized in a previous review (Danan & Teschke, 2015). An etiology study in mainland China suggested that HILI contributed to more than 26% of the 25,927 DILI cases from 308 medical centers (Shen et al., 2019). Herbals and dietery supplements were ranked first among 11 classes of implicated drugs in DILI. Similar results were found in a study from Korea (Byeon, Kil, Ahn, & Son, 2019). A recent review by He et al. analyzed 335 hepatotoxic medicinal plants and 296 hepatotoxic ingredients then provided insights of the phylogenetic- and structure-toxicity relationships (He et al., 2019). Briefly, their results suggest that distribution of hepatotoxic plants in the phylogenetic tree showed a significant cluster pattern. Medicinal plants in certain orders and families may have higher hepatotoxic risk than other plants. Alkaloids, followed by flavonoids and quinones, were suggested as the dominant categories of hepatotoxic phytochemicals, based on frequency. The authors further identified several structural alerts for hepatotoxicity using a QSAR (quantitative structure-activity relationship) method, which will help to predict hepatotoxic risk of bioactive compounds in TCM herbal products based on chemical structure.

5.1 *Radix Bupleuri* (RB)

One of the most famous TCM safety incidences is liver toxicity induced by RB containing "Xiao Chai Hu Tang" in Japan. An RUCAM based clinical study in Germany involving 21,470 patients suggested that RB is one of the most implicated TCM herbals in TCM-related liver injury (Melchart et al., 2017). RB is the dry root of *Bupleurum chinense* DC. (Apiaceae) and *Bupleurum scorzonerifolium* Willd. It is one of the most widely used TCM drugs in the treatment of cold, fever and hepatitis, based on its anti-inflammatory and immunoregulative activities. RB was categorized as the "top grade" in *Shen Nong Ben Cao Jing* and was considered for a very long time to be non-toxic (Li, Li, et al., 2018; Li et al., 2017). Several studies suggested that overdose is the primary risk for RB-induced liver toxicity (Li, Li, et al., 2018). Dysregulation of hepatic lipid metabolism and oxidative stress by saikosaponins are plausible underlying mechanisms.

5.2 *Polygonum multiflorum* (PM)

PM is another representative non-toxic TCM drug that has been reported in the past decades to have potential toxicity. Due to continuous and increasing consumption, PM-induced inflammation-associated idiosyncratic liver injury contributed to about 30% of drug-induced liver injury in China (Lei et al., 2015). However, PM-induced liver injury is usually unpredictable and dose-independent in both clinical and experimental studies. Moreover, the molecular mechanisms underlying are still unknown. Until recently, a clinical-based study suggested that the human leukocyte antigen-B (HLA-B)*35:01 allele is a genetic risk factor and a potential biomarker for predicting PM-liver injury in humans (Li, Rao, et al., 2019). This finding provided new insights into the prediction of TCM-induced undesired toxicity and highlighted the necessity of personalized medicine.

5.3 Adulterated or contaminated herbals

Additionally, some severe TCM toxicity incidences are attributed to the unexpected use of "fake" or incorrect herbals. *Radix Notogingseng* or *Radix pseudo-ginseng* (San Qi) is a commonly used TCM herbal drug to promote hemostasis. Gynura segetum or Gynura Rhizome (Tu San Qi), which has similar morphology as "San Qi," were occasionally misused clinically. The rate of "Tu San Qi"-induced Hepatic veno-occlusive disease (HVOD) has continuously increased in China in recent years (Wang, Qiao, et al., 2018). HVOD is characterized by sinusoid damage and stenosis or occlusion of hepatic veins and is associated with a significant level of mortality (Wang, Qiao, et al., 2018). Pyrrolizidine alkaloids (PAs) have been identified as the primary toxic compounds responsible for "Tu San Qi"-induced severe liver injury (Zhang et al., 2019). Metabolic toxification, disturbance of energy metabolism, and TGF-β-Smad3 related inflammatory signaling pathways were theorized to be involved in PAs-mediated toxicity (Ebmeyer et al., 2019; Ning, Chen, & Rietjens, 2019; Qiu et al., 2018; Zhang, Zhou, et al., 2019).

6. Managing undesired toxicity of TCM drugs

Based on the connection between toxicity and pharmacological effects, managing undesired toxicity without affecting its therapeutic potential is an ongoing topic in the practice and development of TCM. As shown in Fig. 1, in the TCM system all preparation procedures, from the processing of the raw materials, decoction, and drug compatibility, to the identification of the patient's constitution and adjustment of remedies, aim to enhance the therapeutic efficacy and reduce toxicity at the same time. Modern phytochemistry, pharmacokinetic and toxicokinetic studies have begun to reveal the underlying mechanisms. TCM processing is a unique pharmaceutical technique to transfer raw materials into the form that can be used in decoction. By using different adjuvants, such as vinegar, wine or honey, TCM processing contributes significantly to the change in chemical profile and, inevitably, the change of pharmacological effects and toxicity of TCM drugs (Wu et al., 2018). For instance, the process of decomposing higher toxic DDAs into less toxic MDAs is critical for the detoxification of "Fu Zi." The concentration of DDAs was decreased about 50–100-fold (Wang, He, et al., 2016; Wang, Yang, et al., 2016).

Decocting is the most common pharmaceutical procedure for TCM preparations. Water and high temperature will significantly alter the composition of bioactive compounds in the decoction. Decocting is also a critical factor for the safe use of "Fu Zi." Prolonged decoction significantly reduces the stability of ester-diterpenoid alkaloids, resulting in the

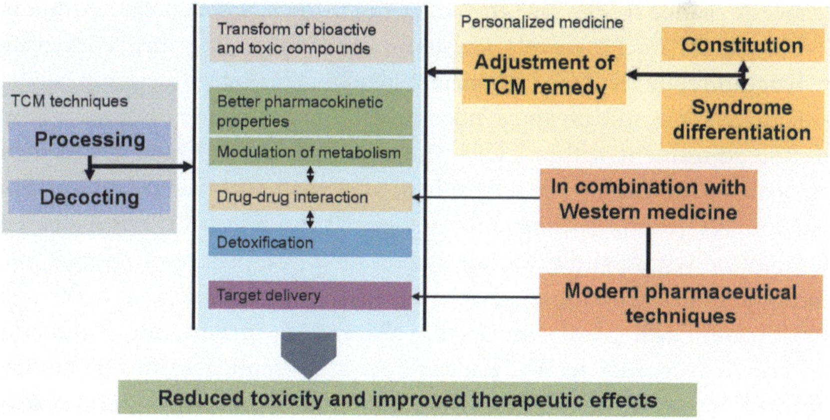

Fig. 1 Managing undesired toxicity of TCM products.

transformation of DDAs into MDAs and eventually UDAs (Zhou et al., 2015). In addition to reducing toxicity, a recent study demonstrated that decocting resulted in the self-assembling of nanostructures containing berberine and flavonoid glycosides and significantly enhanced the pharmaceutical effects against bacteria (Li et al., 2019). This interesting finding provided novel insights into understanding the transformations of bioactive chemicals during decocting.

For the compatibility art of TCM, several molecular mechanisms have been identified. The first is to modify the pharmacokinetics of the bioactive compounds of other components in the remedy. In TCM preparations, almost all "Fu Zi" preparations are in conjugation with *Radix glycyrrhizae* (Licorice). As well-known detoxification agent, *Radix glycyrrhizae* contains bioactive compounds such as glycyrrhizic acid and licoflavone, which are not only implicated in absorption, but also the CYP enzymes-induced metabolism of the ingredients in "Fu Zi" and, consequently, the reduced toxicity of "Fu Zi" (Li, Sun, & Liu, 2019). In addition, natural products also promote the metabolism and elimination of TP and thus protect their multi-organ toxicity (Li, Sun, et al., 2019). The second molecular mechanism is to directly target the toxicological pathways. Bioactive compounds in licorice, again, alleviate TCM-induced oxidative stress and apoptosis by direct activation of Nrf2- and Sirtuin 1 (SIRT1)-dependent anti-oxidant responses (Li, Sun, et al., 2019). The third is to improve the organ-specific targeting of TCM drugs, which is referred to as "Yin Jing" in TCM theory. Glycyrrhetinic acid, a bio-transformed metabolite of glycyrrhizic acid that has been identified to have liver targeting properties, was extensively studied for development of liver-specific targeting drug delivery systems with liposomes or nanoparticles in the treatment of hepatocellular carcinoma (Cai et al., 2016). However, a systemic study regarding this mechanism-mediated directly by TCM drugs is still lacking.

Patients' constitution and syndrome differentiation are critical for composition adjustment within TCM remedies and are the Chinese version of personalized medicine. The scientific connotation of a patient's constitution may contain genetic background, epigenetic modification, homeostasis of the immune system and hormone system, and intestinal microbiota. Combining all of these physiological or pathophysiological conditions of the individual patient will greatly impact the absorption, metabolism, elimination and body's responses to TCM drugs. As a consequence, the therapeutic effects of the same TCM remedy will vary among patients, and the toxicity on different people will also be unpredictable. Systemic studies are urgently required to elucidate the connection between the patient's constitution and unpredictable toxicity of certain widely used TCM drugs.

7. Conclusion

In summary, there is a long history applying TCMs, including TTCMs, to treat human diseases. Great efforts have been dedicated to improving the safety and efficacy of TCM drugs. With the development of modern medicine, several well-known TTCM drugs have been adopted to treat various diseases due to the identification of their novel pharmaceutical effects or improvement of their toxicity management. On the other hand, several widely used non-toxic TCM drugs have been reported to possess potential toxicity. Systemic and mechanistic studies regarding the connection between pharmacological effects and toxicity of TCM-based drugs will not only improve the safety of TCM in clinical use but also promote the drug discovery and development of TCM-based natural products.

Acknowledgments

This work was supported by grants from the National Natural Science Foundation of China (Grant Nos. 81773997, 81073148, 30672649, 81374059); the Key Research and Development Program of Shandong Province, China (Grant Nos. 2017CXGC130, 2016ZDJS07A23, 2016GSF202039); the National Major Fundamental Research Program of China (Grant No. 2009CB522802); the Key Project of Shandong Natural Science Foundation of China (Grant No. ZR2011HZ005); the National Specific Grant for the Research and Development of Traditional Chinese Medicine (201507004-03-04, 201507004-04-04). R. Sun is supported by research fund "Traditional Chinese medicine pharmacology and toxicology expert (No. ts201511107)" from Taishan Scholar Project of Shandong Province; Independent Innovation and Achievement Conversion Project in Shandong Province (2014ZZCX02104); The National Basic Research Program-973 Program (2009CB522802).

Conflict of interest

None.

References

Alam, F., Khan, G. N., & Asad, M. (2018). Psoralea corylifolia L: Ethnobotanical, biological, and chemical aspects: A review. *Phytotherapy Research*, *32*(4), 597–615. https://doi.org/10.1002/ptr.6006.

Bao, F., & Tu, A. (2000). Poisoning and successful rescue of nux vomica powder: A case report. *Chinese Journal of Hospital Pharmacy*, *03*, 59–60.

Bao, H., Zhao, J., Song, J., & Li, Z. (2011). Research on long term toxicity of ethanol extracts of Curculigo or chioides Gaertn. *Pharmacology and Clinics of Chinese Materia Medica*, *27*(03), 70–73.

Bryzgalov, A. O., Romanov, V. E., Tolstikova, T. G., & Shults, E. E. (2013). Lappaconitine: Influence of halogen substituent on the antiarrhythmic activity. *Cardiovascular & Hematological Agents in Medicinal Chemistry*, *11*(3), 211–217.

Byeon, J. H., Kil, J. H., Ahn, Y. C., & Son, C. G. (2019). Systematic review of published data on herb induced liver injury. *Journal of Ethnopharmacology*, *233*, 190–196. https://doi.org/10.1016/j.jep.2019.01.006.

Cai, X., Meng, N., & Yang, B. (2006). Analysis of a case of poisoning caused by overdose of Evodia rutaecarpa. *Beijing Journal of Traditional Chinese Medicine*, *03*, 171–172.

Cai, Y., Xu, Y., Chan, H. F., Fang, X., He, C., & Chen, M. (2016). Glycyrrhetinic acid mediated drug delivery carriers for hepatocellular carcinoma therapy. *Molecular Pharmaceutics*, *13*(3), 699–709. https://doi.org/10.1021/acs.molpharmaceut.5b00677.

Cao, L. J., Li, H. D., Yan, M., Li, Z. H., Gong, H., Jiang, P., et al. (2016). The protective effects of isoliquiritigenin and glycyrrhetinic acid against triptolide-induced oxidative stress in HepG2 cells involve Nrf2 activation. *Evidence-based Complementary and Alternative Medicine*, *2016*, 8912184. https://doi.org/10.1155/2016/8912184.

Chellian, R., Pandy, V., & Mohamed, Z. (2017). Pharmacology and toxicology of alpha- and beta-Asarone: A review of preclinical evidence. *Phytomedicine*, *32*, 41–58. https://doi.org/10.1016/j.phymed.2017.04.003.

Chen, S. R., Dai, Y., Zhao, J., Lin, L., Wang, Y., & Wang, Y. (2018). A mechanistic overview of triptolide and celastrol, natural products from Tripterygium wilfordii Hook F. *Frontiers in Pharmacology*, *9*, 104. https://doi.org/10.3389/fphar.2018.00104.

Chen, C. H., Dickman, K. G., Huang, C. Y., Moriya, M., Shun, C. T., Tai, H. C., et al. (2013). Aristolochic acid-induced upper tract urothelial carcinoma in Taiwan: Clinical characteristics and outcomes. *International Journal of Cancer*, *133*(1), 14–20. https://doi.org/10.1002/ijc.28013.

Chen, Y., Dong, J., Li, F., & Yuan, J. (2017). Reviews and thinking on the toxicity of Evodia rutaecarpa. *Lishizhen Medicine and Materia Medica Research*, *28*(09), 2215–2217.

Chen, F., Gao, X., & Shilatifard, A. (2015). Stably paused genes revealed through inhibition of transcription initiation by the TFIIH inhibitor triptolide. *Genes & Development*, *29*(1), 39–47. https://doi.org/10.1101/gad.246173.114.

Chen, X., Guo, H., Li, Q., Zhang, Y., Liu, H., Zhang, X., et al. (2018). Protective effect of berberine on aconiteinduced myocardial injury and the associated mechanisms. *Molecular Medicine Reports*, *18*(5), 4468–4476. https://doi.org/10.3892/mmr.2018.9476.

Chen, C. N., Tsai, Y. T., & Lai, J. N. (2019). 8years post-marketing surveillance between Asari Radix and hepatocellular carcinoma: Nationwide population-based evidence against an association. *Journal of Ethnopharmacology*, *243*, 112094. https://doi.org/10.1016/j.jep.2019.112094.

Chen, X., Wang, J., & Du, G. (2018). Historical cognition and modern research on toxicity of Melia toosendan. *Pharmacology and Clinics of Chinese Materia Medica*, *34*(04), 189–191.

Chen, Q., & Yan, S. (2012). Advances in pharmacological action and toxic reaction of Rhizoma Paris. *Herald of Medicine*, *31*(07), 886–888.

Chien, K. J., Yang, M. L., Tsai, P. K., Su, C. H., Chen, C. H., Horng, C. T., et al. (2018). Safrole induced cytotoxicity, DNA damage, and apoptosis in macrophages via reactive oxygen species generation and Akt phosphorylation. *Environmental Toxicology and Pharmacology*, *64*, 94–100. https://doi.org/10.1016/j.etap.2018.09.012.

Cohen, S. M., Arnold, L. L., Eldan, M., Lewis, A. S., & Beck, B. D. (2006). Methylated arsenicals: The implications of metabolism and carcinogenicity studies in rodents to human risk assessment. *Critical Reviews in Toxicology*, *36*(2), 99–133.

Cui, Y., Han, J., Ren, J., Chen, H., Xu, B., Song, N., et al. (2019). Untargeted LC-MS-based metabonomics revealed that aristolochic acid I induces testicular toxicity by inhibiting amino acids metabolism, glucose metabolism, beta-oxidation of fatty acids and the TCA cycle in male mice. *Toxicology and Applied Pharmacology*, *373*, 26–38. https://doi.org/10.1016/j.taap.2019.04.014.

Danan, G., & Teschke, R. (2015). RUCAM in drug and herb induced liver injury: The update. *International Journal of Molecular Sciences*, *17*(1), 14. https://doi.org/10.3390/ijms17010014.

Debelle, F. D., Vanherweghem, J. L., & Nortier, J. L. (2008). Aristolochic acid nephropathy: A worldwide problem. *Kidney International*, *74*(2), 158–169. https://doi.org/10.1038/ki.2008.129.

Deng, M., Huang, L., Ning, B., Wang, N., Zhang, Q., Zhu, C., et al. (2016). beta-Asarone improves learning and memory and reduces acetyl cholinesterase and beta-amyloid 42 levels in APP/PS1 transgenic mice by regulating Beclin-1-dependent autophagy. *Brain Research*, *1652*, 188–194. https://doi.org/10.1016/j.brainres.2016.10.008.

Deng, X. H., Liu, J. J., Sun, X. J., Dong, J. C., & Huang, J. H. (2019). Benzoylaconine induces mitochondrial biogenesis in mice via activating AMPK signaling cascade. *Acta Pharmacologica Sinica*, *40*(5), 658–665. https://doi.org/10.1038/s41401-018-0174-8.

Ding, T., Luo, J. Y., Han, X., Yang, S. H., Lin, R. C., & Yang, M. H. (2016). Advances of toxicity evaluation of cinnabar and compatibility necessity analysis. *Zhongguo Zhong Yao Za Zhi*, *41*(24), 4533–4540. https://doi.org/10.4268/cjcmm20162409.

Dong, G., Wang, J., Guo, P., Wei, D., Yang, M., & Kong, L. (2015). Toxicity assessment of Arisaematis Rhizoma in rats by a (1)H NMR-based metabolomics approach. *Molecular BioSystems*, *11*(2), 407–417. https://doi.org/10.1039/c4mb00583j.

Du, X., Nyagblordzro, M., An, L., Gao, X., Du, L., Wang, Y., et al. (2018). Pharmacokinetic and toxicological characteristics of tripterigium glycosides and their derivatives. *Current Drug Metabolism*, *19*(7), 605–627. https://doi.org/10.2174/1389200219666180302152752.

Du, H., Zhang, A., & Zhao, X. (2013). Research progress on toxicity and detoxification methods of bitter almond. *Heilongjiang Journal of Traditional Chinese Medicine*, *42*(04), 58–59.

Ebmeyer, J., Braeuning, A., Glatt, H., These, A., Hessel-Pras, S., & Lampen, A. (2019). Human CYP3A4-mediated toxification of the pyrrolizidine alkaloid lasiocarpine. *Food and Chemical Toxicology*, *130*, 79–88. https://doi.org/10.1016/j.fct.2019.05.019.

Fan, X. X., Li, N., Wu, J. L., Zhou, Y. L., He, J. X., Liu, L., et al. (2014). Celastrol induces apoptosis in gefitinib-resistant non-small cell lung cancer cells via caspases-dependent pathways and Hsp90 client protein degradation. *Molecules*, *19*(3), 3508–3522. https://doi.org/10.3390/molecules19033508.

Fan, S., Li, J., Xiao, H., & Lin, L. (2003). Toxicity and usage of natural star. *ZhongGuo ZhongYiYao XinXi ZaZhi*, *07*, 76–77.

Fan, Y., Liu, S., Chen, X., Feng, M., Song, F., & Gao, X. (2018). Toxicological effects of Nux Vomica in rats urine and serum by means of clinical chemistry, histopathology and (1)H NMR-based metabonomics approach. *Journal of Ethnopharmacology*, *210*, 242–253. https://doi.org/10.1016/j.jep.2017.06.027.

Fan, W., & Mei, Q. (2012). Classification and analysis of toxic traditional chinese medicines from Guangdong real estate. *Lishizhen Medicine and Materia Medica Research*, *23*(10), 2655–2658.

Fields, C. A., Borak, J., & Louis, E. D. (2017). Persistence of mercury-induced motor and sensory neurotoxicity: Systematic review of workers previously exposed to mercury vapor. *Critical Reviews in Toxicology*, *47*(10), 845–866. https://doi.org/10.1080/10408444.2017.1342599.

Fu, Q., Jiang, Z. Z., & Zhang, L. Y. (2013). Impairment of triptolide on liver mitochondria in isolated liver mitochondria and HL7702 cell line. *Chinese Journal of Integrative Medicine*, *19*(9), 683–688. https://doi.org/10.1007/s11655-012-1265-x.

Fu, W., Wang, J., Li, W., Wang, L., & Du, G. (2019). The historical cognition and evaluation of the toxicity of picrasmaeramulus et folium. *Pharmacology and Clinics of Chinese Materia Medica*, *35*(02), 154–156.

Graziose, R., Lila, M. A., & Raskin, I. (2010). Merging traditional Chinese medicine with modern drug discovery technologies to find novel drugs and functional foods. *Current Drug Discovery Technologies*, 7(1), 2–12.

Gu, Y., Li, Y., Jiang, X., Fan, H., Liu, J., Wu, W., et al. (2011). Toxicity on fertility and early embryo development by intragastrical administration of cinnabaris in rat. *Chinese Journal of Experimental Traditional Medical Formulae*, *17*(09), 226–231.

Han, Z., & He, Y. (2008). Advances in pharmacological action and toxicity of total glucosides of paeony. *Journal of Ningxia Medical University*, *04*, 538–541.

Han, B., Qu, M., Ma, X., Cao, S., & Wang, M. (2013). Advances in toxicity and processing of Stellera chamaejasme. *Journal of Chinese Medicinal Materials*, *36*(02), 330–333.

He, Q. L., Titov, D. V., Li, J., Tan, M., Ye, Z., Zhao, Y., et al. (2015). Covalent modification of a cysteine residue in the XPB subunit of the general transcription factor TFIIH through single epoxide cleavage of the transcription inhibitor triptolide. *Angewandte Chemie (International Ed. in English)*, *54*(6), 1859–1863. https://doi.org/10.1002/anie.201408817.

He, X., Yu, L., Yang, X., & Du, G. (2018). Historical textual research and modern research on morning glory poisoning. *Pharmacology and Clinics of Chinese Materia Medica*, *34*(04), 194–196.

He, S., Zhang, C., Zhou, P., Zhang, X., Ye, T., Wang, R., et al. (2019). Herb-induced liver injury: Phylogenetic relationship, structure-toxicity relationship, and herb-ingredient network analysis. *International Journal of Molecular Sciences*, *20*(15). https://doi.org/10.3390/ijms20153633.

Hoang, M. L., Chen, C. H., Chen, P. C., Roberts, N. J., Dickman, K. G., Yun, B. H., et al. (2016). Aristolochic acid in the etiology of renal cell carcinoma. *Cancer Epidemiology, Biomarkers & Prevention*, *25*(12), 1600–1608. https://doi.org/10.1158/1055-9965.EPI-16-0219.

Hou, Z. Y., Tong, X. P., Peng, Y. B., Zhang, B. K., & Yan, M. (2018). Broad targeting of triptolide to resistance and sensitization for cancer therapy. *Biomedicine & Pharmacotherapy*, *104*, 771–780. https://doi.org/10.1016/j.biopha.2018.05.088.

HU, W., Wang, H., Zhang, S., & Sun, N. (2016). The research progress of chemical composition, medicinal properties and toxicity of Pinellia. *China Resources Comprehensive Utilization*, *34*(10), 57–59.

Huang, J., Dai, Z., & Ma, S. (2015). Research progress on Typhonii Rhizoma. *Chinese Traditional and Herbal Drugs*, *46*(18), 2816–2822.

Huang, X., Yang, Q., Huang, X., & Yang, Z. (2017). Study on acute toxicity of different extracts of Sishu Jiulixiang. *Chinese Journal of Ethnomedicine and Ethnopharmacy*, *26*(21), 33–35.

Huang, G., Yang, L., Zhou, W., Tang, X., Wang, Y., Ma, Z., et al. (2018). Study on cardiotoxicity and mechanism of "Fuzi" extracts based on metabonomics. *International Journal of Molecular Sciences*, *19*(11), 3506. https://doi.org/10.3390/ijms19113506.

Jelakovic, B., Dika, Z., Arlt, V. M., Stiborova, M., Pavlovic, N. M., Nikolic, J., et al. (2019). Balkan endemic nephropathy and the causative role of aristolochic acid. *Seminars in Nephrology*, *39*(3), 284–296. https://doi.org/10.1016/j.semnephrol.2019.02.007.

Jian, X. X., Tang, P., Liu, X. X., Chao, R. B., Chen, Q. H., She, X. K., et al. (2012). Structure-cardiac activity relationship of C19-diterpenoid alkaloids. *Natural Product Communications*, 7(6), 713–720.

Jiang, Y., Gao, J., Tian, C., Peng, D., & Xia, D. (2016). Literature analysis of 165 cases of poisoning adverse events induced by Datura metel L. *Chinese Journal of Pharmacovigilance*, *13*(04), 233–235 + 239.

Joshi, P., Vishwakarma, R. A., & Bharate, S. B. (2017). Natural alkaloids as P-gp inhibitors for multidrug resistance reversal in cancer. *European Journal of Medicinal Chemistry*, *138*, 273–292. https://doi.org/10.1016/j.ejmech.2017.06.047.

Kashyap, D., Sharma, A., Tuli, H. S., Sak, K., Mukherjee, T., & Bishayee, A. (2018). Molecular targets of celastrol in cancer: Recent trends and advancements. *Critical Reviews in Oncology/Hematology*, *128*, 70–81. https://doi.org/10.1016/j.critrevonc.2018.05.019.

Khairul, I., Wang, Q. Q., Jiang, Y. H., Wang, C., & Naranmandura, H. (2017). Metabolism, toxicity and anticancer activities of arsenic compounds. *Oncotarget*, *8*(14), 23905–23926. https://doi.org/10.18632/oncotarget.14733.

Kitchin, K. T. (2001). Recent advances in arsenic carcinogenesis: Modes of action, animal model systems, and methylated arsenic metabolites. *Toxicology and Applied Pharmacology*, *172*(3), 249–261. https://doi.org/10.1006/taap.2001.9157.

Kong, L., Li, L., & Du, G. (2018). Research progress of toxicity of Garden Balsam Seed. *Pharmacology and Clinics of Chinese Materia Medica*, *34*(05), 155–156.

Lei, X., Chen, J., Ren, J., Li, Y., Zhai, J., Mu, W., et al. (2015). Liver damage associated with Polygonum multiflorum thunb.: A systematic review of case reports and case series. *Evidence-based Complementary and Alternative Medicine*, *2015*, 459749. https://doi.org/10.1155/2015/459749.

Li, B. (2006). Caution against allergy to traditional Chinese medicine. *Liaoning Journal of Traditional Chinese Medicine*, *01*, 86.

Li, J., Du, J., Ma, L., Dai, B., Li, C., Yang, Y., et al. (2018). Anti-malarial efficacy and acute toxicity of Dichroa alkali salt by intragastric administration. *Chinese Journal of Experimental Traditional Medical Formulae*, *24*(13), 141–146.

Li, Y., Han, L., Huang, C., Dai, W., Tian, G., Huang, F., et al. (2018). New contributions to asarum powder on immunology related toxicity effects in lung. *Evidence-based Complementary and Alternative Medicine*, *2018*, 1054032. https://doi.org/10.1155/2018/1054032.

Li, X. J., Jiang, Z. Z., & Zhang, L. Y. (2014). Triptolide: Progress on research in pharmacodynamics and toxicology. *Journal of Ethnopharmacology*, *155*(1), 67–79. https://doi.org/10.1016/j.jep.2014.06.006.

Li, D., Lei, G., Yan, Y., & Luo, F. (2008). Experimental study on acute toxicity of raw and processed products of Panax ginseng. In *Paper presented at the Papers Collection of the First National Academic Conference on Traditional Chinese Medicine Commodity, 中国山东青岛即墨*.

Li, X., Li, X., Huang, N., Liu, R., & Sun, R. (2018). A comprehensive review and perspectives on pharmacology and toxicology of saikosaponins. *Phytomedicine*, *50*, 73–87. https://doi.org/10.1016/j.phymed.2018.09.174.

Li, X., Li, X., Lu, J., Huang, Y., Lv, L., Luan, Y., et al. (2017). Saikosaponins induced hepatotoxicity in mice via lipid metabolism dysregulation and oxidative stress: A proteomic study. *BMC Complementary and Alternative Medicine*, *17*(1), 219. https://doi.org/10.1186/s12906-017-1733-0.

Li, M., Li, H., Wang, X., & Ma, J. (2016). Progress of experimental research on cardiotoxicity of Chansu. *Chinese Journal of Pharmacology and Toxicology*, *30*(05), 605–610.

Li, S., Li, R., Zeng, Y., Meng, X., Wen, C., & Zheng, S. (2019). Chemical components and pharmacological action of Aconiti Radix. *China Journal of Chinese Materia Medica*, *44*(12), 2433–2443.

Li, P., & Liu, H. (2018). Toxic effects of nitidine choride and sesamin on zebrafish embryos. *Pharmacology and Clinics of Chinese Materia Medica*, *34*(01), 101–104.

Li, C., Rao, T., Chen, X., Zou, Z., Wei, A., Tang, J., et al. (2019). HLA-B*35:01 allele is a potential biomarker for predicting Polygonum multiflorum-induced liver injury in humans. *Hepatology*, *70*(1), 346–357. https://doi.org/10.1002/hep.30660.

Li, X., Sun, R., & Liu, R. (2019). Natural products in licorice for the therapy of liver diseases: Progress and future opportunities. *Pharmacological Research*, *144*, 210–226. https://doi.org/10.1016/j.phrs.2019.04.025.

Li, Y., Wang, Y., & Du, G. (2018). The historical cognition and evaluation of realgar toxicity. *Pharmacology and Clinics of Chinese Materia Medica*, *34*(04), 196–198.

Li, T., Wang, P., Guo, W., Huang, X., Tian, X., Wu, G., et al. (2019). Natural berberine-based chinese herb medicine assembled nanostructures with modified antibacterial application. *ACS Nano*, *13*(6), 6770–6781. https://doi.org/10.1021/acsnano.9b01346.

Li, Y., & Yao, G. (2011). Review on pharmacological effects and toxicity of Phytolaccae. *Chinese Journal of Experimental Traditional Medical Formulae, 17*(13), 248–251.

Liang, Q., Ni, C., Yan, X., Xie, M., Zhang, Y., Zhang, Q., et al. (2010). Comparative study on metabonomics and on liver and kidney toxicity of Aristolochia fangchi and Stephania tetrandra. *China Journal of Chinese Materia Medica, 35*(21), 2882–2888.

Liang, G., Zhao, F., Bao, S., Yang, Y., & Liu, M. (2017). Studies on acute toxicity experiment of Buthus martensii Karsch superfine powder. *Journal of Modern Medicine & Health, 33*(16), 2418–2419 + 2424.

Liao, L. Z., Chen, Y. L., Lu, L. H., Zhao, Y. H., Guo, H. L., & Wu, W. K. (2013). Polysaccharide from Fuzi likely protects against starvation-induced cytotoxicity in H9c2 cells by increasing autophagy through activation of the AMPK/mTOR pathway. *The American Journal of Chinese Medicine, 41*(2), 353–367. https://doi.org/10.1142/S0192415X13500262.

Lin, Y., Xiao, R., Yin, L. Z., Wu, P., Liu, Y. X., Li, C., et al. (2019). Developing spectrum-toxicity relationship with rough set theory for hepatotoxicity material basis of Polygonum multiflorum. *Zhongguo Zhong Yao Za Zhi, 44*(3), 509–517. https://doi.org/10.19540/j.cnki.cjcmm.20181114.001.

Liu, Z. (2012). Clinical analysis of 10 cases of acute sulfur poisoning. *Chinese Community Doctors, 14*(28), 124.

Liu, F., Han, X., Li, N., Liu, K., & Kang, W. (2019). Aconitum alkaloids induce cardiotoxicity and apoptosis in embryonic zebrafish by influencing the expression of cardiovascular relative genes. *Toxicology Letters, 305*, 10–18. https://doi.org/10.1016/j.toxlet.2019.01.002.

Liu, X. X., Jian, X. X., Cai, X. F., Chao, R. B., Chen, Q. H., Chen, D. L., et al. (2012). Cardioactive C(1)(9)-diterpenoid alkaloids from the lateral roots of Aconitum carmichaeli "Fu Zi" *Chemical & Pharmaceutical Bulletin (Tokyo), 60*(1), 144–149.

Liu, X., Li, X., Chen, Y., Luo, Q., Ge, C., Wang, C., et al. (2016). Acute toxicity and genotoxicity of dipsaci radix water extract liquid in mice. *Chinese Journal of Experimental Traditional Medical Formulae, 22*(05), 160–165.

Liu, Y., Liu, Y., Feng, L., Guo, D., & Liu, M. (2018). Research progress on the snake venom of Agkistrodonacutus. *Sheng Wu Hua Gong, 4*(06), 137–141.

Liwei, M. A., Fan, L., Shiyu, N., Yu, H., Zhou, L., Chen, Z., et al. (2018). Study on single drug toxicity of Euphorbia fischeriana Steud Powder and Decoction of Compatibility of Euphorbia fischeriana Steud and Jujubae. *China Medical Herald*, 15(02), 4–8 + 18.

Lou, J., Wu, H., Wang, L., Zhao, L., Li, X., Kang, Y., et al. (2018). Taurine-magnesium coordination compound, a potential anti-arrhythmic complex, improves aconitine-induced arrhythmias through regulation of multiple ion channels. *Toxicology and Applied Pharmacology, 356*, 182–190. https://doi.org/10.1016/j.taap.2018.08.008.

Lu, D., & Zhang, C. (2013). Study on sub- chronic toxicity evaluation on Gleditsia Cctlrllct Rats. *Journal of Hubei University of Chinese Medicine, 15*(06), 16–19.

Luo, L., Liu, H., Zhou, B., & Song, J. (2018). Research of toxicity of Herba Leonuri. *Jilin Journal of Chinese Medicine, 38*(09), 1082–1086.

Luo, W., Lu, J., Chen, X., & Wang, Y. (2016). The pharmacological effect and its underlying mechanisms of toosendanin: A review. *Pharmacology and Clinics of Chinese Materia Medica, 32*(04), 161–164.

Luo, F., Ma, X., & Lin, F. (2014). Study on the long-term toxicity of anticancer drug in rats Chelidonium majus. *Carcinogenesis, Teratogenesis & Mutagenesis, 26*(06), 459–462.

Man, Y. L., Rui, H. L., Chen, Y. P., Wang, G. Q., Sun, L. J., & Cheng, H. (2017). Aristolochic acid-induced autophagy promotes epithelial-to-myofibroblast transition in human renal proximal tubule epithelial cells. *Evidence-based Complementary and Alternative Medicine, 2017*, 9596256. https://doi.org/10.1155/2017/9596256.

Melchart, D., Hager, S., Albrecht, S., Dai, J., Weidenhammer, W., & Teschke, R. (2017). Herbal traditional chinese medicine and suspected liver injury: A prospective study. *World Journal of Hepatology*, *9*(29), 1141–1157. https://doi.org/10.4254/wjh.v9.i29.1141.

Miao, X., Zhang, X., Liu, D., Ma, Z., Xing, H., & Li, G. (2018). Research on toxicities and related models of Aconiti Kusnezoffii Radix. *Traditional Chinese Drug Research and Clinical Pharmacology*, *29*(06), 836–839.

Michl, J., Bello, O., Kite, G. C., Simmonds, M. S. J., & Heinrich, M. (2017). Medicinally used asarum species: High-resolution LC-MS analysis of aristolochic acid analogs and in vitro toxicity screening in HK-2 cells. *Frontiers in Pharmacology*, *8*, 215. https://doi.org/10.3389/fphar.2017.00215.

Miller, W. H., Jr. (2002). Molecular targets of arsenic trioxide in malignant cells. *The Oncologist*, 7(Suppl. 1), 14–19. https://doi.org/10.1634/theoncologist.7-suppl_1-14.

Naranmandura, H., Xu, S., Koike, S., Pan, L. Q., Chen, B., Wang, Y. W., et al. (2012). The endoplasmic reticulum is a target organelle for trivalent dimethylarsinic acid (DMAIII)-induced cytotoxicity. *Toxicology and Applied Pharmacology*, *260*(3), 241–249. https://doi.org/10.1016/j.taap.2012.02.017.

Ng, A. W. T., Poon, S. L., Huang, M. N., Lim, J. Q., Boot, A., Yu, W., et al. (2017). Aristolochic acids and their derivatives are widely implicated in liver cancers in Taiwan and throughout Asia. *Science Translational Medicine*, *9*(412), eaan6446. https://doi.org/10.1126/scitranslmed.aan6446.

Ni, S., Qi, Q., Ma, H., & Wang, X. (2014). Acute aconite poisoning: A case report. *China's Naturopathy*, *22*(06), 59.

Nie, A., Gao, M., Jia, W., Zhu, C., Zhang, X., Zhou, Z., et al., (2019). Discussion on safety of Xanthii Fructus and consideration on its rational use. *China Journal of Chinese Materia Medica*, 1–9.

Nie, A., Zhao, X., Gao, M., Chao, Y., Li, X., Gui, X., et al. (2018). Discussion and consideration on safety of Sophorae Tonkinensis Radix et Rhizoma and its rational use. *Chinese Traditional and Herbal Drugs*, *49*(17), 4152–4161.

Ning, J., Chen, L., & Rietjens, I. (2019). Role of toxicokinetics and alternative testing strategies in pyrrolizidine alkaloid toxicity and risk assessment; state-of-the-art and future perspectives. *Food and Chemical Toxicology*, *131*, 110572. https://doi.org/10.1016/j.fct.2019.110572.

Ning, B., Zhang, Q., Wang, N., Deng, M., & Fang, Y. (2019). beta-Asarone regulates ER stress and autophagy via inhibition of the PERK/CHOP/Bcl-2/Beclin-1 pathway in 6-OHDA-induced parkinsonian rats. *Neurochemical Research*, *44*(5), 1159–1166. https://doi.org/10.1007/s11064-019-02757-w.

Qiang, G., Fang, L., & Du, G. (2019). The historical cognition and evaluation of centipedetoxicity. *Pharmacology and Clinics of Chinese Materia Medica*, *35*(02), 151–154.

Qiu, H., & Wang, Q. (2015). Risk assessment for clinical external application of calomel. *Zhongguo Zhong Yao Za Zhi*, *40*(14), 2706–2710.

Qiu, S., Zhang, H., Fei, Q., Zhu, F., Wang, J., Jia, X., et al. (2018). Urine and plasma metabolomics study on potential hepatoxic biomarkers identification in rats induced by Gynura segetum. *Journal of Ethnopharmacology*, *216*, 37–46. https://doi.org/10.1016/j.jep.2018.01.017.

Rajput, S. B., Tonge, M. B., & Karuppayil, S. M. (2014). An overview on traditional uses and pharmacological profile of Acorus calamus Linn. (Sweet flag) and other Acorus species. *Phytomedicine*, *21*(3), 268–276. https://doi.org/10.1016/j.phymed.2013.09.020.

Rao, Y., Li, R., & Zhang, D. (2013). A drug from poison: How the therapeutic effect of arsenic trioxide on acute promyelocytic leukemia was discovered. *Science China Life Sciences*, *56*(6), 495–502. https://doi.org/10.1007/s11427-013-4487-z.

Ren, H. (2009). The influence of traditional Chinese medicine on development of ovary and uterus in experimental study in mice. *Journal of Clinical and Experimental Medicine*, *8*(10), 3–4.

Rosenquist, T. A., & Grollman, A. P. (2016). Mutational signature of aristolochic acid: Clue to the recognition of a global disease. *DNA Repair (Amst)*, *44*, 205–211. https://doi.org/10.1016/j.dnarep.2016.05.027.

Sanz, M. A., Fenaux, P., Tallman, M. S., Estey, E. H., Lowenberg, B., Naoe, T., et al. (2019). Management of acute promyelocytic leukemia: Updated recommendations from an expert panel of the European LeukemiaNet. *Blood*, *133*(15), 1630–1643. https://doi.org/10.1182/blood-2019-01-894980.

Shan, X. L., Yu, H. L., Wu, H., Wang, W., Zhang, Y. B., Cheng, Z. Y., et al. (2018). Intestinal toxicity of different processed products of Crotonis fructus and effect of processing on fatty oil and total protein. *Zhongguo Zhong Yao Za Zhi*, *43*(23), 4652–4658. https://doi.org/10.19540/j.cnki.cjcmm.20181105.005.

Shen, T., Liu, Y., Shang, J., Xie, Q., Li, J., Yan, M., et al. (2019). Incidence and etiology of drug-induced liver injury in Mainland China. *Gastroenterology*, *156*(8), 2230–2241. e2211 https://doi.org/10.1053/j.gastro.2019.02.002.

Singhuber, J., Zhu, M., Prinz, S., & Kopp, B. (2009). Aconitum in traditional Chinese medicine: A valuable drug or an unpredictable risk? *Journal of Ethnopharmacology*, *126*(1), 18–30. https://doi.org/10.1016/j.jep.2009.07.031.

Stegmuller, S., Schrenk, D., & Cartus, A. T. (2018). Formation and fate of DNA adducts of alpha- and beta-asarone in rat hepatocytes. *Food and Chemical Toxicology*, *116*(Pt. B), 138–146. https://doi.org/10.1016/j.fct.2018.04.025.

Sun, R., & Wang, C. (2009). Research development on toxicity of Rhizoma Menispermi. *Chinese Journal of Pharmacovigilance*, *6*(09), 546–549.

Sun, R., Wang, H., Huang, W., Chi, X., & Miao, D. (2010). Experimental comparison study on mice's acute toxicity of different composition in Folium Artemisiae Argyi. *Chinese Journal of Pharmacovigilance*, 7(07), 392–396.

Sun, R., & Yang, Q. (2010). Research development on toxicity of fructus bruceae based on efficacy and material basis. *Chinese Journal of Pharmacovigilance*, 7(03), 159–161.

Szegezdi, E., Logue, S. E., Gorman, A. M., & Samali, A. (2006). Mediators of endoplasmic reticulum stress-induced apoptosis. *EMBO Reports*, 7(9), 880–885. https://doi.org/10.1038/sj.embor.7400779.

Tan, W., Yang, X., Zhang, L., & Du, G. (2019). The historical cognition and evaluation of Papaverispericarpium. *Pharmacology and Clinics of Chinese Materia Medica*, *35*(02), 159–162.

Tao, G., Irie, Y., Li, D. J., & Keung, W. M. (2005). Eugenol and its structural analogs inhibit monoamine oxidase A and exhibit antidepressant-like activity. *Bioorganic & Medicinal Chemistry*, *13*(15), 4777–4788. https://doi.org/10.1016/j.bmc.2005.04.081.

Tian, J., Tian, Z., Qin, S. L., Zhao, P. Y., Jiang, X., & Tian, Z. (2017). Anxiolytic-like effects of alpha-asarone in a mouse model of chronic pain. *Metabolic Brain Disease*, *32*(6), 2119–2129. https://doi.org/10.1007/s11011-017-0108-z.

Vanherweghem, J. L., Depierreux, M., Tielemans, C., Abramowicz, D., Dratwa, M., Jadoul, M., et al. (1993). Rapidly progressive interstitial renal fibrosis in young women: Association with slimming regimen including Chinese herbs. *Lancet*, *341*(8842), 387–391. https://doi.org/10.1016/0140-6736(93)92984-2.

Vispe, S., DeVries, L., Creancier, L., Besse, J., Breand, S., Hobson, D. J., et al. (2009). Triptolide is an inhibitor of RNA polymerase I and II-dependent transcription leading predominantly to down-regulation of short-lived mRNA. *Molecular Cancer Therapeutics*, *8*(10), 2780–2790. https://doi.org/10.1158/1535-7163.MCT-09-0549.

Wang, H., Bao, Q., Yi, H., & Xia, Q. (2019). The evaluation of embryotoxicity of Ligusticum chuanxiong on mice and embryonic stem cells. *Journal of Ethnopharmacology*, *239*, 111895. https://doi.org/10.1016/j.jep.2019.111895.

Wang, S., Gong, N., Duan, C., Lv, Y., & Du, G. (2019). Historical cognition and modern evaluation on the toxicity of aconitum-derived Chinese traditional medicines. *Pharmacology and Clinics of Chinese Materia Medica*, *35*(02), 149–151.

Wang, L., He, Y., Zhang, Y., Zhou, H., Yu, L., Yang, J., et al. (2016). Effects of active components of Fuzi and Gancao compatibility on Bax, Bcl-2, and Caspase-3 in chronic heart failure rats. *Evidence-based Complementary and Alternative Medicine*, *2016*, 7686045. https://doi.org/10.1155/2016/7686045.

Wang, M., Huang, J., Fan, H., He, D., Zhao, S., Shu, Y., et al. (2018). Treatment of rheumatoid arthritis using combination of methotrexate and tripterygium glycosides tablets-A quantitative plasma pharmacochemical and pseudotargeted metabolomic approach. *Frontiers in Pharmacology*, *9*, 1051. https://doi.org/10.3389/fphar.2018.01051.

Wang, X., Jia, S., & Li, J. (2012). the toxic injury study of arsenic exposure from different origin Angelica sinensis exposure in hepatic and kidney of mice. *Chinese Journal of Pharmacovigilance*, *9*(10), 577–580.

Wang, D., Jia, D. X., Li, Z. Z., Yao, J. K., Zhang, L., Sun, X. B., et al. (2018). Safety evaluation and risk control measures for Aconiti Kusnezoffii Radix. *Zhongguo Zhong Yao Za Zhi*, *43*(15), 3093–3100. https://doi.org/10.19540/j.cnki.cjcmm.20180516.006.

Wang, X. Y., Lin, R. C., Dong, S. F., Guan, J., Sun, L., & Huang, J. M. (2017). Toxicity of mineral Chinese medicines containing mercury element. *Zhongguo Zhong Yao Za Zhi*, *42*(7), 1258–1264. https://doi.org/10.19540/j.cnki.cjcmm.20170224.002.

Wang, L., Liu, N., Xue, X., & Zhou, S. (2019). The effect of overexpression of the enhancer of zeste homolog 1 (EZH1) gene on aristolochic acid-induced injury in HK-2 human kidney proximal tubule cells in vitro. *Medical Science Monitor*, *25*, 801–810. https://doi.org/10.12659/MSM.911611.

Wang, S., Lu, J., Meng, L., & Ji, S. (2014). Volatile toxic constituents of Toxicodendri Resina by headspace GC/MS. *Chinese Traditional Patent Medicine*, *36*(03), 567–571.

Wang, Y., Qiao, D., Li, Y., & Xu, F. (2018). Risk factors for hepatic veno-occlusive disease caused by Gynura segetum: A retrospective study. *BMC Gastroenterology*, *18*(1), 156. https://doi.org/10.1186/s12876-018-0879-7.

Wang, J., Wang, L., Lou, G. H., Zeng, H. R., Hu, J., Huang, Q. W., et al. (2019). Coptidis Rhizoma: A comprehensive review of its traditional uses, botany, phytochemistry, pharmacology and toxicology. *Pharmaceutical Biology*, *57*(1), 193–225. https://doi.org/10.1080/13880209.2019.1577466.

Wang, N. N., Wang, J., Tan, H. L., Wang, Y. G., Gao, Y., & Ma, Z. C. (2019). Aconitine ameliorates cardiomyocyte hypertrophy induced by angiotensin. *Zhongguo Zhong Yao Za Zhi*, *44*(8), 1642–1647. https://doi.org/10.19540/j.cnki.cjcmm.20190117.002.

Wang, C., Wang, X., & Zhu, N. (2018). Neurobehavioral toxicity of aconitine on embryos and juvenile fish. *Chinese Journal of Laboratory Diagnosis*, *22*(08), 1432–1435.

Wang, L., Yang, W., Li, Y., & Li, C. (2016). Chemical constituents of Cortex Periplocae Radicis and its main toxic ingredients: Research advances. *Journal of International Pharmaceutical Research*, *43*(06), 1067–1075.

Wang, L., Zhang, X., Kong, L., & Du, G. (2018). Historical cognition and evaluation of the toxicity of three traditional Chinese medicines (CurculiginisRhizoma, Psammosilenes Radix and Periplocae Cortex) with the activity of expelling wind-evil and removing wetness. *Pharmacology and Clinics of Chinese Materia Medica*, *34*(05), 157–160.

Wei, M., Liu, L., Li, D., & Liu, H. (2009). Protection in vitro of aFGF on human liver cell L-02 and human kidney cell 293 caused by nitidine chloride. *Chinese Traditional Patent Medicine*, *31*(09), 1338–1341.

Wei, W., Wu, S., Wang, X., Sun, C. K., Yang, X., Yan, X., et al. (2014). Novel celastrol derivatives inhibit the growth of hepatocellular carcinoma patient-derived xenografts. *Oncotarget*, *5*(14), 5819–5831. https://doi.org/10.18632/oncotarget.2171.

Wei, L., Yan, Z., Liu, L., & Zhao, L. (2011). Study on determination of the levels of DNA damage induced by aconitum using high performance liquid chromatography. *Journal of Instrumental Analysis*, *30*(07), 755–759.

Wu, J. J., Guo, Z. Z., Zhu, Y. F., Huang, Z. J., Gong, X., Li, Y. H., et al. (2018). A systematic review of pharmacokinetic studies on herbal drug Fuzi: Implications for Fuzi as personalized medicine. *Phytomedicine*, *44*, 187–203. https://doi.org/10.1016/j.phymed.2018.03.001.

Wu, X., Ma, F., Zheng, G., Liang, Y., Chen, H., & Liu, D. (2016). Toxicity research progress on indole alkaloids of strychni semen. *Pharmacology and Clinics of Chinese Materia Medica*, *32*(06), 231–235.

Wu, C., Wang, J., Cheng, J., Zhao, J., & Li, Y. (2017). Simutaneous determination of three anthraquinone components in Knoxia valerianoides by HPLC. *China Pharmacist*, *20*(06), 1120–1122.

Wu, X., Wang, S., Lu, J., Jing, Y., Li, M., Cao, J., et al. (2018). Seeing the unseen of Chinese herbal medicine processing (Paozhi): Advances in new perspectives. *Chinese Medicine*, *13*, 4. https://doi.org/10.1186/s13020-018-0163-3.

Xi, C., Peng, S., Wu, Z., Zhou, Q., & Zhou, J. (2017). Toxicity of triptolide and the molecular mechanisms involved. *Biomedicine & Pharmacotherapy*, *90*, 531–541. https://doi.org/10.1016/j.biopha.2017.04.003.

Xin, Y., Sun, W., Long, K., Wang, C., & Cheng, Y. (2014). Toxicity and usage of flying grass. *Henan Traditional Chinese Medicine*, *34*(11), 2270–2271.

Yan, Z., Lu, Z., Yuan, J., An, P., Fang, C., Ren, N., et al. (2017). Analysis on two cases of castor seed poisoning. *Chinese Journal of Industrial Medicine*, *30*(03), 184–185.

Yang, Y. (2002). Progress in experimental research on efficacy of woodlouse worm. *Journal of Chinese Medicinal Materials*, *02*, 150–152.

Yang, M., Ji, X., & Zuo, Z. (2018). Relationships between the toxicities of radix aconiti lateralis preparata (Fuzi) and the toxicokinetics of its main diester-diterpenoid alkaloids. *Toxins (Basel)*, *10*(10), 391. https://doi.org/10.3390/toxins10100391.

Yang, L., Su, T., Li, X. M., Wang, X., Cai, S. Q., Meng, L. Q., et al. (2012). Aristolochic acid nephropathy: Variation in presentation and prognosis. *Nephrology, Dialysis, Transplantation*, *27*(1), 292–298. https://doi.org/10.1093/ndt/gfr291.

Yang, Y., Wang, W., Xiong, Z., Kong, J., Qiu, Y., Shen, F., et al. (2016). Activation of SIRT3 attenuates triptolide-induced toxicity through closing mitochondrial permeability transition pore in cardiomyocytes. *Toxicology In Vitro*, *34*, 128–137. https://doi.org/10.1016/j.tiv.2016.03.020.

Yang, X., Xia, D., Tian, C., Li, L., & Sun, Y. (2017). Literature analysis of 508 cases reports of adverse reactions induced by Aconiti Lateralis Radix praeparata. *Chinese Journal of Pharmacovigilance*, *14*(10), 615–621.

Yang, A. H., Zhang, L., Zhi, D. X., Liu, W. L., Gao, X., & He, X. (2018). Identification and analysis of the reactive metabolites related to the hepatotoxicity of safrole. *Xenobiotica*, *48*(11), 1164–1172. https://doi.org/10.1080/00498254.2017.1399227.

Ye, K., Han, D., Mao, P., Wang, Z., Huang, J., Luan, H., et al. (2019). Comparative study on toxicity of Aconiti Kusnezoffii Radix cocta formula granule and decoctum on H9c2 myocardial Cell. *Chinese Journal of Modern Applied Pharmacy*, *36*(13), 1622–1626.

Yen, C.-C., Huang, C.-F., Lee, W.-J., Hsu, M.-J., Liu, S.-H., & Lin-Shiau, S.-Y. (2008). Studies on mercuric sulfide, a component of cinnabar, a Chinese herbal medicine, on cellular functions in mouse lung and fibroblasts. *Toxicological & Environmental Chemistry*, *90*(1), 181–201.

Yi, P., Melnyk, S., Pogribna, M., Pogribny, I. P., Hine, R. J., & James, S. J. (2000). Increase in plasma homocysteine associated with parallel increases in plasma S-adenosylhomocysteine and lymphocyte DNA hypomethylation. *The Journal of Biological Chemistry*, *275*(38), 29318–29323. https://doi.org/10.1074/jbc.M002725200.

Yu, H., & Yu, D. (2019). Literature review of adverse drug reactions induced by Mylabris. *Chinese Journal of Pharmacovigilance, 16*(01), 47–51 + 57.

Zan, K., Wang, J., Lu, J., Guo, L., Zheng, J., & Ma, s. (2018). Content determination of four diester diterpenoid alkaloids in leaves of Aconitum kusnezoffii by HPLC. *China Journal of Chinese Materia Medica, 43*(04), 766–771.

Zhang, X. (2014). Research progress of toxicity and detoxification mechanism of Euphorbia kansui. *Chinese Journal of Hospital Pharmacy, 34*(18), 1611–1615.

Zhang, L., Bao, Z., Huang, Y., Huang, W., Zhang, Y., & Sun, R. (2011). Experimental study on the "dosage-time-toxicity" relationship of acute hepatotoxicity induced by water extraction from Rhizoma Pinelliae in mice. *Chinese Journal of Pharmacovigilance, 8*(01), 11–15.

Zhang, F., Cai, L., Zhang, J., Qi, X., & Lu, C. (2018). Aconitine-induced cardiac arrhythmia in human induced pluripotent stem cell-derived cardiomyocytes. *Experimental and Therapeutic Medicine, 16*(4), 3497–3503. https://doi.org/10.3892/etm.2018.6644.

Zhang, Y., Kang, L., Guo, L., & Zhou, A. (2017). Herbalogical study of mugwort leaves and research advances in its application. *Shanghai Journal of Acupuncture, 36*(03), 245–255.

Zhang, L., Li, L., & Du, G. (2018). Historical cognition and modern research of Strychnos venom. *Pharmacology and Clinics of Chinese Materia Medica, 34*(04), 191–194.

Zhang, M., & Shen, Y. (2018). Research progress on toxicity of matrine-type alkaloids. *Drug Evaluation Research, 41*(04), 682–691.

Zhang, J., Wang, Y., Wang, J., Wang, L., & Li, H. (2007). Toxic effects of aconitine on rat sertoli cells. *Modern Preventive Medicine,* (07), 1221–1223 + 1227.

Zhang, C., Wu, W., & Tang, J. (2011). Detection of genotoxicity of Cinnabaris by using micronucleus assay and comet assay. *Chinese Journal of Experimental Traditional Medical Formulae, 17*(17), 228–233.

Zhang, X. W., Yan, X. J., Zhou, Z. R., Yang, F. F., Wu, Z. Y., Sun, H. B., et al. (2010). Arsenic trioxide controls the fate of the PML-RARalpha oncoprotein by directly binding PML. *Science, 328*(5975), 240–243. https://doi.org/10.1126/science.1183424.

Zhang, L., Zhang, J., Fan, Q., Su, Z., Chen, C., Peng, L., et al. (2018). Hepatoxicity of epimedii folium in rat model based on uniform design and regression analysis. *Chinese Journal of Experimental Traditional Medical Formulae, 24*(06), 189–197.

Zhang, H. M., Zhao, X. H., Sun, Z. H., Li, G. C., Liu, G. C., Sun, L. R., et al. (2019). Recognition of the toxicity of aristolochic acid. *Journal of Clinical Pharmacy and Therapeutics, 44*(2), 157–162. https://doi.org/10.1111/jcpt.12789.

Zhang, F., Zhou, Y., Yang, X., Xiong, A. Z., Wang, Z. T., & Yang, L. (2019). Gynura Rhizoma containing pyrrolizidine alkaloids induces the hepatic sinusoidal obstruction syndrome in mice via upregulating fibrosis-related factors. *Acta Pharmacologica Sinica, 40*(6), 781–789. https://doi.org/10.1038/s41401-018-0155-y.

Zhao, Q., & Sun, R. (2014). Research development on toxicity of Psoralea corylifolia L. related to efficacy and chemical material basis. *Chinese Journal of Pharmacovigilance, 11*(08), 482–484.

Zhao, J., & Wei, X. (2016). Thyroidectomy induced hepatic toxicity and possible amelioration by Ginkgo biloba leaf extract. *Journal of Qiqihar Medical University, 37*(20), 2525–2527.

Zhou, Q., Jin, R., & Yao, G. (2012). Preliminary study on hepatocytes and nephrocytes toxicity induced by dauricine. *Chinese Journal of Pharmacovigilance, 9*(10), 580–583.

Zhou, Q., Pei, J., Poon, J., Lau, A. Y., Zhang, L., Wang, Y., et al. (2019). Worldwide research trends on aristolochic acids (1957–2017): Suggestions for researchers. *PLoS One, 14*(5). e0216135https://doi.org/10.1371/journal.pone.0216135.

Zhou, H., Sun, Y., Li, Y., Wang, B., & Liu, D. (2007). Progress in studies on chemical constituents and pharmacological effect of anemone raddeana regel. *Lishizhen Medicine and Materia Medica Research, 05*, 1239–1241.

Zhou, Q., Sun, P., Xiao, L., Liu, Q., & Zhang, L. (2019). Effect of processing with vinegar on hepatorenal toxicity of dichloromethane site of Genkwa Flos. *Chinese Journal of Experimental Traditional Medical Formulae*, *25*(02), 35–39.

Zhou, G., Tang, L., Zhou, X., Wang, T., Kou, Z., & Wang, Z. (2015). A review on phytochemistry and pharmacological activities of the processed lateral root of Aconitum carmichaelii Debeaux. *Journal of Ethnopharmacology*, *160*, 173–193. https://doi.org/10.1016/j.jep.2014.11.043.

Zhu, H. H., Hu, J., Lo Coco, F., & Jin, J. (2019). The simpler the better: Oral arsenic for acute promyelocytic leukemia. *Blood*, *134*, 597–605. https://doi.org/10.1182/blood.2019000760.

Zhu, H. H., Wu, D. P., Du, X., Zhang, X., Liu, L., Ma, J., et al. (2018). Oral arsenic plus retinoic acid versus intravenous arsenic plus retinoic acid for non-high-risk acute promyelocytic leukaemia: A non-inferiority, randomised phase 3 trial. *The Lancet Oncology*, *19*(7), 871–879. https://doi.org/10.1016/S1470-2045(18)30295-X.

Zhuang, P., Huang, Y., Lu, Z., Yang, Z., Xu, L., Sun, F., et al. (2016). cAMP-PKA-CaMKII signaling pathway is involved in aggravated cardiotoxicity during Fuzi and Beimu Combination Treatment of Experimental Pulmonary Hypertension. *Scientific Reports*, *6*, 34903. https://doi.org/10.1038/srep34903.

Zong, X., Yan, X., Wu, J. L., Liu, Z., Zhou, H., Li, N., et al. (2019). Potentially cardiotoxic diterpenoid alkaloids from the roots of Aconitum carmichaelii. *Journal of Natural Products*, *82*(4), 980–989. https://doi.org/10.1021/acs.jnatprod.8b01039.

FSC
www.fsc.org
MIX
Papier | Fördert gute Waldnutzung
FSC® C083411

Kolibri 360 GmbH
Ferdinand-Jühlke-Straße 7
99095 Erfurt, Deutschland
produktsicherheit@kolibri360.de